Gestational Diabetes During and After Pregnancy

Catherine Kim • Assiamira Ferrara (Editors)

Gestational Diabetes During and After Pregnancy

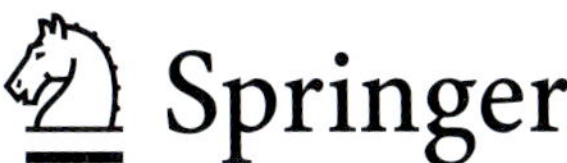

Springer

Dr. Catherine Kim
Department of Obstetrics
and Gynecology,
University of Michigan,
Ann Arbor, MI,
USA

Dr. Assiamira Ferrara
Division of Research,
Kaiser Permanente Northern California,
Oakland, CA,
USA

ISBN: 978-1-84882-119-4 e-ISBN: 978-1-84882-120-0
DOI: 10.1007/978-1-84882-120-0
Springer Dordrecht Heidelberg London New York

A catalogue record for this book is available from the British Library

Library of Congress Control Number: 2010933596

Cover design: eStudio Calamar, Figueres/Berlin

Printed on acid-free paper

Springer is part of Springer Science+Business Media (www.springer.com)

We dedicate this book to Bob Knopp, a pioneer in GDM. He died unexpectedly, shortly after the completion of his chapter. His work is especially relevant now, given the increasing recognition that lipids play a crucial role in the effects of GDM upon the offspring. We would also acknowledge Yeong, Sofia, Sam, Stephen and Stella.

Many thanks to Samantha Ehrlich for her patience and thoroughness in assisting with this book.

Preface

Gestational diabetes (GDM), or glucose intolerance first identified during pregnancy, is a disease of our times. While diabetes as a disease has been recognized for thousands of years, GDM is a relatively new condition that has been identified as recently as the nineteenth century. Recognition of the full impact of GDM is only possible because of the declines in maternal and child mortality, increases in obesity and chronic disease, and increased delivery of prenatal care, GDM screening, and infertility services that are unique to modern society.

One of the reasons that GDM fascinates us is that it represents the intersection of both the mother's and her child's health trajectory, and the management of it can affect not only perinatal health but also the development of disease even decades into the future. Our understanding of these relationships has grown over the past several decades, fed by progress made in other areas of diabetes research, particularly genetics, diabetes prevention in high-risk populations, and inflammatory biomarkers.

This book is our attempt to summarize the exciting developments in our understanding of this unique entity. Our book begins with an overview by Dr. Jack Kitzmiller, who guides us through the changing face of GDM over the past several decades. His chapter delves into the randomized trials published over the past several years and the diagnostic strategies advocated as recently as 2009. This overview is followed by a detailed description of the landmark Hyperglycemia and Adverse Pregnancy Outcome (HAPO) study, unique in its size and international setting. The current state of GDM screening worldwide is summarized by Dr. Agarwal, who provides a comprehensive overview of the several coexisting guidelines.

The next section discusses the current burden that GDM poses and the reasons why we expect that GDM will affect ever larger portions of the population. Dr. Lawrence discusses the prevalence of GDM and its overlap with diabetes which preceded pregnancy. Dr. Zhang gives a detailed summary of risk factors for GDM, informed by her extensive work in cohort studies, most notably the Nurses' Health Study. Importantly, GDM is not a "western" condition but has increasing importance for rapidly industrializing countries. Drs. Yang and Shou discuss how GDM has increased in China, a matter of particular concern considering the million-plus births which occur in China annually.

Our understanding of the genetics and pathophysiology of GDM has grown rapidly over the past decade. The role of the placenta, a powerful but still poorly understood endocrine organ, is discussed by Drs. Desoye and Hiden in their chapter. Drs. Buchanan and

Xiang review their key insulin clamp studies in GDM women, which furthered our understanding of the overlap between GDM and type 2 diabetes. Drs. McCurdy and Friedman discuss their work on insulin resistance during GDM, particularly in skeletal muscles. Drs. Knopp and colleagues review their lipid work and also introduce several exciting new findings regarding the evolution of lipids during pregnancy. The coexistence of hypertensive disorders of pregnancy and carbohydrate intolerance of pregnancy has long been recognized and is summarized by Drs. Sibai and Habli in the following chapter.

As the number of women with GDM increases, so do perinatal comorbidities. Dr. Nicholson reviews obesity during pregnancy and its impact on perinatal complications, particularly for the GDM pregnancy. Her chapter is followed by a detailed discussion of the other obstetrical complications that accompany GDM by Drs. Kjos and Guberman. Dr. Dabelea reviews how GDM can have longer-term complications through "imprinting" in the intrauterine environment, exemplifying how GDM continues to affect child health even years after delivery.

Thus, we have set the stage for current management options of GDM, both during and after pregnancy. Drs. Artal, Zavorsky, and Catanzaro discuss current exercise recommendations and studies illustrating the strength of evidence behind physical activity limitations during pregnancy. Drs. King and Sacks extend this to a valuable review of the myriad recommendations regarding nutrition and weight management during the GDM pregnancy. This section on management is accompanied by Dr. Langer's chapter on pharmacologic treatment options, both regarding oral medications and insulin.

GDM was first defined by O'Sullivan and Mahan by maternal diabetes risk, and Dr. Kim discusses this risk and other factors contributing this risk in the next chapter. Dr. Hedderson reviews the interaction between hormonal and non-hormonal family planning with GDM in the following chapter. Dr. Gunderson discusses the fascinating literature regarding breast-feeding, a behavior that affects chronic disease risk decades into the future, even when engaged in over only several months.

Interventions to prevent GDM and to target GDM for future diabetes prevention are few. Dr. Chasan-Taber reviews her own work on GDM prevention during pregnancy, followed by Dr. Ferrara and Dr. Ehrlich, who review intervention science for diabetes prevention in GDM women.

Our book concludes with a discussion of where key medical organizations stand on management of GDM. The lack of uniformity across organizations leaves room for improvement. Consensus would aid in a more effective plan to address the many health implications raised by GDM and the multiple areas for future research raised in these chapters.

There are several obvious problems caused by the lack of uniform GDM definitions, tracking, and management recommendations. Given the extensive overlap between GDM and diabetes, the advances in diabetes pathophysiology, epidemiology, and healthcare delivery could serve as a template for further development of GDM infrastructure. In the United States, the fragmentation of health care and its accompanying variation in GDM screening strategies hamper the compilation of a large cohort of GDM women. Globally, this fragmentation is accompanied by variation between countries. In turn, this has hampered genetic studies, which require larger numbers particularly for genome-wide association work. National tracking systems or registries are currently limited regarding their sensitivity and specificity for GDM, and more work should be done to refine these tools. It has also limited our understanding of how future diabetes develops in these women and their children. Cohort studies which acknowledge the onset of time between GDM development and future disease are difficult, but could be modeled on prospective cohort studies that have examined cardiovascular risk. Such studies would need to follow children as well as mothers.

Ann Arbor, MI, USA Catherine Kim
Oakland, CA, USA Assiamira Ferrara

Contents

Contributors

Mukesh M. Agarwal, MD FCAP
Department of Pathology,
UAE University, Al Ain,
United Arab Emirates

Raul Artal, M.D.
Department of Obstetrics,
Gynecology and Women's Health,
Saint Louis University,
Saint Louis, MO, USA

Bartolome Bonet, MD
Northwest Lipid Research Clinic,
Division of Metabolism,
Endocrinology and Nutrition,
Division of Cardiology,
University of Washington,
Seattle, WA, USA

Thomas A. Buchanan, MD
Departments of Medicine,
Obstetrics and Gynecology, and
Physiology and Biophysics,
Keck School of Medicine,
University of Southern California,
Los Angeles, CA, USA

Rosemary B. Catanzaro, MS RD
Department of Obstetrics,
Gynecology and Women's Health,
Saint Louis University,
Saint Louis, MO, USA

Elizabeth Chan, MD
Northwest Lipid Research Clinic,
Division of Metabolism,
Endocrinology and Nutrition,
Division of Cardiology,
University of Washington,
Seattle, WA, USA

Lisa Chasan-Taber, ScD
Department of Public Health,
University of Massachusetts Amherst,
Amherst, MA, USA

Donald R. Coustan, MD
Department of Obstetrics and Gynecology,
Women and Infant's Hospital of Rhode
Island, Providence, RI, USA

Dana Dabelea, MD, PhD
Department of Epidemiology,
Colorado School of Public Health,
University of Colorado Denver,
Aurora, CO, USA

Gernot Desoye, PhD
Department of Obstetrics and Gynecology,
Medical University of Graz, Graz,
Austria

Alan R. Dyer, PhD
Department of Preventive Medicine,
Northwestern University Feinberg School
of Medicine, Chicago, IL, USA

Samantha F. Ehrlich, MPH
Division of Research, Kaiser Permanente
Northern California, Oakland, CA, USA

Assiamira Ferrara, MD PhD
Division of Research, Kaiser Permanente
Northern California,
Oakland, CA, USA

Jacob E. Friedman, PhD
Department of Biochemistry and
Molecular Genetics,
University of Colorado Denver,
School of Medicine,
Aurora, CO, USA

Cristiane Guberman, MD
Department of Obstetrics and Gynecology,
University of Kentucky,
Lexington, KY, USA

Erica P. Gunderson, PhD
Division of Research,
Epidemiology and Prevention Section,
Kaiser Permanente Northern California,
Oakland, CA, USA

Mounira A. Habli, MD
Department of Obstetrics and Gynecology,
University of Cincinnati
College of Medicine,
Cincinnati, OH, USA

David R. Hadden, MD
Royal Jubilee Maternity Hospital,
Belfast, Northern Ireland

Monique Hedderson, PhD
Kaiser Permanente Northern California's,
Divison of Research,
Oakland, CA, USA

Ursula Hiden, MS PhD
Department of Obstetrics and Gynecology,
Medical University of Graz,
Graz, Austria

Moshe Hod, MD
Helen Schneider Hospital for Women,
Rabin Medical Center and Sackler Faculty
of Medicine, Tel-Aviv University,
Petah-Tiqva, Isreal

Lois Jovanovic, MD
Department of Research,
Sansum Diabetes Research Institute,
Santa Barbara, CA, USA

Catherine Kim, MD MPH
Department of Obstetrics and Gynecology,
University of Michigan,
Ann Arbor, MI, USA

Janet C. King, PhD
Children's Hospital Oakland
Research Institute,
Oakland, CA, USA

John L. Kitzmiller, MD
Maternal-Fetal Medicine,
Santa Clara Valley Health Center,
San Jose, CA, USA

Siri L. Kjos, MD MS Ed
Department of Obstetrics and Gynecology,
Harbor UCLA Medical Center,
Torrance, CA, USA

Robert H. Knopp, MD
Northwest Lipid Research Clinic,
Division of Metabolism,
Endocrinology and Nutrition,
Division of Cardiology,
University of Washington,
Seattle, WA, USA

Oded Langer, MD PhD
Department of Obstetrics and Gynecology,
St Luke's-Roosevelt Hospital Center,
University Hospital of Columbia University,
New York, NY, USA

Jean M. Lawrence, ScD, MPH, MSSA
Department of Research and Evaluation,
Kaiser Permanente Southern California,
Pasadena, CA, USA

Lynn P. Lowe, PhD
Department of Preventive Medicine,
Northwestern University Feinberg
School of Medicine,
Chicago, IL, USA

Carrie E. McCurdy, PhD
Department of Pediatrics,
University of Colorado Denver,
School of Medicine,
Aurora, CO, USA

Boyd E. Metzger, MD
Division of Endocrinology,
Metabolism and Molecular Medicine,
Northwestern University Feinberg
School of Medicine,
Chicago, IL, USA

Wanda K. Nicholson, MD MPH MBA
Department of Obstetrics and Gynecology,
Centre for Women's Health Research,
University of North Carolina at Chapel Hill,
Chapel Hill, MD, USA

Scott C. Nickel, BS
Sansum Diabetes Research Institute,
Santa Barbara, CA, USA

Jeremy J.N. Oats, MD
Royal Women's Hospital,
University of Melbourne,
Victoria, Australia

Bengt E.H. Persson, MD PhD
Department of Women and Child Health,
Karolinska Institute,
Stockholm, Sweden

Pathmaja Paramsothy, MD
Northwest Lipid Research Clinic,
Division of Metabolism,
Endocrinology and Nutrition,
Division of Cardiology,
University of Washington,
Seattle, WA, USA

Ravi Retnakaran, MD MSc FRCPC
Leadership Sinai Centre for Diabetes,
Toronto, ON, Canada

David A. Sacks, MD
Department of Research and Evaluation,
Southern California Permanente
Medical Group, Bellflower,
CA, USA

Chong Shou, MD
Department of Obstetrics and Gynecology,
Peking University First Hospital,
Beijing, P.R. China

Baha Sibai, MD
Department of Obstetrics and Gynecology,
University of Cincinnati
College of Medicine,
Cincinnati, OH, USA

Elisabeth R. Trimble, MD FRCPath
Diabetes Research Group,
Queen's University Belfast,
Belfast, Northern Ireland

Richard M. Watanabe, PhD
Department of Preventive Medicine,
Keck School of Medicine,
University of Southern California,
Los Angeles, CA, USA

Anny H. Xiang, PhD
Department of Preventive Medicine,
University of Southern California,
Keck School of Medicine,
Los Angeles, CA, USA

Huixia Yang
Department of Obstetrics and Gynecology,
Peking University First Hospital,
Beijing, P.R. China

Gerald S. Zavorsky PhD
Department of Obstetrics,
Gynecology and Women's Health
and Department of Pharmacological
and Physiological Science,
Saint Louis University,
Saint Louis, MO, USA

Cuilin Zhang, PhD MD MPH
Division of Epidemiology,
Statistics and Prevention Research,
Eunice Kennedy Shriver National Institute
of Child Health and Human Development,
National Institutes of Health,
Rockville, MD, USA

Xiaodong Zhu, MD
Northwest Lipid Research Clinic,
Division of Metabolism, Endocrinology
and Nutrition, Division of Cardiology,
University of Washington,
Seattle, WA, USA

An Overview of Problems and Solutions in the Diagnosis and Treatment of Gestational Diabetes

1

John L. Kitzmiller

1.1 Introduction

The present volume presents exciting advances in the knowledge of the pathophysiology, epidemiology, and management of gestational diabetes (GDM), and the maternal-fetal-placental-neonatal effects of metabolic imbalance. GDM is also described as temporary hyperglycemia during pregnancy, or glucose intolerance in pregnancy, that impairs perinatal outcome. However, we now know that abnormalities in insulin sensitivity and insulin secretion[1, 2] are detectable before pregnancy in women with GDM and that the abnormalities often persist afterwards.[3] GDM predicts increased risk of later diabetes in the mother and metabolic abnormalities in the offspring (as reviewed in chapters in this book), so there is nothing temporary about it. GDM was actually first known as *prediabetes*.

Since insulin resistance and glucose intolerance in women are associated with excess cardiovascular disease later in life, and pregnant women are usually motivated to improve health behaviors, pregnancy is a good time to educate women with GDM. The long-term effects of GDM, available postpartum prevention trials, and the need for further research are well covered in this book. Effects of glucose intolerance on pregnancy outcome and the debate as to whether the effects are independent of confounders or preventable, have been more controversial.

1.2 Controversy Regarding Screening

My purpose is to give a personal view of the evidence relating to the diagnosis and treatment of GDM. As recently as May 2008 the U. S. Preventive Services Task Force (USPSTF) concluded[4, 5]:

- Current evidence is insufficient to assess the balance between the benefits and harms of screening women for GDM either before or after 24 weeks gestation.

J.L. Kitzmiller
Maternal-Fetal Medicine, Santa Clara Valley Health Center,
750 South Bascom, Suite 340, San Jose, CA 95128, USA
e-mail: john.kitzmiller@hhs.sccgov.org

C. Kim and A. Ferrara (eds.), *Gestational Diabetes During and After Pregnancy*,
DOI: 10.1007/978-1-84882-120-0_1, © Springer-Verlag London Limited 2010

- Harms of screening include short-term anxiety in some women with positive screening results; [there is] inconvenience to many women and medical practices because most positive screening test results are probably false positive [as is true with prenatal genetic risk screening].
- The extent to which these interventions [dietary modification, medication, support from diabetes educators and nutritionists, increased surveillance in prenatal care] improve health outcomes is uncertain.
- Until there is better evidence, clinicians should discuss screening for GDM with their patients and make case-by-case decisions. This discussion should include information about the uncertain benefits and harms as well as the frequency and uncertain meaning of a positive screening test result.
- Nearly all pregnant women should be encouraged to achieve moderate weight gain based on their prepregnancy body mass index and to participate in physical activity.

The Task Force cited prior recommendations of the American College of Obstetricians and Gynecologists,[6] the American Academy of Family Physicians,[7] and the American Diabetes Association[8] that asymptomatic low-risk pregnant women need not be screened with glucose testing. Low risk was defined as (a) age younger than 25 years, (b) not a member of a racial/ethnic group with increased risk for developing type 2 diabetes, (c) body mass index (BMI) of 25 kg/m^2 or less, (d) no previous history of abnormal glucose tolerance or adverse obstetrics outcomes usually associated with GDM, and (e) no known history of diabetes in a first-degree relative. There is also no consensus on routine diagnosis in other countries, as reviewed in this book. The USPSTF did point to ongoing large prospective studies that would provide helpful information, and the results are now available.

1.3 History of GDM Screening

In the 1940–1950s, it was recognized that women developing type 2 diabetes had excess perinatal mortality and very large infants in their prior pregnancies. Therefore, investigators began to study glucose levels in nondiabetic women during pregnancy in relation to pregnancy outcome and to long-term development of maternal diabetes. In the USA, O'Sullivan pioneered the use of 100-g oral glucose tolerance testing during pregnancy.[9] He conducted a randomized controlled trial in 599 women classified as "potentially diabetic," comparing diet management and a small dose of Neutral Protamine Hagedorn (NPH) insulin vs. routine prenatal care. A normal control group was also included. The study demonstrated a significant reduction in babies with birth weight above 4,090 g (4.3 vs. 13.1 vs. 3.7%, $p<0.05$) but no difference in preterm delivery (8.5 vs. 7.8 vs. 7.7%) or perinatal mortality (3.8 vs. 4.9 vs. 1.9%).[10] The randomized controlled trial was conducted prior to the availability of glucose monitoring or fetal surveillance.

So then, what is the importance of reducing fetal macrosomia? Macrosomia (variously defined by absolute birth weight) or large birth weight for gestational age and gender (LGA) have been considered major indicators of the effects of hyperglycemia during pregnancy.[11–14]

The association of fetal macrosomia and excess adiposity with fetal hyperglycemia and hyperinsulinemia is strong[15–18] and is supported by experiments in pregnant monkeys.[19] Fetal macrosomia and adiposity may also be related to maternal triglyceridemia and free fatty acids, as reviewed in this book. The intuitive risks of difficult delivery and maternal/neonatal damage associated with fetal macrosomia[20] are confirmed in recent large data sets.[21–23] The long-term risks of fetal macrosomia (independent of confounders) in infants of women with GDM include increased childhood overweight[24–27] and association with metabolic factors that are expected to increase risk of cardiovascular disease.[28–31] Since there are many causes of high birth weight and childhood obesity or later diabetes, it might be assumed that their associations have not been universal.[32–37] It may be preferable to include fetal insulin or neonatal adiposity or lipid markers as indicators of the quality of treatment for maternal glucose intolerance or as predictors of problems with childhood development.[18, 38–42]

In the decades following O'Sullivan's work, there was uncertainty about the methods of screening and the diagnostic glucose values to use for GDM, as reviewed in this book. Many investigators found that maternal glucose levels lower than those used to indicate treatment of GDM were associated with increased perinatal complications.[25, 43–57] However, associations do not prove cause and effect, and observational studies may be biased in many ways. Although the evidence is strong that marked fasting and postprandial hyperglycemia in early and later pregnancy is linked to excess risk of congenital malformations, fetal death, and costly neonatal morbidity,[58–62] large randomized controlled trials have been needed to prove or disprove that treatment is indicated for women with mild GDM.

1.4
Recent Randomized Controlled Trials-Australia

The first multicenter randomized controlled trial was conducted in Australia and the United Kingdom during 1993–2003 in women with risk factors or a 50-gram (g) 1-hour (h) oral glucose challenge >140 mg/dL (>7.8 mM).[63] GDM diagnosis was based on fasting plasma glucose (FPG) <140 mg/dL (<7.8 mM) and 2-h plasma glucose (2-h PG) 140–198 mg/dL (7.8–11.0 mM) on a 75-g glucose tolerance test (GTT) at 24–34 weeks gestation. As the trial moved along, the FPG exclusion threshold was lowered to 126 mg/dL (7.0 mM), when the World Health Organization changed the definition of diabetes.[63] Median entry gestational age was 29 weeks and 25% were beyond 30 weeks gestation; 24.8% were nonwhite. Average GTT FPG was 86.4±12.6 mg/dL (4.8±0.7 mM) and median 2-h PG was 154 mg/dL (8.55 mM) for subjects enrolled in the trial.

Women with GDM were randomized to intervention (n=490) with "individualized dietary advice from a qualified dietitian, which took into consideration a woman's prepregnancy weight, activity level, dietary intake, and weight gain; instructions on how to self-monitor glucose levels, which the woman was then asked to do four times daily until the levels had been in the recommended range for 2 weeks (fasting blood glucose (BG) 63–99 mg/dL (3.5–5.5 mM), 2-h postprandial BG <126 mg/dL (<7.0 mM), followed by daily monitoring at rotating times during the day)".[63] Insulin therapy was required in only 20%, "if there were two capillary-blood glucose results during the 2-week period in which the fasting level was at least 99 mg/dL (5.5 mM) or the postprandial level was at least 126 mg/dL (7.0 mM) at 35 weeks gestation or less; or if there was one BG at least 162 mg/dL (9.0 mM)".[63] Higher postprandial values were used to indicate insulin therapy >35 weeks gestation (144 mg/dL; 8.0 mM).

Women with glucose intolerance randomized to routine prenatal care ($n=510$) and their caregivers were not aware of the diagnosis. Very few women in this group required a physician clinic visit after enrollment (median antenatal clinic visits 5.2), but 10.5% had a visit to a dietitian or a diabetes educator and 3% used insulin based on attending clinician suspicion of diabetes.[63] There were five perinatal deaths (three stillborn, two neonatal) among infants born to women in the routine-care group, but none in the intervention group ($p=0.06$). The rate of serious perinatal complications (death, shoulder dystocia, bone fracture, and nerve palsy) was less in the intervention group (1 vs. 4%; relative risk adjusted for maternal age, race or ethnic group, and parity, 0.33; 95% CI 1.03–1.23; $p=0.01$). Statistical analysis was based on intention to treat. Secondary outcomes are presented in Table 1.1. The authors concluded that treatment of GDM reduces serious perinatal morbidity; the number needed to treat to benefit was 34 (95% CI, 20–103). Intervention also reduced gestational weight gain, gestational hypertension, and fetal macrosomia.[63]

The "clinical cost" of intervention in this trial was a higher rate of induction of labor (39 vs. 29%) and of admission to neonatal nursery (71 vs. 61%), possibly since clinicians were aware of the GDM intervention.[63] However, intervention was not associated with increased cesarean sections (31 vs. 32%) or small-for-gestational age infants <10th percentile on Australian charts (7 vs. 7%).[64] The frequency of antenatal admission was similar (29 vs. 27%), the interquartile gestational age at birth was 38–40 weeks gestation for both groups, and the interquartile length of postnatal stay was 3–5 days for both groups. Maternal anxiety score was not increased during the intervention or 3 months postpartum and several quality of life measures were consistent with improved health status in the intervention group. Postnatal depression was reduced in the intervention group (8 vs. 17%; relative risk 0.46, 95% CI 0.29–0.73; $p=0.001$).[63]

Subsequent economic costs-consequences evaluation of data in this trial showed that the incremental cost per additional serious perinatal complication prevented was $27,503 (2002 Australian dollar = 0.74 U.S, dollar, 0.48 UK pounds or 0.66 Euros), per perinatal death prevented was $60,506, and per discounted life-year gained was $2,988. The authors concluded that, "it is likely that the general public in high-income countries such as Australia would find reductions in perinatal mortality and in serious perinatal complications sufficient to justify additional health service and personal monetary charges. Over the whole lifespan, the incremental cost per extra life-year gained is highly favorable".[65]

1.5 Recent Randomized Controlled Trials-United States

The second multicenter randomized controlled trial was conducted during 2002–2007 in 16 maternal-fetal medicine units in the USA.[66] Women at 24–30 weeks gestation with 50-g 1-h glucose challenge results of 135–200 mg/dL (7.5–11.1 mM) and gestational age confirmed by ultrasound and no prior history of GDM, hypertension, or stillbirth were invited to

Table 1.1 Pregnancy outcomes in mild GDM: randomized controlled trials of medical nutrition therapy and self-monitoring of blood glucose (with insulin treatment as necessary) compared to routine prenatal care with blinding of GTT results

Characteristics, outcomes	Crowther et al 2005[63]		Landon et al 2009[66]	
Groups	Intervention	Routine care	Intervention	Routine care
Number of subjects	490	510	485	473
Required insulin (%)	20	3	7.8	0.6
Perinatal death	0	5 *p* 0.07	0	0
Pregnancy hypertensive disorder	12%	18% *p* 0.02	8.6%	13.6% *p* 0.01
Induction of labor	39%	29% *p* 0.003	27.3%	26.8%
Gestational age at birth (week)	39.0	39.3	39.0±1.8	38.9±1.8
Cesarean delivery	31%	32%	26.9%	33.8% *p* 0.02
Shoulder dystocia	1%	3% *p* 0.08	1.5%	4.0% *p* 0.02
Birth trauma	0	2	3/476	6/455 *p* 0.33
Birth weight >4,000 g	10%	21% *p* 0.001	5.9%	14.3% *p* 0.001
Large for gestational age	13%	22% *p* 0.001	7.1%	14.5% *p* 0.001
Small for gestational age (%)	7	7	7.5	6.4
Admission to intensive neonatal observation	71%	61% *p* 0.01	9.0%	11.6%
Respiratory distress syndrome (%)	5	4	1.9	2.9
Hypoglycemia requiring intravenous treatment (%)	7	5	5.3	6.8
Hyperbilirubinemia requiring phototherapy or >95th percentile	9%	9%	9.6%	12.9% *p* 0.12
Maternal anxiety score at 6 weeks after enrollment	11.2±3.7	11.5±4.0		
Depression at 3 months postpartum	8%	17% *p* 0.001		

participate in the study; 7,381 women consented. Then a 100-g 3-h oral GTT was performed. If the FPG was ≥95 mg/dL (<5.3 mM) the subject was excluded from the trial. If 2 of 3 post-load levels were >180 mg/dL (>10 mM) at 1-h, >155 mg/dL (>8.6 mM) at 2-h, >140 mg/dL (>7.8 mM) at 3-h, the glucose intolerant subjects were randomized to usual prenatal care, blinded to glucose results ($n=473$), *or* to formal nutritional counseling and diet therapy with self-monitoring of blood glucose ($n=485$), and insulin if necessary (only 7.6%). Insulin was prescribed if the majority of capillary glucose values between visits exceeded 95 mg/dL fasting or 120 mg/dL 2-h postprandial. If there was clinical suspicion of hyperglycemia in a routine care subject and a random PG of ≥160 mg/dL was detected, the patient's caregiver initiated treatment of some kind. Results were analyzed on the basis of intention to treat.[66]

Mean gestational age at randomization was 28±1.6 weeks gestation for both groups. Maternal age, parity, BMI, and ethnicity did not differ in the two groups. Hispanic race/ethnicity was claimed by 58% in the treatment group and 56% in the routine care group. Mean GTT FPG was 86±5.7 mg/dL (4.8±0.3 mM) in both groups, mean 1-h PG was 192 vs. 193±22–20 mg/dL in the two groups, mean 2-h PG was 173±20 mg/dL in the two groups, and mean 3-h on the GTT was 137 vs. 134±29–31.5 mg/dL in the two groups (a non-significant difference).[66]

After randomization, there were seven prenatal visits on average in the treatment group, compared to an average of five visits in the routine care group. Weight gain from enrollment to delivery was less in the treatment group, 2.8±4.5 kg vs. 5.0±3.3 kg, ($p < 0.001$). Capillary blood glucose treatment targets were largely achieved: for the diet-treated subgroup, the interquartile self-monitored fasting BG levels were 76–86 mg/dL, 90.5–104 mg/dL after breakfast, 96–109 mg/dL after lunch, and 102–115 mg/dL after dinner. Treatment values were about 10 points higher in the small group of 37 requiring insulin treatment. Two subjects in the routine care group ended up with insulin treatment, although glucose monitoring was not used in this group.[66]

Women in both groups assessed fetal movements daily, and there were no perinatal deaths in either group. The primary outcome was a composite of the neonatal complications hyperbilirubinemia, hypoglycemia, hyperinsulinemia, and birth trauma (32.4% in the treatment group, 37.0% in the routine treatment group; a non-significant difference).[66] Predetermined secondary outcomes are presented in Table 1.1. Shoulder dystocia, cesarean delivery, birth weight >4,000 g, frequency of LGA infants, estimated neonatal fat mass, and preeclampsia were all significantly reduced by intervention. Intervention did not increase induction of labor, preterm birth, the frequency of small-for-gestational age infants, or admission to the neonatal intensive care unit. The authors concluded that risks associated with fetal overgrowth are most sensitive to treatment of mild GDM, and that inclusion of patients with more severe hyperglycemia is probably necessary to demonstrate reduction in perinatal death and neonatal morbidities.[66]

Thus, we have proof of benefit that medical nutrition therapy and self-monitoring of blood glucose enhance short-term outcomes from two similar large, well-conducted intervention trials in women with mild GDM. Insulin treatment was needed in a minority of subjects in both trials. It is hoped that subjects will be followed to determine if there are long-term benefits from such intervention during pregnancy. The evidence regarding different treatment modalities for the management of GDM is covered in chapters of this book. Given the difficulties of conducting blinded studies and withholding proven treatments from pregnant women, it is not likely we will have more randomized trials of treatment compared to no treatment. Since the benefit was much stronger than the harm of treatment, it is worthwhile to diagnose GDM during pregnancy. The diagnostic entry criteria were somewhat different in the two trials, and the question remains of the best way to diagnose women with GDM.

1.6
Current Screening Criteria

In January 2009, the American Diabetes Association recommended: "Screen for GDM using risk factor analysis and, if appropriate, use of an OGTT".[67] The ADA further stated: "because of the risks of GDM to the mother and neonate, screening and diagnosis are warranted… Women at very high risk for GDM should be screened as soon as possible after the confirmation of pregnancy." Criteria for very high risk are:

- Severe obesity
- Prior history of GDM or delivery of LGA infant
- Presence of glycosuria
- Diagnosis of polycystic ovarian syndrome
- Strong family history of type 2 diabetes

The ADA also noted that screening/diagnosis at this stage of pregnancy should use standard diagnostic testing, i.e., an FPG ≥126 mg/dL (7.0 mM) *or* random PG ≥200 mg/dL (11.1 mM) *or* 2-h 75-g GTT value ≥200 mg/dL (11.1 mM).[67]

The ADA also recommended that women at greater than low risk of GDM, including those above not found to have diabetes early in pregnancy, should undergo GDM testing at 24–28 weeks of gestation.[67] Low risk status, which does not require GDM screening, is defined as women with ALL of the following characteristics:

- Age < 25 years
- Weight normal before pregnancy
- Member of a racial/ethnic group with a low prevalence of diabetes
- No known diabetes in first-degree relatives
- No history of abnormal glucose tolerance
- No history of poor obstetrical outcome

Many clinicians have opined that few women satisfy all these low-risk exclusion criteria in US clinics today. Many of the criteria are not specifically defined, which allows clinicians some latitude in judgment.

In 2009, the ADA recommended[67] either of two approaches to GDM diagnostic testing according to the 2004 ADA Position Statement on GDM[8]: (1) *two-step approach* with 50-g 1-h PG screen ≥140 mg/dL (7.8 mM) or ≥130 mg/dL (7.2 mM) (better sensitivity), followed by the 100-g 3-h GTT; *or* (2) a *one step approach* "which may be preferred in clinics with high prevalence of GDM". To make a diagnosis of GDM, at least two of the following plasma glucose values must be found: fasting ≥95 mg/dL (5.3 mM), 1-h ≥180 mg/dL (10 mM), 2-h ≥155 mg/dL (8.6 mM), 3-h ≥140 mg/dL (7.8 mM). It should be noted that the Proceedings of the ADA-sponsored Fifth International Workshop-Conference on Gestational Diabetes Mellitus published in 2007 had recommended use of *either* the 100-g 3-h *or* the 75-g 2-h oral GTT, with the same glucose thresholds.[68]

1.7 Diagnostic Screening Cutpoints and HAPO

Due to the inconsistencies around the world and in the USA regarding diagnosis of GDM, the National Institutes of Health and other organizations sponsored a large-scale (23,216 pregnant women ≥18 years of age) multinational epidemiologic study of the relationship of 75-g GTT values at 24–28 weeks gestation to perinatal outcome measures – the Hyperglycemia and Pregnancy Outcomes study.[69] The GTT results were blinded to subjects and caregivers. Such a large study was necessary to control for confounders like age, weight, ethnicity, family history and geographic region. Women with FPG >105 mg/dL (5.8 mM), 2-h PG >200 mg/dL (11.1 mM), any PG <45 mg/dL (2.5 mM), or subsequent random PG >160 mg/dL (8.9 mM) at 34–37 weeks gestation were unblinded and treated as deemed locally appropriate. Thus, this was a huge study of untreated mild glucose intolerance. The results and implications of the HAPO study are discussed in detail in this book in the chapter by Lowe, Metzger, Dyer et al.[18, 69]

The major conclusion of the HAPO investigators was that the risk of adverse pregnancy outcomes (maternal, fetal, and neonatal) *continuously* increased as a result of maternal fasting or postload glycemia at 24–28 weeks gestation, at levels previously considered normal, and no obvious glucose thresholds were detected for most outcomes.[69] Importantly, the relationships were independent and not confounded by risk factors like maternal age, obesity, race/ethnicity, and family history. That is not to say that the risk factors are not real, but that low risk women also have significant relationships between their test glucose levels and key outcomes. The investigators showed a continuous glucose relationship with fetal macrosomia, cord C-peptide, and neonatal adiposity assessed either by skinfolds or by derived percent body fat, supporting the determining role of fetal hyperinsulinemia.[18,70] The continuous maternal glucose relationship with fetal macrosomia is similar to that seen in smaller scale observational studies.[47, 48, 50, 71–74] Since there were no apparent maternal glucose thresholds to predict risk, the HAPO investigators concluded that consensus methods were needed to set global diagnostic standards for GDM. The standardization will assist interpretation of clinical research studies in which investigators use different diagnostic approaches, and should allay confusion among clinicians and health plan managers.

To help achieve that aim, a global conference sponsored by the International Association of Diabetes and Pregnancy Study Groups (IADPSG) was convened in Pasadena, California in June 2008. After complete interactive presentation of the many aspects of the HAPO results, some other relevant studies, and poster presentations, eleven caucuses representing the major international and US stakeholder organizations and attending clinicians and investigators from all continents discussed the implications of the data. The caucus recommendations were then considered by a 50-person IADPSG Consensus Panel representing the whole group, the health organizations, and the IADPSG members unable to attend.[75] The Consensus Panel concluded that (1) single-step testing should be used for all pregnant women at 24–28 weeks gestation, (2) the 75-g GTT should be used as the test for GDM with any one abnormal value counting as the diagnosis, and (3) criteria and methods should be developed to identify marked hyperglycemia early in pregnancy, since many women have undiagnosed diabetes when they become pregnant, and they have increased risks of fetal malformations and maternal vascular complications for which extended testing is indicated. The task remained for the IADPSG Consensus Panel to develop the glucose threshold criteria to use to make these diagnoses.[75]

During the subsequent 15 months, the IADPSG Consensus Panel used online and writing group conference call communications to develop the recommendations, with open presentations of the pros and cons at many international conferences, including at least three major ones in the USA. The review paper appears in *Diabetes Care.*[75] Panel members agreed to use glucose values with odds ratios of 1.75 for the various perinatal risks, compared to mean glucose values at each testing time. The chosen thresholds represent a compromise between users of glucose measurement as mg/dL or mM, choosing numbers that should be easy to remember. For GDM diagnosis at 24–28 weeks gestation, the recommended plasma glucose thresholds are fasting ≥92 mg/dL (5.1 mM) *or* 1-h ≥180 mg/dL (10 mM) *or* 2-h ≥153 mg/dL (8.5 mM).

For diagnosis of marked hyperglycemia in early pregnancy that may represent undiagnosed diabetes, the panel members agreed to use standardized hemoglobin A1c (HbA1c) ≥6.5 *or* FPG ≥126 mg/dL (7.0 mM) *or* random PG ≥200 mg/dL (11.1 mM), with abnormal results to be confirmed by subsequent testing. The panel recommended that local conditions should determine if the early pregnancy screening should be universal or selective. It is of interest that an international panel has recommended use of standardized HbA1c ≥6.5 for the diagnosis of diabetes in general.[76] High-risk women with negative early tests should undergo a 75-g 2-h GTT at 24–28 weeks gestation.

It is anticipated that concerned health care organizations in different countries will adopt these recommendations. Do they represent an "inconvenient truth" with reference to the concerns of the 2008 USPSTF? Yes, because the projected prevalence of GDM according to the HAPO data will be ±16% of pregnancies. That figure will vary in different communities. The prevalence is in agreement with the increasing rates of obesity and prediabetes found in all parts of the world.

Managers and planners are concerned these numbers will overly burden existing prenatal care facilities and personnel. An ethical consideration of not using the new criteria is whether it is right to deny women diagnosis and treatment that has been shown to benefit them and their offspring, at some cost. Undoubtedly, some triage methods will be developed to decide the intensity of treatment regimens offered to the women diagnosed with GDM. We may take heart that the excellent randomized controlled trials show that medical nutrition therapy, physical activity, and self-monitoring of blood glucose and fetal activity are sufficient to achieve good outcomes in most cases. It should be possible to find ways of delivering this care at reasonable cost.

References

1. Barbour LA, McCurdy CE, Hernandez TL, Kiewan JP, Catalano PM, Friedman JE. Cellular mechanisms for insulin resistance in normal pregnancy and gestational diabetes. *Diabetes Care*. 2007;30:S112-S119.

2. Buchanan TA, Xiang A, Kjos SL, Watanabe R. What is gestational diabetes? *Diabetes Care.* 2007;30:S105-S111.
3. Catalano PM, Kirwan JP, Haugel-de Mouzon S, King J. Gestational diabetes and insulin resistance: role in short- and long-term implications for mother and fetus. *J Nutr.* 2003;133: 1674S-1683S.
4. Hillier TA, Vesco KK, Pedula KL, Beil TL, Whitlock EP, Pettitt D. Screening for gestational diabetes mellitus: a systematic review for the U.S. Preventive Services Task Force. *Ann Intern Med.* 2008;148:766-775.
5. United States Preventive Services Task Force. Screening for gestational diabetes mellitus: U.S. Preventive Services Task Force recommendation statement. *Ann Intern Med.* 2008;148: 759-765.
6. ACOG Practice Bulletin. Clinical management guidelines for obstetrician-gynecologists. *Obstet Gynecol.* 2001;98:525-538.
7. American Academy of Family Physicians. *Policy Action. Summary of Recommendations for Clinical Preventive Services; Revision 6.4.* Leawood, KS: American Academy of Family Physicians; 2007.
8. American Diabetes Association. Gestational diabetes mellitus. *Diabetes Care.* 2004;27:S88-S90.
9. O'Sullivan JB, Mahan CM. Criteria for the oral glucose tolerance test in pregnancy. *Diabetes.* 1964;13:278-285.
10. O'Sullivan JB, Gellis SS, Dandrow RV, Tenney BO. The potential diabetic and her treatment in pregnancy. *Obstet Gynecol.* 1966;27:683-689.
11. Jang HC, Cho NH, Min YK, Han IK, Jung KB, Metzger BE. Increased macrosomia and perinatal morbidity independent of maternal obesity and advanced age in Korean women with GDM. *Diabetes Care.* 1997;20:1582-1588.
12. Yang X, Hsu-Hage B, Zhang H, Zhang C, Zhang Y, Zhang C. Women with impaired glucose tolerance during pregnancy have significantly poor pregnancy outcomes. *Diabetes Care.* 2002;25:1619-1624.
13. Langer O, Yogev Y, Most O, Xanakis EMJ. Gestational diabetes: the consequences of not treating. *Am J Obstet Gynecol.* 2005;192:989-997.
14. Suhonen L, Hiilesmaa V, Kaaja R, Teramo K. Detection of pregnancies with high-risk fetal macrosomia among women with gestational diabetes mellitus. *Acta Obstet Gynecol Scand.* 2008;87:940-945.
15. Heding LG, Persson B, Stangenberg M. Beta-cell function in newborn infants of diabetic mothers. *Diabetologia.* 1980;19:427-432.
16. Metzger BE, Silverman BL, Freinkel N, Sl D, Ogata ES, Green O. Amniotic fluid insulin concentration as a predictor of obesity. *Arch Dis Child.* 1990;65:1050-1052.
17. Weiss PA, Haeusler M, Tamussino K, Haas J. Can glucose tolerance test predict fetal hyperinsulinism? *Br J Obstet Gynecol.* 2000;107:1480-1485.
18. HAPO Study Cooperative Research Group. Hyperglycemia and Pregnancy Outcome Study: Associations with neonatal anthropometrics. *Diabetes.* 2009;58:453-459.
19. Susa JB, Schwartz R. Effects of hyperinsulinemia in the primate fetus. *Diabetes.* 1985;34:36-41.
20. Spellacy WN, Miller S, Winegar A, Peterson PQ. Macrosomia-maternal characteristics and infant complications. *Obstet Gynecol.* 1985;66:158-161.
21. Boulet SL, Alexander GR, Salihu HM, Pass M. Macrosomic births in the United States: determinants, outcomes, and proposed grades of risk. *Am J Obstet Gynecol.* 2003;188:1372-1378.
22. Zhang X, Decker A, Platt RW, Kramer MS. How big is too big? The perinatal consequences of fetal macrosomia. *Am J Obstet Gynecol.* 2008;198:517.
23. Esakoff TF, Cheng YW, Sparks TN, Caughey AB. The association between birthweight 4000 grams or greater and perinatal outcomes in patients with and without gestational diabetes mellitus. *Am J Obstet Gynecol.* 2009;200:672.e671-672.e674.
24. Vohr BR, McGarvey ST, Tucker R. Effects of maternal gestational diabetes on offspring adiposity at 4-7 years of age. *J Mat Fetal Neonat Med.* 1999;21:149-157.

25. Hillier TA, Pedula KL, Schmidt MM, Mullen JA, Charles M, Pettitt DJ. Childhood obesity and metabolic imprinting: the ongoing effects of maternal hyperglycemia. *Diabetes Care*. 2007;30:2287-2292.
26. Murtaugh M, Jacobs DR, Moran A, Steinerger J, Sinaiko AR. Relation of birth weight to fasting insulin, insulin resistance, and body size in adolescence. *Diabetes Care*. 2003;26:187-192.
27. Schaefer-Graf UM, Pawliczak J, Passow D, et al. Birth weight and parental BMI predict overweight in children from mothers with gestational diabetes. *Diabetes Care*. 2005;28:1745-1750.
28. Dabelea D, Pettitt D, Hanson R, Imperatore G, Bennett P, Knowler W. Birth weight, type 2 diabetes, and insulin resistance in Pima Indian children and young adults. *Diabetes*. 1999;22:944-950.
29. Hypponen E, Power C, Smith GD. Prenatal growth, BMI, and risk of type 2 diabetes by early midlife. *Diabetes Care*. 2003;26:2512-2517.
30. Wei J, Sung F, Li C, et al. Low birth weight and high birthweight infants are both at increased risk to have type 2 diabetes among school children in Taiwan. *Diabetes Care*. 2003;26:343-348.
31. Boney CM, Verma A, Tucker R, Vohr BR. Metabolic syndrome in childhood: association with birth weight, maternal obesity, and gestational diabetes mellitus. *Pediatrics*. 2005;115:e290-e296.
32. Whitaker RC, Pepe MS, Seidel KD, Wright JA, Knopp RH. Gestational diabetes and the risk of offspring obesity. *Pediatrics*. 1998;101:91-97.
33. Clausen TD, Mathiesen ER, Hansen T, et al. High prevalence of type 2 diabetes and pre-diabetes in adult offspring of women with gestational diabetes mellitus or type 1 diabetes. *Diabetes Care*. 2008;31:340-346.
34. Clausen TD, Mathiesen ER, Hansen T, et al. Overweight and the metabolic syndrome in adult offspring of women with diet-treated gestational diabetes mellitus or type 1 diabetes. *J Clin Endocrinol Metab*. 2009;94:2464-2470.
35. Gillman M, Rifas-Shiman S, Berkey C, Field A, Colditz G. Maternal gestational diabetes, birth weight and adolescent obesity. *Pediatrics*. 2003;111:221-226.
36. Hediger ML, Overpeck MD, McGlynn A, Kuczmarski RJ, Maurer KR, Davis WW. Growth and fatness at three to six years of age of children born small- or large-for-gestational-age. *Pediatrics*. 1999;104:e33.
37. Hadden DR. Prediabetes and the big baby. *Diabet Med*. 2008;25:1-10.
38. Kohlhoff R, Doerner G. Perinatal hyperinsulinism and perinatal obesity as risk factors for hyperinsulinemia in later life. *Exp Clin Endocrinol*. 1990;96:105-108.
39. Catalano PM, Thomas AJ, Huston LP, Fung CM. Effect of maternal metabolism on fetal growth and body composition. *Diabetes Care*. 1998;21:B85-B90.
40. Roach VJ, Fung H, Corckram CS, Lau TK, Rogers MS. Evaluation of glucose intolerance in pregnancy using biochemical markers of fetal hyperinsulinemia. *Gynecol Obstet Invest*. 1998;45:175-176.
41. Pirc LK, Owens JA, Crowther CA, Willson KJ, De Blasio M, Robinson JS. Mild gestational diabetes in pregnancy and the adipoinsulin axis in babies born to mothers in the ACHOIS randomized controlled trial. *BMC Pediatrics*. 2007;7:18.
42. Leipold H, Kautzky-Willer A, Ozbal A, Bancher-Todesca D, Worda C. Fetal hyperinsulinism and maternal one-hour postload plasma glucose level. *Obstet Gynecol*. 2004;104:1301-1306.
43. Tallarigo L, Giampietro O, Penno G, Miccoli R, Gregori G, Navalesi R. Relation of glucose tolerance to complications of pregnancy in nondiabetic women. *N Engl J Med*. 1986;315:989-992.
44. Langer O, Anyaegbunam A, Brustman L, Divon M. Management of women with one abnormal oral glucose tolerance value reduces adverse outcome in pregnancy. *Am J Obstet Gynecol*. 1989;161:593-599.
45. Lindsay MK, Graves W, Klein L. The relationship of one abnormal glucose tolerance test value and pregnancy complications. *Obstet Gynecol*. 1989;73:103-106.
46. Magee MS, Walden CE, Benedetti TJ, Knopp RH. Influence of diagnostic criteria on the incidence of gestational diabetes and perinatal morbidity. *JAMA*. 1993;269:609-615.

47. Sacks DA, Greenspoon JS, Abu-Fadil S, Henry HM, Wolde-Tsadik G, Yao JFF. Toward universal criteria for gestational diabetes: the 75 gram glucose tolerance test in pregnancy. *Am J Obstet Gynecol.* 1995;172:607-614.
48. Sermer M, Naylor CD, Gare DJ, et al. Impact of increasing carbohydrate intolerance on maternal-fetal outcomes in 3637 women without gestational diabetes. The Toronto Tri-Hospital Gestational Diabetes Project. *Am J Obstet Gynecol.* 1995;173:146-156.
49. Schaefer-Graf UM, Dupak J, Vogel M, et al. Hyperinsulinism, neonatal obesity, and placental immaturity in infants born to women with one abnormal glucose tolerance test value. *J Perinat Med.* 1998;26:27-36.
50. Jensen DM, Damm P, Sorensen B, et al. Clinical impact of mild carbohydrate intolerance in pregnancy: a study of 2904 nondiabetic Danish women with risk factors for gestational diabetes mellitus. *Am J Obstet Gynecol.* 2001;185:413-419.
51. Hedderson MM, Ferrara A, Sacks DA. Gestational diabetes mellitus and lesser degrees of pregnancy hyperglycemia: association with increased risk of spontaneous preterm birth. *Obstet Gynecol.* 2003;102:850-856.
52. Ostlund I, Hanson U, Bjorklund A, et al. Maternal and fetal outcomes if gestational impaired glucose tolerance is not treated. *Diabetes Care.* 2003;26:2107-2111.
53. Ferrara A, Weiss NS, Hedderson MM, et al. Pregnancy plasma glucose levels exceeding the American Diabetes Association thresholds, but below the National Diabetes Data Group thresholds for gestational diabetes mellitus, are related to the risk of neonatal macrosomia, hypoglycaemia, and hyperbilirubinaemia. *Diabetologia.* 2007;50:298-306.
54. Lapolla A, Dalfra MG, Bonomo M, et al. Can plasma glucose and HbA1c predict fetal growth in mothers with different glucose tolerance levels? *Diabetes Res Clin Pract.* 2007;77(3):465-470.
55. Ju H, Rumbold AR, Willson KJ, Crowther CA. Borderline gestational diabetes mellitus and pregnancy outcomes. *BMC Pregnancy Childbirth.* 2008;8:31.
56. Kautzky-Willer A, Bancher-Todesca D, Weitgasser R, et al. The impact of risk factors and more stringent diagnostic criteria of gestational diabetes on outcomes in central European women. *J Clin Endocrinol Metab.* 2008;93:1689-1695.
57. Corrado F, Bendetto AD, Cannata ML, et al. A single abnormal value of the glucose tolerance test is related to increased adverse perinatal outcome. *J Matern Fetal Neonatal Med.* 2009;22: 597-601.
58. de Veciana M, Major CA, Morgan MA, et al. Postprandial versus preprandial blood glucose monitoring in women with gestational diabetes mellitus requiring insulin therapy. *N Engl J Med.* 1995;333:1237-1241.
59. Schaefer-Graf UM, Songster G, Xiang A, Berkowitz K, Buchanan TA, Kjos SL. Congenital malformations in offspring of women with hyperglycemia first detected during pregnancy. *Am J Obstet Gynecol.* 1997;177:1165-1171.
60. Adams KM, Li H, Nelson RL, Ogburn PL Jr, Danilenko-Dixon DR. Sequelae of unrecognized gestational diabetes. *Am J Obstet Gynecol.* 1998;178:1321-1332.
61. Allen VM, Armson BA, Wilson RD, et al. Teratogenicity associated with pre-existing and gestational diabetes. *J Obstet Gynecol Can.* 2007;29:927-944.
62. Kitzmiller JL, Block JM, Brown FM, et al. *Managing Preexisting Diabetes and Pregnancy. Technical Reviews and Consensus Recommendations for Care.* Alexandria, VA: American Diabetes Association; 2008.
63. Crowther CA, Hiller JE, Moss JR, et al. Effect of treatment of gestational diabetes mellitus on pregnancy outcomes. *N Engl J Med.* 2005;352:2477-2486.
64. Roberts G. Shoulder dystocia. *Br J Obstet Gynaecol.* 1999;106:610.
65. Moss JR, Crowther CA, Hiller JE, Willson KJ, Robinson JS, The Australian Carbohydrate Intolerance Study in Pregnant Women (ACHOIS) Trial Group. Costs and consequences of treatment for mild gestational diabetes mellitus-evaluation from the ACHOIS randomized trial. *BMC Pregnancy Childbirth.* 2007;7:27.

66. Landon MB, Spong CY, Thom E, et al. A multicenter, randomized trial of treatment of mild gestational diabetes. *N Engl J Med*. 2009;361:1339-1348.
67. American Diabetes Association. Standards of medical care in diabetes: position statement. *Diabetes Care*. 2009;32:S13-S61.
68. Metzger BE, Buchanan TA, Coustan DR, et al. Summary and recommendations of the Fifth International Workshop-Conference on Gestational Diabetes Mellitus. *Diabetes Care*. 2007; 30:S251-S260.
69. HAPO Study Cooperative Research Group. Hyperglycemia and adverse pregnancy outcomes. *N Engl J Med*. 2008;358:1991-2002.
70. Lindsay RS. Many HAPO returns. Maternal glycemia and neonatal adiposity: new insights from the Hyperglycemia and Adverse Pregnancy Outcomes (HAPO) study. *Diabetes*. 2009;58: 302-303.
71. Jensen DM, Korsholm L, Ovesen P, Beck-Nielsen H, Molsted-Pedersen L, Damm P. Adverse pregnancy outcome in women with mild glucose intolerance: is there a clinically meaningful threshold value for glucose? *Acta Obstet Gynecol Scand*. 2008;87:59-62.
72. Retnakaran R, Qi Y, Sermer M, Connelly PW, Hanley AJG, Zinman B. The antepartum glucose values that predict neonatal macrosomia differ from those that predict postpartum prediabetes or diabetes: implications for the diagnostic criteria for gestational diabetes. *J Clin Endocrinol Metab*. 2009;94:840-845.
73. Riskin-Mashiah S, Younes G, Damti A, Auslender R. First-trimester fasting hyperglycemia and adverse pregnancy outcome. *Diabetes Care*. 2009;32:1639-1643.
74. Voldner N, Qvigstad E, Froslie KF, Godang K, Henriksen T, Bollderslev J. Increased risk of macrosomia among overweight women with high gestational rise of fasting glucose. *J Mat Fetal Neonat Med*. 2009;1:1-8.
75. IADSPG Consensus Panel. International Association of Diabetes and Pregnancy Study Groups recommendations on the diagnosis and classification of hyperglycemia in pregnancy. *Diabetes Care*. 2010;33:676-682.
76. International Expert Committee. International Expert Committee report on the role of the A1c assay in the diagnosis of diabetes. *Diabetes Care*. 2009;32:1327-1334.

Section I

Screening for and Identification of GDM During Pregnancy

Hyperglycemia and Adverse Pregnancy Outcome (HAPO) Study: An Overview

2

Lynn P. Lowe, Boyd E. Metzger, Alan R. Dyer, Donald R. Coustan, David R. Hadden, Moshe Hod, Jeremy J. N. Oats, Bengt Persson, Elisabeth R. Trimble G and the HAPO Study Cooperative Research Group

2.1 Rationale for the HAPO Study

Gestational diabetes mellitus (GDM), defined as "glucose intolerance with onset or first recognition during pregnancy"[1, 2] has been the subject of considerable controversy. The initial criteria for the diagnosis of GDM that were established more than 40 years ago[3] remain in use today, with only minor modifications. The criteria were chosen to identify women at high risk for the development of diabetes following pregnancy,[4] or were derived from adaptation of criteria used for non-pregnant persons,[5] not to identify pregnant women at increased risk for adverse perinatal outcome. There is consensus that overt diabetes mellitus (DM) during pregnancy, whether or not accompanied by symptoms or signs of metabolic decompensation, is associated with a significant risk of adverse perinatal outcome; the risk of such outcomes associated with degrees of hyperglycemia less severe than overt DM is controversial. A number of factors contribute to this longstanding controversy.

The lack of international uniformity in the approach to ascertainment and diagnosis of GDM has been a major hurdle.[2] Some have attributed the risk of adverse outcomes associated with GDM to confounding characteristics such as obesity, advanced maternal age of subjects with GDM, or other medical complications, rather than glucose intolerance.[6–8] Bias of the caregiver toward the expectation of adverse outcomes may increase the likelihood of morbidity due to increased intervention.[9] Other reports suggest that the criteria currently used for the diagnosis of GDM[1] are too restrictive and that lesser degrees of hyperglycemia increase the risk of adverse perinatal outcomes.[10–15] Conversely, others believe that all systematic efforts to identify the condition should be stopped unless more data become available to link significant morbidities to specific degrees of glucose intolerance.[7] Finally, questions have been raised regarding the benefit of treating GDM. However, two recently reported randomized controlled trials found that treatment, achieved primarily by diet/lifestyle modification, resulted in reduced frequency of large-for-gestational age

B.E. Metzger (✉)
Division of Endocrinology, Metabolism and Molecular Medicine,
Northwestern University Feinberg School of Medicine,
645 N. Michigan Avenue Suite 530-22, Chicago, IL, 60611, USA
e-mail: bem@northwestern.edu

C. Kim and A. Ferrara (eds.), *Gestational Diabetes During and After Pregnancy*,
DOI: 10.1007/978-1-84882-120-0_2,

births and pre-eclampsia.[16,17] Notably, the most recent recommendations of the US Preventive Services Task Force, the UK National Health Service, and the Canadian Task Force on the Periodic Health Examination assert that there is not sufficient high level evidence to make a recommendation for, or against, screening for GDM.[18–20]

The objective of the Hyperglycemia and Adverse Pregnancy Outcome (HAPO) Study was to clarify the risk of adverse outcome associated with degrees of maternal glucose intolerance less severe than overt DM during pregnancy. Glucose tolerance was measured in a large, heterogeneous, multinational, multicultural, ethnically diverse cohort of women at 24–32 weeks gestation with medical caregivers "blinded" to status of glucose tolerance (except when predefined thresholds were met).[21]

In 1952, Jorgen Pedersen[22] postulated that maternal hyperglycemia led to fetal hyperglycemia that, in turn, evoked an exaggerated fetal insulin response. Fetal hyperinsulinemia was then responsible for the typical diabetic fetopathy such as macrosomia, neonatal hypoglycemia, perinatal trauma, and death. The hypothesis has represented the context in which associations between maternal glycemia and adverse perinatal outcome have been viewed for more than 50 years. In analyzing and reporting the results of the HAPO study, we considered the associations between maternal glycemia and the primary outcomes of increased size at birth, delivery by cesarean section, neonatal hypoglycemia and the presence of fetal hyperinsulinism within the framework of the Pedersen Hypothesis. Additional outcomes in HAPO included preterm delivery, shoulder dystocia and/or birth injury, sum of skinfolds >90th percentile, percent body fat >90th percentile, intensive neonatal care, hyperbilirubinemia, and pre-eclampsia.

2.2 Design of the HAPO Study

2.2.1 Participants and Exclusion Criteria

Participants were enrolled between July 2000 and April 2006. All pregnant women at each of 15 field centers in nine countries were eligible to participate unless they had one or more of the following exclusion criteria: age less than 18 years, planned delivery at a non-field center hospital, date of last menstrual period (LMP) not certain and no ultrasound (US) estimation from 6 to 24 weeks of gestational age available, unable to complete the oral glucose tolerance test (OGTT) within 32 weeks gestation, multiple pregnancy, conception using gonadotropin ovulation induction or by in vitro fertilization, glucose testing prior to recruitment or a diagnosis of diabetes during this pregnancy, diagnosis of diabetes antedating pregnancy requiring treatment with medication, participation in another study which might interfere with HAPO, known to be HIV positive or to have hepatitis B or C, prior participation in HAPO, or inability to converse in the languages used in field center forms without the aid of an interpreter. Age and education level attained were ascertained for those women who declined to participate in the study.

Gestational age and the expected date of delivery (EDD) were determined from the date of the LMP, if the participant was certain of her dates. If the participant was unsure, the EDD was determined from an US performed between 6 and 24 weeks gestation. The final

EDD was also determined from US if: (1) the gestational dating from LMP differed from the US dating by more than 5 days, when the US was performed between 6 and 13 weeks gestation, or (2) if the dating differed by more than 10 days when the US was done between 14 and 24 weeks gestation.

2.2.2 Procedures

2.2.2.1 Glucose Testing

Participants underwent a standard 75-g OGTT between 24 and 32 weeks gestation and as close to 28 weeks as possible, following an overnight fast (8–14 h) and after at least 3 days of unrestricted diet and normal physical activity. Height, weight, and blood pressure were measured at the time of the OGTT. Data concerning smoking and use of alcohol during pregnancy, first degree family history of hypertension and/or diabetes, and demographic data were collected using standardized questionnaires. Race/ethnicity was self-identified by participants from a list read to them.

As a safety measure, a sample for random plasma glucose (RPG) was collected at 34–37 weeks gestation to reduce the unlikely possibility that undiagnosed diabetes may have evolved in late gestation. Participants could be retested under the blinded HAPO protocol at any time the managing clinician so requested.

2.2.2.2 Glucose Analysis

Glucose concentrations were measured by enzymatic methods on aliquots of plasma. The procedures used to assure comparability of results across the 15 field centers and the Central Laboratory were previously reported.[23] Samples were analyzed at the local field center laboratory for purposes of clinical decision making with respect to blinding or unblinding. To avoid confounding effects of center-to-center analytical variation, aliquots of all OGTT plasma glucose (PG) specimens (fasting, 1-, and 2-h) were analyzed at the Central Laboratory and these results were used in this report. Results subsequently obtained at the Central Laboratory did not reveal any bias in inclusion or exclusion due to methodological variations across the 15 field center laboratories.[23]

2.2.2.3 Unblinding

Aliquots of the fasting and 2-h OGTT plasma samples and the RPG sample were analyzed at the field center laboratory and values were unblinded only if the fasting plasma glucose (FPG) level exceeded 105 mg/dL (5.8 mmol/L), if the 2-h OGTT PG sample exceeded 200 mg/dL (11.1 mmol/L), if the RPG level was greater than or equal to 160 mg/dL

(8.9 mmol/L), or if any PG value was less than 45 mg/dL (2.5 mmol/L). Otherwise, the woman, her caregivers, and HAPO Study staff (except for laboratory personnel) remained blinded to her glucose values. Only women whose results were within these limits, with no additional glucose testing outside the HAPO protocol, were included in these analyses.

2.2.2.4 Prenatal Care and Delivery

Participants received prenatal care according to the usual practice at their field center. The timing of delivery was determined by standard practice for the individual field center. None of the field centers arbitrarily delivered their patients before full term or routinely performed cesarean delivery at a specified maternal or gestational age.

2.2.2.5 Cord Plasma Glucose and Serum C-Peptide Samples

Cord blood was collected at delivery for assessment of fetal β-cell function (C-peptide) and for glucose measurement. The samples were collected as soon as possible after the cord was clamped. The sample for cord PG measurement was placed in a tube containing sodium fluoride and placed in ice water to minimize glycolysis. The samples were separated within 60 min of collection. Aliquots of plasma from the glucose sample and serum from the C-peptide sample were prepared and frozen. These were analyzed at the Central Laboratory. A "Vitros 750" analyzer was used for glucose analysis and serum C-peptide was assayed on an Autodelfia instrument.[23] Fetal hyperinsulinism is typically assessed by measurements of insulin concentration in amniotic fluid or in cord blood serum or plasma. We used cord serum C-peptide (secreted in equimolar concentrations with insulin) as our index rather than insulin for the following reasons: first, insulin degradation is known to be increased in the presence of even small amounts of hemolysis; second, approximately 15% of cord samples show detectable hemolysis when serum or plasma is separated; and third, the concentration of C-peptide is not altered by hemolysis.[23]

2.2.2.6 Neonatal Care and Follow-Up

After delivery, customary routine neonatal care was carried out at each field center. Measurements of neonatal PG were performed at the field center for clinical indications at the discretion of the attending physician, if signs or symptoms suggested sustained or later development of hypoglycemia. Such measurements were performed without blinding in the local field center laboratory using a glucose enzymatic method. The need for other assessments, e.g., bilirubin and status of respiratory function, was determined by clinical indications.

Medical records were abstracted to obtain data regarding the prenatal, labor and delivery, postpartum, and newborn course. A questionnaire was administered to the participant between 4 and 6 weeks after delivery to collect follow-up information, including readmission of the mother or baby to the hospital.

2.2.2.7 Neonatal Anthropometrics

Neonatal anthropometrics were obtained within 72 h of delivery. Anthropometric measurements included weight, length, head circumference, and skinfold thickness at three sites (flank, subscapular, triceps). Two measurements were made; if results differed by more than a pre-specified amount (>10 g for weight, 0.5 cm for length and head circumference, or 0.5 mm for skinfolds, respectively), a third was done. For these analyses, the average of the two measurements was used, unless a third measurement was taken. In that case, if two of three measurements differed by less than the pre-specified amount, the average of those two was used; otherwise the average of all three was used.

Birth weight was obtained without diaper using a calibrated electronic scale. Length was measured on a standardized plastic length board constructed for use in the HAPO study. Head circumference was measured with a standard plastic measuring tape across the occipital fontanel. Skinfold thickness was measured with Harpenden (Baty, UK) skinfold calipers. Flank skinfold was measured on the left side just above the iliac crest on a diagonal fold on the mid axillary line. Triceps measurement was taken at the vertical fold over the triceps muscle half the distance between the acromion process and olecranon, and subscapular just below the lower angle of the scapula at about a 45° angle to the spine.

Mean coefficients of variation for anthropometric measurements were 0.04% for birth weight, 0.17% for length, 0.16% for head circumference, 2.91% for flank skinfold, 2.57% for subscapular skinfold, and 2.73% for triceps skinfold.

2.2.3 Outcomes

2.2.3.1 Primary Outcomes

a. *Birthweight >90th percentile for gestational age*: This was defined based on gender, ethnicity (Caucasian or other, Black, Hispanic, Asian), field center, gestational age (30–44 weeks only), and parity, using separate 90th percentile regression analyses for each of eight HAPO newborn gender-ethnic groups. A newborn was considered to have a birth weight >90th percentile, if the birth weight was greater than the estimated 90th percentile for HAPO newborns of the same gender, gestational age, ethnicity, field center, and maternal parity. Otherwise, the newborn was considered to have a birth weight ≤90th percentile.
b. *Primary cesarean delivery*: A cesarean delivery was defined as primary if it was the woman's first cesarean delivery.
c. *Clinical neonatal hypoglycemia*: Babies were categorized as having clinical neonatal hypoglycemia if the medical record contained a notation of neonatal hypoglycemia and there were symptoms and/or treatment with a glucose infusion or a local laboratory report of a glucose value ≤30.6 mg/dL (1.7 mmol/L) in the first 24 h and/or ≤45 mg/dL (2.5 mmol/L) after the first 24 h.[24]
d. *Hyperinsulinemia*: A cord serum C-peptide value >90th percentile of values for the total cohort of participants (1.7 ug/L) was defined as hyperinsulinemia.

2.2.3.2
Other Outcomes

a. *Preterm delivery*: Delivery prior to 37 weeks gestation was defined as preterm.
b. *Shoulder dystocia and/or birth injury*: Instances of shoulder dystocia and birth injury were reviewed without knowledge of glucose values and those that were confirmed were defined as having this outcome.
c. *Sum of skinfolds >90th percentile for gestational age*: 90th percentiles for gestational age (36–44 weeks only) were determined from 90th percentile regression analyses using eight newborn gender-ethnic groups (Caucasian or other, Black, Hispanic, Asian), with adjustment for field center, and parity (0, 1, 2+). A newborn was considered to have a sum of skinfolds >90th percentile if the sum was greater than the estimated 90th percentile for the baby's gender, gestational age, ethnicity, field center, and maternal parity. Otherwise, the newborn was considered to have a sum ≤90th percentile.
d. *Percent body fat >90th percentile for gestational age*: Fat mass was calculated from birthweight, length, and flank skinfold according to the equation given in Catalano et al[25] that was based on measurements of total body electrical conductivity (TOBEC). The derived formula was also prospectively validated with estimates of fat mass by TOBEC. Percent body fat was then calculated as 100 × fat mass/birthweight. Percent body fat >90th percentile for gestational age (36–44 weeks only) was defined using the same methods as for sum of skinfolds >90th percentile.
e. *Intensive neonatal care*: Admission to any type of unit for care more intensive than normal newborn care was classified as intensive neonatal care when the duration was greater than 24 h, or the baby died or was transferred to another hospital. Admissions where the only reason(s) for admission was (a) possible sepsis and sepsis was ruled out; (b) observation; or (c) feeding problems were not included.
f. *Hyperbilirubinemia*: If there was treatment with phototherapy after birth, or at least one laboratory report of a bilirubin level ≥20 mg/dL, or readmission for hyperbilirubinemia, the baby was categorized as having hyperbilirubinemia.
g. *Pre-eclampsia*: Hypertension present prior to 20 weeks that did not progress to pre-eclampsia was classified as chronic hypertension. After 20 weeks gestation, hypertension disorders in pregnancy were categorized according to International Society for the Study of Hypertension (ISSHP) guidelines.[26] Pre-eclampsia = systolic BP ≥140 mmHg and/or diastolic BP ≥90 mmHg on two or more occasions a minimum of 6 h apart with proteinuria of ≥1+ dipstick or ≥300 mg/24 h. If the criteria for elevated BP but not proteinuria were met, this was classified as gestational hypertension.
h. *Birthweight <10th percentile for gestational age*: This was defined using the same methods that were used for birthweight >90th percentile for gestational age.

2.2.3.3
Possible Severe Adverse Outcomes

The field centers were asked to abstract additional data whenever a possible severe adverse event such as death, shoulder dystocia, birth injury, or major malformation was identified.

These data were reviewed by a subcommittee of the HAPO Steering Committee, blinded to the glycemic status of the mother. They confirmed whether the event was present. Perinatal deaths were classified according to the guidelines given in the "Australia and New Zealand Antecedent Classification of Perinatal Mortality".[27] Major malformations were classified according to ICD 10 coding.[28] The HAPO external Data Monitoring Committee also reviewed the adverse outcomes and deaths, but with full details of the OGTT and RPG levels.

2.2.4 Statistical Analyses

For unadjusted analyses of associations of glycemia with primary outcomes each glucose measurement was divided into seven categories, so that approximately 50% of all values were in the two lowest categories, and 3 and 1% were in the two highest categories, respectively. The smaller numbers in the higher categories for glucose variables were designed to allow us to assess whether or not there was a threshold effect with regard to each glycemia-outcome association, since we did not know, a priori, whether associations would be continuous and graded or whether risk might be increased only above a specific threshold. Thus, for these analyses FPG was categorized as <75, 75–79, 80–84, 85–89, 90–94, 95–99, and ≥100 mg/dL; 1-h PG as <105, 106–132, 133–155, 156–171, 172–193, 194–211, and ≥212 mg/dL; and 2-h PG as ≤90, 91–108,109–125, 126–139, 140–157, 158–177, ≥178 mg/dL (for cut-offs, see Fig. 2.1).

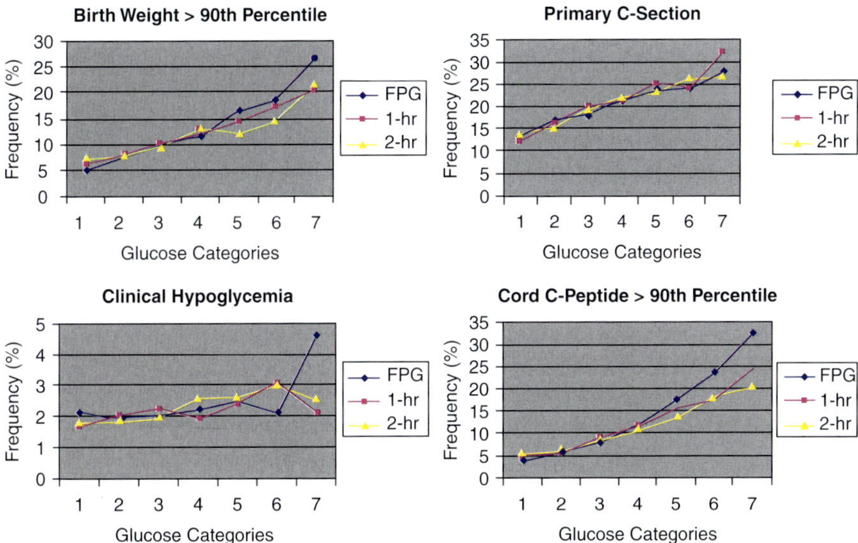

Fig. 2.1 Frequency of primary outcomes across categories of glucose. Fasting: Category 1=<75, 2=75–79, 3=80–84, 4=85–89, 5=90–94, 6=95–99, 7=≥100 mg/dL. One hour oral glucose tolerance test (OGTT): Category 1=≤105, 106–132, 133–155, 156–171, 172–193, 194–211, ≥212. Two hour OGTT: Category 1=≤90, 91–108, 109–125, 126–139, 140–157, 158–177, ≥178

To make categorical analyses of neonatal anthropometric outcomes for cord serum C-peptide comparable to those that had previously been done for maternal glycemia, we also divided cord serum C-peptide into seven categories so that approximately 50% of the values were in the two lowest categories, and 3 and 1% were in the two highest categories respectively.[29] Thus, for these analyses cord serum C-peptide was categorized as ≤0.5, 0.6–0.8, 0.9–1.2, 1.3–1.5, 1.6–2.1, 2.2–3.0, ≥3.1 ug/L. In these analyses, the lowest cord serum C-peptide category was used as the referent category.

Each glucose measure was also considered as a continuous variable in multiple logistic regression analyses, with odds ratios calculated for each of the three glucose determinations (fasting, 1-, and 2-h PG) increased by one standard deviation. To assess whether or not the log of the odds of each outcome was linearly related to glucose, we added squared terms in each glucose measure. We also examined cord C-peptide as a continuous variable with both linear and squared terms for each outcome. However, because the squared term was significant ($p < 0.001$) for each anthropometric outcome, indicating significant nonlinearity, only categorical multiple logistic analyses are reported here for cord C-peptide.

For the results of the multiple logistic analyses reported here, associations with outcomes for each glycemia measure and cord serum C-peptide were adjusted for field center, maternal age, maternal body mass index (BMI) and height calculated from measurements taken at the OGTT visit, smoking and alcohol use during pregnancy, hospital admission during the prenatal period (except in the analyses for pre-eclampsia), family history of diabetes, mean arterial blood pressure at the OGTT (except in the analyses for pre-eclampsia), gestational age at the OGTT, parity (except in the analyses for cesarean delivery), gender of the neonate, maternal urinary tract infection and family history of high blood pressure for the outcome of pre-eclampsia, and cord PG for the outcome of fetal hyperinsulinemia. Ethnicity was not included as an additional potential confounder in these analyses except for the fetal adiposity measures in which it was included in the definition, since there was strong overlap with field center, and there was little or no contribution of ethnicity for the other outcomes when dummy variables for field center were included. In the continuous glucose analyses, we also tested for interactions of glucose with field center, age, BMI, and maternal height in relation to outcomes. In the analyses of the relationship between maternal glucose and delivery by primary cesarean, women who delivered by repeat cesarean were excluded altogether.

2.3 Results

2.3.1 Research Participants

A total of 53,295 women were found to be eligible and of these 28,562 (54%) agreed to participate between July 2000 and April 2006. The average age of participants was 29.0 years, compared with 28.5 among those who declined; the average number of years of education was 12.9 vs. 12.5 among those who agreed and declined, respectively. These differences, although statistically significant, were small. A total of 25,505 women underwent an OGTT and of these, 746 or 2.9% were unblinded for at least one PG result outside of the threshold ranges (OGTT or RPG values) and excluded from the main study. A total of 1,412 women were dropped from the study due mainly to non-HAPO glucose testing or delivery in a non-field center hospital. Thirty-one women were excluded due to missing data on birth weight, gestational age at delivery, maternal age, BMI, mean arterial pressure at the OGTT, or 1- or 2-h PG, or for having a gestational age >44 weeks at delivery (which was assumed to be erroneous). A total of 23,316 women remained in the main study and this is the group for which results have been reported.[29, 30]

Selected characteristics of HAPO participants and their newborns are shown in Table 2.1. In this cohort of blinded participants, the mean FPG was 80.9 mg/dL (4.5 mmol/L); the mean 1-h PG was 134.1 mg/dL (7.4 mmol/L) and the mean 2-h PG was 111 mg/dL (6.2 mmol/L). Of the participants, 48.3% were white, non-Hispanic. The remainder were from several other ethnic groups. Approximately 23% reported a first degree family history of diabetes and 36% reported a first degree family history of hypertension.

The mean gestational age at delivery was 39.4 weeks. Mean birthweight of the newborns was 3,292 g (standard deviation 529 g) and the mean varied by more than 400 g among the field centers (data not shown). The mean cord glucose was 81.5 mg/dL (4.5 mmol/L). A total of 51.5% of the babies were male, and 6.9% were delivered preterm (prior to 37 weeks).

There were two maternal deaths, one due to pulmonary embolism and the other to respiratory failure secondary to pneumonia. In the postpartum period, 187 or 0.8% of mothers experienced a major hemorrhage requiring transfusion or operative treatment. A total of 26 women required transfer to intensive care for treatment and 172 or 0.74% of mothers were readmitted to hospital after initial post delivery discharge. There were 130 perinatal deaths among the 23,316 deliveries, or 5.6/1,000. These were comprised of 89 fetal and 41 neonatal/infant deaths.

2.3.2 Glycemia and Outcomes

The frequency of each primary outcome across categories of glucose is shown in Fig. 2.1. With higher levels of maternal glycemia, the frequency of each primary outcome rose, although to a lesser extent for clinical neonatal hypoglycemia than for the other outcomes. Using FPG categories as an example, frequencies in the lowest and highest categories were: birthweight above the 90th percentile 5.3 and 26.3%; primary cesarean section 13.3 and 27.9%; clinical neonatal hypoglycemia 2.1 and 4.6%; and C-peptide above the 90th percentile 3.7 and 32.4%.

Results for glucose as a continuous variable with adjustment for confounders for both primary and other outcomes are shown in Table 2.2. For primary outcomes, odds ratios for glucose higher by 1 standard deviation were largest for birthweight and cord C-peptide and ranged from 1.38 to 1.46 for birthweight >90th percentile and from 1.37 to 1.55 for cord C-peptide >90th percentile. For primary cesarean section and clinical neonatal hypoglycemia, associations were weaker and the associations of clinical neonatal hypoglycemia with FPG and 2-h PG were not statistically significant.

Table 2.1 Characteristics of HAPO participants and frequency of outcomes

Maternal characteristics	*N*	*Mean*	*SD*
Age (years)	23,316	29.2	5.8
Body mass index (BMI)[a]	23,316	27.7	5.1
Mean arterial pressure (MAP) (mmHg)[a]	23,316	80.9	8.3
Fasting plasma glucose (FPG) (mg/dL)[a]	23,316	80.9	6.9
1-h plasma glucose (PG) (mg/dL)[a]	23,316	134.1	30.9
2-h plasma glucose (mg/dL)[a]	23,316	111.0	23.5
Gestational age* (weeks)	23,316	27.8	1.8
	N	%	
Ethnicity			
White, non-Hispanic	11,265	48.3	
Black, non-Hispanic	2,696	11.6	
Hispanic	1,984	8.5	
Asian/oriental	6,757	29.0	
Other or unknown	614	2.6	
Prenatal smoking (any)	1,581	6.8	
Prenatal alcohol use (any)	1,612	6.9	
Family history of diabetes	5,282	22.7	
Parity (prior delivery ≥20 weeks)	12,233	52.5	
Prenatal urinary tract infection	1,655	7.1	
Hospitalization prior to delivery	3,271	14.0	
Newborn characteristics	*N*	*Mean*	*SD*
Gestational age (weeks)	23,316	39.4	1.7
Birthweight (g)	23,267	3,292	529
Cord serum C-peptide (ug/L)	19,885	1.0	0.6
Cord plasma glucose (mg/dL)	19,859	81.5	19.6
	N	%	
Sex – Male	12,003	51.5	
Obstetric outcomes	*N*	%	
Cesarean section delivery			
Primary	3,731	16.0	
Repeat	1,792	7.7	
Hypertension[2]			
Chronic hypertension	582	2.5	
Gestational hypertension	1,370	5.9	
Pre-eclampsia	1,116	4.8	
Newborn outcomes	*N*	%	
Birthweight >90th percentile[3]	2,221	9.6	
Clinical neonatal hypoglycemia[4]	480	2.1	
Cord C-peptide >90th percentile[5]	1,671	8.4	
Preterm delivery (before 37 weeks)	1,608	6.9	
Shoulder dystocia and/or birth injury	311	1.3	
Intensive neonatal care[6]	1,855	8.0	
Hyperbilirubinemia[7]	1,930	8.3	

[a]Measured at the OGTT

[b]Hypertension: Hypertension present prior to 20 weeks which did not progress to pre-eclampsia was classified as chronic hypertension. After 20 weeks gestation, hypertension disorders in

pregnancy were categorized according to International Society for the Study of Hypertension (ISSHP) guidelines (26). Pre-eclampsia = systolic BP > 140 mmHg and/or diastolic BP > 90 mmHg on 2 or more occasions a minimum of 6 hours apart and proteinuria of > 1+ dipstick or > 300 mg per 24 hours. If the criteria for elevated BP but not proteinuria were met, this was classified as gestational hypertension.

[c]Birthweight > 90th percentile: 90th percentiles for gestational age (30-44 weeks only) were determined using quantile regression analyses for each of 8 newborn gender-ethnic groups (Caucasian or Other, Black, Hispanic, Asian), with adjustment for gestational age, field center, and parity (0, 1, 2+). A newborn was considered to have a birthweight > 90th percentile if the birthweight was greater than the estimated 90th percentile for the baby's gender, gestational age, ethnicity, field center, and maternal parity. Otherwise, the newborn was considered to have a birthweight < 90th percentile.

[d]Clinical neonatal hypoglycemia: Clinical neonatal hypoglycemia was defined as present if there was notation of neonatal hypoglycemia in the medical record and there were symptoms and/or treatment with a glucose infusion or a local laboratory report of a glucose value < 30.6 mg/dL (1.7 mmol/L) in the first 24 hours and/or < 45 mg/dL (2.5 mmol/L) after the first 24 hours after birth (24).

[e]Cord C-Peptide > 90th %ile: Defined from the total HAPO cohort with a C-peptide result.

[f]Intensive Neonatal Care: Admission to any type of unit for care more intensive than normal newborn care when the duration was greater than 24 hours, or the baby died or was transferred to another hospital. Admissions for only: (a) possible sepsis and sepsis was ruled out; (b) observation; or (c) feeding problems were excluded.

[g]Hyperbilirubinemia: Treatment with phototherapy after birth, or at least 1 laboratory report of a bilirubin level > 20mg/dL, or readmission for hyperbilirubinemia.

Table 2.2 Adjusted[a] odds ratios and 95% confidence intervals for associations between maternal glucose as a continuous variable and perinatal outcomes

Outcome	FPG		1-h PG		2-h PG	
	OR[b]	95% CI	OR	95% CI	OR	95% CI
Birthweight >90th percentile	1.38	(1.32–1.44)	1.46	(1.39–1.53)	1.38	(1.32–1.44)
Primary cesarean delivery[c]	1.11	(1.06–1.15)	1.10	(1.06–1.15)	1.08	(1.03–1.12)
Clinical neonatal hypoglycemia	1.08[d]	(0.98–1.19)	1.13	(1.03–1.26)	1.10	(1.00–1.12)
Cord C-peptide >90th percentile	1.55	(1.47–1.64)	1.46	(1.38–1.54)	1.37	(1.30–1.44)
Preterm delivery (<37 weeks)	1.05	(0.99–1.11)	1.18	(1.12–1.25)	1.16	(1.10–1.23)
Shoulder dystocia and/or birth injury	1.18	(1.04–1.33)	1.23	(1.09–1.38)	1.22	(1.09–1.37)
Sum of skinfolds >90th percentile	1.39	(1.33–1.47)	1.42	(1.35–1.49)	1.36	(1.30–1.43)
Percent body fat >90th percentile	1.35	(1.28–1.42)	1.44	(1.37–1.52)	1.35	(1.29–1.42)

Table 2.2 (continued)

Outcome	FPG		1-h PG		2-h PG	
	OR[b]	95% CI	OR	95% CI	OR	95% CI
Intensive neonatal care	0.99	(0.94–1.05)	1.07	(1.02–1.13)	1.09	(1.03–1.14)
Hyperbilirubinemia	1.00	(0.95–1.05)	1.11	(1.05–1.17)	1.08	(1.02–1.13)
Pre-eclampsia	1.21	(1.13–1.29)	1.28	(1.20–1.37)	1.28	(1.20–1.37)

[a]Associations were adjusted for field center, age, BMI, height, smoking status, alcohol use, family history of diabetes, gestational age at OGTT, infant's gender, hospitalization prior to delivery, mean arterial pressure, parity (not included in the model for primary cesarean delivery), cord plasma glucose (included in the model for cord serum C-peptide >90th percentile only), pre-eclampsia did not include adjustment for hospitalization or mean arterial pressure, and family history of hypertension and prenatal urinary tract infection were included only in the model for pre-eclampsia

[b]Odds ratios for glucose higher by 1 standard deviation (6.9 mg/dL for FPG, 30.9 mg/dL for 1-h PG, 23.5 mg/dL for 2-h PG) (mmol/L = mg/dL/18)

[c]Excluding those with a prior cesarean section

[d]Nonlinear relationship

There were also strong associations with pre-eclampsia, where the odds ratios for each 1 standard deviation increase in each glucose measure ranged from 1.21 to 1.28; corresponding odds ratios for shoulder dystocia and/or birth injury were approximately 1.2. Premature delivery, intensive neonatal care, and hyperbilirubinemia were significantly related to 1- and 2-h PG, but not to FPG.

Odds ratios for associations of glycemia with percent body fat >90th percentile and sum of skinfolds >90th percentile were similar in size to those for birthweight >90th percentile.

2.3.3 Cord C-peptide and Neonatal Anthropometrics

Associations between cord C-peptide and neonatal anthropometrics are shown in Table 2.3. With higher levels of cord C-peptide, frequency of each measure of size and adiposity rose. For example, the frequency of birthweight >90th percentile ranged from 4.5 to 25.6% across categories of cord C-peptide. With adjustment only for field center, odds ratios for the three measures ranged from 5.97 to 7.31 in the highest category of cord C-peptide (data not shown). In the fully adjusted logistic regression models, odds ratios were modestly attenuated, but strong graded associations remained.

When cord C-peptide was examined in relationship to birthweight, sum of skinfolds, percent body fat and fat free mass as continuous dependent variables in multiple regression analyses, mean differences between the highest and lowest categories for cord C-peptide were 345 g for birth weight, 2.0 mm for sum of skinfolds, 2.7% for percent fat, and 221 g for fat free mass (all $p < 0.001$) (data not shown).

Table 2.3 Relationship between cord C-peptide and neonatal anthropometrics

Cord C-peptide (ug/L)	*N*	#	%	OR[a]	95% CI
Birthweight >90th percentile[b]					
≤0.5	2,911	131	4.5	1.00	(1.03–1.55)
0.6–0.8	6,530	392	6.0	1.26	(1.82–2.70)
0.9–1.2	5,899	614	10.4	2.21	(2.32–3.60)
1.3–1.5	2,077	283	13.6	2.89	(3.77–5.82)
1.6–2.1	1,639	333	20.3	4.68	(4.31–7.33)
2.2–3.0	571	140	24.5	5.62	(4.75–9.51)
≥3.1	242	62	25.6	6.72	
Total	19,869	1,955	9.8		
Sum of skinfolds >90th percentile[b]					
≤0.5	2,412	117	4.9	1.00	(1.03–1.58)
0.6–0.8	5,647	369	6.5	1.27	(1.56–2.37)
0.9–1.2	5,145	513	10.0	1.92	(2.26–3.57)
1.3–1.5	1,821	267	14.7	2.84	(2.97–4.72)
1.6–2.1	1,409	265	18.8	3.74	(2.99–5.36)
2.2–3.0	485	101	20.8	4.00	(3.78–8.21)
≥3.1	181	46	25.4	5.57	
Total	17,100	1,678	9.8		
Percent body fat >90th percentile[b]					
≤0.5	2,399	119	5.0	1.00	(1.00–1.54)
0.6–0.8	5,630	370	6.6	1.24	(1.52–2.31)
0.9–1.2	5,140	513	10.0	1.87	(2.30–3.62)
1.3–1.5	1,817	276	15.2	2.88	(2.99–4.75)
1.6–2.1	1,403	269	19.2	3.77	(3.79–6.66)
2.2–3.0	485	121	25.2	5.02	(3.41–7.52)
≥3.1	181	43	23.8	5.06	
Total	17,050	1,726	10.0		

[a]Associations were adjusted for the variables used in estimating 90th percentiles, age, BMI, height, mean arterial blood pressure, gestational age at the OGTT, smoking, alcohol use, hospitalization prior to delivery, any family history of diabetes

[b]Defined based on gender, ethnicity, field center, gestational age (36–44 weeks for skinfolds and body fat), and parity

N total number in the cord C-peptide category (excluding births with gestational age <30 weeks and fetal deaths); # number in the cord C-peptide category with the outcome; % proportion in the cord C-peptide category with the outcome

2.3.4 Frequency of Birthweight >90th and <10th Percentile

Figure 2.2 shows the frequencies of babies with a birthweight <10th percentile and >90th percentile across categories of FPG, 1-, and 2-h PG. The change in the frequency of birthweight <10th percentile shows a smaller decline across increasing categories of glucose, compared with the change in the increased frequency of birthweight >90th percentile across glucose categories.

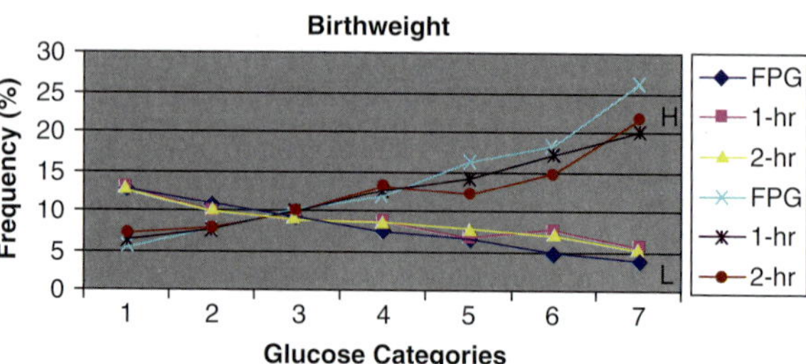

Fig. 2.2 Frequency of birthweight <10th percentile (L) and >90th percentile (H) across categories of glucose

2.4 Clinical Implications

The objective of the HAPO study was to clarify the risk of adverse outcome associated with degrees of maternal glucose intolerance less severe than overt DM. The data published in the initial reports[29,30] demonstrate associations between higher fasting, 1- and 2-h OGTT PG concentrations and birthweight >90th percentile and cord serum C-peptide >90th percentile. Weaker associations were found between glucose levels and primary cesarean delivery and clinical neonatal hypoglycemia. We also found positive associations between increasing PG levels and each of the five secondary outcomes: preterm delivery, shoulder dystocia or birth injury, intensive neonatal care, hyperbilirubinemia, and pre-eclampsia, as well as with newborn adiposity.[30]

The associations were examined with adjustments made for potential confounders that included field center, age, BMI, height, mean arterial pressure measured at the time of the OGTT, gestational age at the OGTT, smoking, drinking, family history of diabetes, parity, hospitalization pre-delivery, and neonatal gender. In general, the adjustments resulted in small to moderate attenuation of most of the field center or unadjusted associations, and associations generally did not differ among field centers. Thus, the influence of maternal glycemia on various maternal/fetal outcomes appears to be a basic biologic phenomenon, and not an epiphenomenon related to the confounders described above. The Pedersen Hypothesis has formed the basis for understanding the pathophysiology of diabetic pregnancy over the past 50+ years. The associations between maternal glucose at concentrations less than those diagnostic of diabetes and outcomes such as birthweight greater than the 90th percentile, fetal hyperinsulinemia (cord C-peptide >90th percentile) and infant adiposity (percent body fat >90th percentile) are strongly supportive of the Pedersen hypothesis.

The lack of differences across field centers for all of the associations described above confirms their applicability to all of the centers. Thus, the results can be used to develop "outcome based" criteria for classifying glucose metabolism in pregnancy that apply globally.

Because the associations of maternal glycemia with perinatal outcomes were continuous with no obvious thresholds at which risks increased, it is evident that a consensus is required to translate these results into clinical practice. Other issues must be addressed as well. For example, is it important to have all three OGTT glucose measurements (fasting, 1-, and 2-h-post load values)? The individual OGTT glucose measures were not highly correlated, and no single measure was clearly superior in predicting the primary outcomes. Can a single glucose value that is equal to or greater than a certain threshold value represent GDM, or must thresholds be met for more than one value? Which of the primary or secondary outcomes should be used to identify the level of glycemia that will be considered GDM, that is to say, the threshold at or above which the risk of adverse outcome is too high?

The International Association of Diabetes and Pregnancy Study Groups (IADPSG) sponsored an "International Workshop Conference on Gestational Diabetes Diagnosis and Classification" in Pasadena, CA on June 11–12, 2008 to initiate the process of consensus development. The IADPSG, an umbrella organization, was formed in 1998 to facilitate collaboration between the various regional and national groups that have a primary or significant focus on diabetes and pregnancy. More than 225 conferees from 40 countries reviewed the published results of the HAPO Study, additional unpublished HAPO Study findings and results of other published and unpublished work that examined associations of maternal glycemia with perinatal and long-term outcomes in offspring. Following the presentation and review of data, conferees held regional caucuses to consider the clinical implications of the large body of information that had been presented.

On the following day, June 13, 2008, the IADPSG Consensus Panel (with representation from the ten member organizations of the IADPSG, together with representatives from other organizations with an interest in diabetes and pregnancy) was convened to begin the process of moving from dialog to consensus. Subsequently, with coordination from the Consensus Panel Steering Committee/Writing Group, the Panel reviewed further HAPO Study results provided by the HAPO Study Data Coordinating Center. Through this process the Consensus Panel has formulated "Recommendations on the Diagnosis and Classification of Hyperglycemia in Pregnancy" which were recently published[31]. These new thresholds for the diagnosis of GDM are shown in Table 2.4. It is expected that this report will be considered by all of the major diabetes organizations and will serve as the basis for internationally endorsed criteria for the diagnosis and classification of diabetes in pregnancy.

Table 2.4 Threshold Values for Diagnosis of GDM and Cumulative Proportion of HAPO Cohort Equaling or Exceeding those Thresholds

Glucose Measure	Glucose Concentration Threshold+		Percent ≥ Threshold
	mmol/l	mg/dl	Cumulative
FPG	5.1	92	8.3
1-h PG	10.0	180	14.0
2-h PG	8.5	153	16.1*

+One or more of these values from a 75-g OGTT must be equaled or exceeded for the diagnosis of GDM.

*In addition, 1.7% of participants in the initial cohort were unblinded because of a FPG >5.8 mmol/l (105 mg/dl) or 2-h OGTT values >11.1 mmol/l (200 mg/dl) bringing the total to 17.8%.

Acknowledgments The study is funded by grants R01-HD34242 and R01-HD34243 from the National Institute of Child Health and Human Development and the National Institute of Diabetes, Digestive, and Kidney Diseases, by the National Center for Research Resources (M01-RR00048, M01-RR00080), and by the American Diabetes Association. Support has also been provided to local field centers by Diabetes UK (RD04/0002756), Kaiser Permanente Medical Center, KK Women's and Children's Hospital, Mater Mother's Hospital, Novo Nordisk, the Myre Sim Fund of the Royal College of Physicians of Edinburgh, and the Howard and Carol Bernick Family Foundation.

2.5 Appendix: HAPO Study Cooperative Research Group

Field Centers: (North American Region) M Contreras, DA Sacks, W Watson (deceased) (Kaiser Foundation Hospital, Bellflower, California); SL Dooley, M Foderaro, C Niznik (Prentice Women's Hospital of Northwestern Memorial Hospital/Northwestern University Feinberg School of Medicine, Chicago, Illinois); J Bjaloncik, PM Catalano, L Dierker, S Fox, L Gullion, C Johnson, CA Lindsay, H Makovos, F Saker (MetroHealth Medical Center/Case Western Reserve University, Cleveland, Ohio); MW Carpenter, J Hunt, MH Somers (Women and Infants Hospital of Rhode Island/Brown University Medical School, Providence, Rhode Island); KS Amankwah, PC Chan, B Gherson, E Herer, B Kapur, A Kenshole, G Lawrence, K Matheson, L Mayes, K McLean, H Owen (Sunnybrook and Women's College Health Sciences Center/University of Toronto, Toronto, Ontario); (*European Region*) C Cave, G Fenty, E Gibson, A Hennis, G McIntyre, YE Rotchell, C Spooner, HAR Thomas (Queen Elizabeth Hospital/School of Clinical Medicine and Research, University of the West Indies, Barbados); J Gluck, DR Hadden, H Halliday, J Irwin, O Kearney, J McAnee, DR McCance, M Mousavi, AI Traub (Royal Jubilee Maternity Hospital, Belfast, Northern Ireland); JK Cruickshank, N Derbyshire, J Dry, AC Holt, A Khan, F Khan, C Lambert, M Maresh, F Prichard, C Townson (St. Mary's Hospital/ Manchester University, Manchester, United Kingdom); TW van Haeften, AMR van de Hengel, GHA Visser, A Zwart (University Hospital/University Medical Center Utrecht, Utrecht, Netherlands); (*Middle Eastern/Asian Region*) U Chaovarindr, U Chotigeat, C Deerochanawong, I Panyasiri, P Sanguanpong (Rajavithi Hospital, Bangkok, Thailand); D Amichay, A Golan, K Marks, M Mazor, J Ronen, A Wiznitzer (Soroka Medical Center/ Ben-Gurion University, Beersheba, Israel); R Chen, D Harel, N Hoter, N Melamed, J Pardo, M Witshner, Y Yogev (Helen Schneider Hospital for Women, Rabin Medical Center/Sackler Faculty of Medicine, Tel-Aviv University, Petah-Tiqva, Israel); (*Austral-Asian Region*) F Bowling, D Cowley, P Devenish-Meares, HG Liley, A McArdle, HD McIntyre, B Morrison, A Peacock, A Tremellen, D Tudehope (Mater Misericordiae Mothers' Hospital/University of Queensland, Brisbane, Australia); KY Chan, NY Chan, LW Ip, SL Kong, YL Lee, CY Li, KF Ng, PC Ng, MS Rogers, KW Wong (Prince of Wales Hospital/Chinese University of Hong Kong, Hong Kong); M Edgar, W Giles, A Gill, R Glover, J Lowe, F Mackenzie, K Siech, J Verma, A Wright (John Hunter Hospital, Newcastle, Australia); YH Cao, JJ Chee, A Koh, E Tan, VJ Rajadurai, HY Wee, GSH Yeo (KK Women's and Children's Hospital, Singapore).

Regional Centers: D Coustan, B Haydon (Providence); A Alexander, DR Hadden (Belfast); O Attias-Raved, M Hod (Petah-Tiqva), JJN Oats, AF Parry (Brisbane).

Clinical Coordinating Center: A Collard, AS Frank, LP Lowe, BE Metzger, A Thomas (Northwestern University Feinberg School of Medicine, Chicago).

Data Coordinating Center: T Case, P Cholod, AR Dyer, L Engelman, M Xiao, L Yang (Northwestern University Feinberg School of Medicine, Chicago).

Clinical Coordinating Center: A Collard, AS Frank, LP Lowe, BE Metzger, A Thomas (Northwestern University Feinberg School of Medicine, Chicago).

Data Coordinating Center: T Case, P Cholod, AR Dyer, L Engelman, M Xiao, L Yang (Northwestern University Feinberg School of Medicine, Chicago).

Central Laboratory: CI Burgess, TRJ Lappin, GS Nesbitt, B Sheridan, M Smye, ER Trimble (Queen's University Belfast, Belfast).

Steering Committee: D Coustan (Providence), AR Dyer (Chicago), DR Hadden (Belfast), M Hod (Petah-Tiqva), BE Metzger (Chicago), LP Lowe, ex officio (Chicago), JJN Oats (Brisbane), B Persson (Stockholm), ER Trimble (Belfast).

Consultants: Y Chen, J Claman, J King.

Data Monitoring Committee: GR Cutter, SG Gabbe, JW Hare, LE Wagenknecht.

References

1. American Diabetes Association. Clinical practice recommendations 2001: gestational diabetes mellitus. *Diabetes Care*. 2001;24(suppl 1):S77-S79.
2. Metzger BE, Coustan DR. Summary and recommendations of the Fourth International Workshop Conference on Gestational Diabetes Mellitus. *Diabetes Care*. 1998;21(suppl 2): B161-B167.
3. O'Sullivan JB, Mahan C. Criteria for oral glucose tolerance test in pregnancy. *Diabetes*. 1964; 13:278-285.
4. Metzger BE, Buchanan TA, Coustan DR, et al. Summary and recommendations of the Fifth International Workshop-Conference on Gestational Diabetes Mellitus. *Diabetes Care*. 2007;30(suppl 2):S251-S260.
5. World Health Organization. WHO Expert Committee on Diabetes Mellitus: second report. *World Health Organ Tech Rep Ser*. 1980;646:1-80.
6. Jarrett RJ. Reflections on gestational diabetes. *Lancet*. 1981;28:1220-1221.
7. Hunter DJS, Keirse MJNC. Gestational diabetes in effective care. In: Chalmers I, Enkin M, Kierse M, eds. *Pregnancy and Childbirth*. Oxford: Oxford University Press; 1989:403-410.
8. Spellacy WN, Miller S, Winegar A, et al. Macrosomia: maternal characteristics and infant complications. *Obstet Gynecol*. 1985;66:158-161.
9. Coustan DR. Management of gestational diabetes: a self-fulfilling prophecy? [editorial]. *JAMA*. 1996;275:1199-1200.
10. Jensen DM, Damm P, Sorensen B, et al. Clinical impact of mild carbohydrate intolerance in pregnancy: a study of 2904 nondiabetic Danish women with risk factors for gestational diabetes. *Am J Obstet Gynecol*. 2001;185:413-419.
11. Yang X, Zhang C, Hsu-Hage B, et al. Women with impaired glucose tolerance during pregnancy have significantly poor pregnancy outcomes. *Diabetes Care*. 2002;25:1619-1624.
12. Vambergue A, Nuttens MC, Verier-Mine O, Dognin C, Cappoen JP, Fontaine P. Is mild gestational hyperglycemia associated with maternal and neonatal complications? The Diagest Study. *Diabet Med*. 2000;17:203-208.

13. Langer O, Brustman L, Anyaegbunam A, Mazze R. The significance of one abnormal glucose tolerance test value on adverse outcome in pregnancy. *Am J Obstet Gynecol.* 1987;157:758-763.
14. Sacks DA, Abu-Fadil S, Greenspoon JS, Fotheringham N. Do the current standards for glucose tolerance testing in pregnancy represent a valid conversion of O'Sullivan's original criteria? *Am J Obstet Gynecol.* 1989;161:638-641.
15. Ferrara A, Weiss NS, Hedderson MM, et al. Elevations in pregnancy plasma glucose levels below the National Diabetes Data group thresholds for gestational diabetes mellitus are associated with an increased risk of neonatal macrosomia, hypoglycemia and hyperbilirubinemia. *Diabetologia*. 2007;50:298-306.
16. Crowther CA, Hiller JE, Moss JR, et al. Effect of treatment of gestational diabetes on pregnancy outcomes. *N Engl J Med.* 2005;352:2477-2486.
17. Landon MB, Spong CY, Thom E, et al. A multicenter randomized trial of treatment for mild gestational diabetes. *N Engl J Med.* 2009;361:1339-1348.
18. U.S. Preventive Services Task Force. Screening for gestational diabetes mellitus: U.S. Preventive Services Task Force Recommendation Statement. *Ann Intern Med.* 2008;148:759-765.
19. Scott DA, Loveman E, McIntyre L, Waugh N. Screening for gestational diabetes: a systematic review and economic evaluation. *Health Technol Assess*. 2002;6(11):1-161.
20. Canadian Task Force on the Periodic Health Examination. *The Canadian Guide to Clinical Preventive Health Care*. Ottawa: Health Canada; 1994:15-23.
21. HAPO Study Cooperative Research Group. The Hyperglycemia and Adverse Pregnancy Outcome (HAPO) Study. *Int J Gynaecol Obstet.* 2002;78:69-77.
22. Pedersen J. *Diabetes and Pregnancy. Blood Sugar of Newborn Infants* [Copenhagen]. 1952:230.
23. Nesbitt GS, Smye M, Sheridan B, Lappin TRJ, Trimble ER for the HAPO Study Cooperative Research Group. Integration of local and central laboratory functions in a worldwide multicentre study. Experience from the Hyperglycemia and Adverse Pregnancy Outcome (HAPO) Study. *Clin Trials*. 2006;3:397-407.
24. Alkalay AL, Sarnat HB, Flores-Sarnat L, Elashoff JD, Farber SJ, Simmons CF. Population meta-analysis of low plasma glucose thresholds in full-term normal newborns. *Am J Perinatol.* 2006;23:115-119.
25. Catalano PM, Thomas AJ, Avallone DA, Amini SB. Anthropometric estimation of neonatal body composition. *Am J Obstet Gynecol.* 1995;173:1176-1181.
26. Brown MA, Lindheimer MD, deSwiet M, Van Assche A, Moutquin JM. The classification and diagnosis of the hypertensive disorders of pregnancy: Society for the Study of Hypertension in Pregnancy (ISSHP). Hypertens Pregnancy 2001;20:ix-xiv.
27. Chan A, King J, Flenady V, Haslam R, Tudehope D. Classification of perinatal deaths: development of the Australian and New Zealand classifications. *J Paediatr Child Health*. 2004; 40:340-347.
28. WHO. *Tenth International Statistical Classification of Diseases and Related Health Problems (ICD-10)*. Geneva, Switzerland: WHO; 1992.
29. Hyperglycemia and Adverse Pregnancy Outcome (HAPO) Study Cooperative Research Group. Hyperglycemia and Adverse Pregnancy Outcome (HAPO) Study: associations with neonatal anthropometrics. *Diabetes*. 2009;58:453-459.
30. Hyperglycemia and Adverse Pregnancy Outcome (HAPO) Study Cooperative Research Group. Hyperglycemia and Adverse Pregnancy Outcomes. *N Engl J Med.* 2008;358:1991-2002.
31 International Association of Diabetes and Pregnancy Study Groups Consensus Panel. International Association of Diabetes and Pregnancy Study Groups Recommendations on the Diagnosis and Classification of Hyperglycemia in Pregnancy. *Diabetes Care* 2010; 33: 676-682.

3 Evolution of Screening and Diagnostic Criteria for GDM Worldwide

Mukesh Agarwal

3.1 Introduction

Despite several international workshops and over four decades of research, there is still no unified global approach to GDM. Most countries have their own diabetes associations; the International Diabetes Federation (IDF) Web site lists 158 countries, each one with 1–3 diabetes societies as an IDF member.[1] These societies often advocate guidelines for GDM, which may be similar or markedly different; often, no guideline is proposed. Most pre-eminent diabetes/health organizations like the American Diabetes Association (ADA),[2] the Australasian Diabetes in Pregnancy Society (ADIPS),[3] the Canadian Diabetes Association (CDA),[4] the European Association for the Study of Diabetes (EASD),[5] the New Zealand Society for the Study of Diabetes, and the World Health Organization (WHO)[6] support screening for GDM. They offer comprehensive guidelines on how to screen, diagnose, treat, and follow-up women with GDM. Many other regional health associations, e.g., the National Institute for Health and the Clinical Excellence (NICE)[7] from the United Kingdom and Clinical Resource Efficiency Support Team (CREST)[8] from Northern Ireland also have guidelines for caregivers to follow. The scourge of GDM is the lack of an international consensus among these organizations.

In countries with guidelines derived from regional and national data (e.g., Japan, Australia, and Brazil), it would be reasonable to expect uniformity in the screening and diagnosis for GDM, at least within the jurisdiction of the health organization. However, there is a wide diversity in the methods used in most of these countries (e.g., the United Kingdom) due to multiple reasons. Health providers often prefer to use alternate criteria; they may choose to follow the recommendation of a diabetes or health organization from another country.[9] Often there is disagreement between the country's national diabetes organization, its local health society, and its regional obstetric organization, with each one recommending a different approach for GDM.

M. Agarwal
Department of Pathology, UAE University, PO Box 17666, Al Ain, United Arab Emirates
e-mail: magarwal7@gmail.com

C. Kim and A. Ferrara (eds.), *Gestational Diabetes During and After Pregnancy*,
DOI: 10.1007/978-1-84882-120-0_3,

In countries without any nationally derived guidelines, the situation would be expected to be more disorderly. But this may not always be the case, as most of these countries have local diabetes organizations that may choose to implement 1 (e.g., Spain) or more of these "international" guidelines. The two most popular international guidelines are those of the WHO[6] and the ADA.[2] However, since both these organizations have changed their approach over the last three decades, some health providers (and/or their advising organizations) have not kept up with the latest changes and updates. Thus, although the practice in the United States has moved from O'Sullivan and Mahan's criteria to the National Diabetes Data Group (NDDG-1979) to the Carpenter and Coustan (C&C) criteria for the diagnosis of GDM, both the NDDG and C&C may still be vogue in the same country/region/county. If more than one international guideline is approved by a national diabetes organization, the inconsistency between the various well-known health organizations (e.g., WHO vs. EASD) is reflected at the ground level within these countries. Thus, similar to countries with national data, the diversity in practice observed remains varied. There are additional problems in some of these countries; often, they have minimal testing for carbohydrate intolerance in pregnancy. A deficiency of resources and poor dissemination of information are some of the reasons for this shortcoming. Many countries in Africa, South America, and Asia suffer from this predicament.

This review is an attempt to get a bird's eye-view of the reasons for dichotomy in the strategies for GDM, globally[10, 11]; it not an encyclopedic endeavor at synthesizing all the practices for GDM the world-over, which are easily available in multiple publications.[12,13] An insight into the evolution of the common criteria for GDM diagnosis used worldwide may help us to find the ideal solution: one single, universal, global guideline for GDM.

3.2 Evolution of the World Health Organization Criteria

Outside of North America, the WHO criteria[6] are the most uniformly accepted for the diagnosis of GDM, in part due to the global reach and influence of the WHO. The WHO guidelines were first published in 1965, one year after the first WHO Expert Committee on Diabetes Mellitus convened in Geneva. It was one of the earliest attempts at an international consensus on the classification of diabetes mellitus. At that time, GDM was defined as "hyperglycemia of diabetic levels occurring during pregnancy." Subsequently, WHO guidelines evolved with bulletins in 1980, 1985, and 1999.

The WHO-1980 guidelines used the 75-g OGTT (for diabetes diagnosis in nonpregnant adults) limiting the requirement to only two (fasting and 2-hour (2-h)) plasma glucose levels, eliminating the need for intermediate readings. Pregnant women who met the WHO criteria for impaired glucose tolerance (IGT) in nonpregnant adults were classified as having GDM. The subsequent WHO-1985 criteria were very similar to the WHO-1980 criteria but for rounding the glucose values to the nearest tenth of a millimole instead of the nearest millimole. The WHO-1999 criteria (Table 3.1) incorporated some of the ADA-1997 recommendations, i.e., the fasting plasma glucose (FPG) was lowered (from 7.8 to 7.0 mmol/L) for the diagnosis of diabetes. However, the WHO has remained ambivalent about the term "impaired fasting glucose" (fasting glucose 5.6–6.9 mmol/L) of the ADA.

Table 3.1 Summary of major international recommendations for the screening and diagnosis of gestational diabetes

Continent	Organization	Screening	Screening method (1-h threshold ≥)	Diagnostic OGTT	Fasting	1-h	2-h	3-h	Abnormal values needed for diagnosis ≥
			a = 50-g GCT (7.8)	*b* = 3-h, 100-g *c* = 2-h, 75-g					
North America	ADA, 2003	All except low-risk	a	b	5.3	10.0	8.6	7.8	2
				c	5.3	10.0	8.6	–	2
	NDDG, 1979	No	a	b	5.8	10.5	9.2	8.0	2
	O'Sullivan and Mahan, 1964	–	–	b	5.0	9.1	8.0	6.9	2
	CDA, 2003	All	a	c	5.3	10.6	8.9	–	2
	SOGC, 2002	Same as ADA	–	–	–	–	–	–	–
South America	BSD, 2007	All	FPG (4.7)	c	–	7.0		7.8	1
Europe	EASD, 1991	NS	NS	c	5.5 or 6.0			9.0	
Asia	JDS, 2002	All	a RPG (5.3)	c	5.5	10.0	8.3	–	2
Australia	ADIPS, 1998	All, unless resources limited	a 75-g (8.0)	c	5.5	–	8.0	–	1
	NZSSD, 1998	All should be offered	a 75-g (8.0)	c	5.5	–	9.0	–	1

(continued)

Table 3.1 (continued)

Continent	Organization	Screening	Screening method (1-h threshold ≥)	Diagnostic OGTT	Fasting	1-h	2-h	3-h	Abnormal values needed for diagnosis ≥
All continents (universal criteria)	WHO, 1999 ADA, 2003 (as above)	–	–	c	7.0		7.8	–	1
	IDF, 2005	All except low risk	Glucose type NS	c	NS	NS	NS	–	–

ADA American Diabetes Organization; *ADIPS* The Australian Diabetes in Pregnancy Society; *BSD* Brazilian Society of Diabetes; *CDA* Canadian Diabetes Association; *EASD* European Association for the Study of Diabetes; *IDF* International Diabetes Federation; *JDS* Japan Diabetes Society; *NDDG*, National Diabetes Data Group; *NZSSSD* New Zealand Society for the Study of Diabetes; *SOGC* Society of Obstetricians and Gynecologists of Canada; *WHO* World Health Organization; *NS* not specified; *FPG* fasting plasma glucose; *RPG* random plasma glucose

Values given in mmol/L

Thus, the WHO has opted to apply the same criteria to the pregnant and nonpregnant state. The WHO criteria for GDM diagnosis were extrapolated to pregnant women from diagnostic cutoffs of the nonpregnant women. However, data from nonpregnant women and men may not be applicable to pregnant women.[14] Conversely, the WHO criteria for GDM are relatively simple to use. Moreover, studies have shown that they predict both maternal and fetal abnormalities in index pregnancy[15] as well as increased risk for type 2 diabetes after delivery.[16]

3.3 Evolution of the American Diabetes Association Criteria

Many countries outside North America use the ADA definition, which is unique in that it relies on the 3-h 100-g OGTT for the diagnosis of GDM. The original diagnostic glucose thresholds were first established by the pioneering studies of John O'Sullivan and Claire Mahan, in 1964.[17] This study used the Nelson-Somogyi glucose assay, which was not specific for glucose, but measured all reducing substances present in whole blood. In 1979, the National Diabetes Data Group (NDDG)[18] converted these whole blood glucose thresholds to the higher (approximately 14%) plasma glucose values, as most of the laboratory instruments by that time had started reporting plasma glucose values instead of whole blood glucose. In 1982, Carpenter and Coustan (C&C)[19] modified the O'Sullivan and Mahan's original glucose thresholds by using two conversion factors, which corrected for the nonglucose reducing substances in blood and converted whole blood glucose to plasma glucose. Therefore, these C&C thresholds are similar to the current "glucose specific" enzymatic methods measuring plasma glucose. The correction proposed by C&C has been validated.[20] In 2000, the ADA endorsed the recommendations of the (1998) Fourth International Workshop-Conference on GDM[21] proposal that until more data became available, the C&C thresholds be used for the interpretation of the 100-g, 3-h OGTT.

There have been criticisms of the ADA criteria. The current ADA criteria for the diagnosis of GDM (C&C) were derived from the original O'Sullivan and Mahan's criteria for the 100-g OGTT, which were originally formulated to predict type 2 diabetes in the future and not to predict maternal and fetal problems in index pregnancy. However, many subsequent studies have substantiated that they can predict perinatal problems of pregnancy.[15] Another criticism of the ADA criteria has been its application of the 100-g OGTT cutoffs to the 75-g OGTT plasma glucose values (Table 3.1).[22]

3.4 Evolution of the European Association for the Study of Diabetes Criteria

The Diabetic Pregnancy Study Group of the EASD was founded in 1969. Its recommendations for GDM were published in 1991.[5] This report analyzed 1,009 pregnant women who underwent the 75-g OGTT in 11 centers across Europe. Glucose was analyzed on different samples i.e., venous whole blood/plasma or capillary whole blood or plasma. Approximately 10% of women exceeded the 2-h cutoff of 8.0 mmol/L (which was close to the WHO-1980 threshold of 7.8 mmol/L) for glucose intolerance. The authors concluded that the prevailing WHO criteria identified an excess of pregnant women of northern European origin with glucose intolerance. Therefore, they recommended that the definition of GDM be limited to women who reached glucose thresholds of diabetes, as defined by the WHO-1965 guidelines. For a diagnosis of "gestational IGT," they proposed that the 2-h plasma glucose equal or exceed 9.0 mmol/L and either the fasting or the 1-h value exceed 7.0 and 11.0 mmol/L, respectively.

In 1996, the Pregnancy and Neonatal Care Group[23] suggested the cutoffs of 6.0 mmol/L and 9.0 mmol/L be used for the fasting and 2-h plasma venous glucose, respectively (either one or both) (Table 3.1). These have been used as the EASD criteria for GDM.[24] Studies have compared perinatal outcomes using WHO and EASD thresholds; however, no definite conclusions about the advantages of one set of criteria over the other could be made.[25] Since the EASD glucose thresholds were derived from pregnant women (unlike the WHO), they are still popular in many centers in Europe.[26] Nevertheless, despite new epidemiological data with the modern advances in glucose standardization and laboratory technology,[27] the EASD recommendations have not changed in nearly two decades.

3.5 Evolution of The Australasian Diabetes in Pregnancy Society Criteria

The ADIPS first published its guidelines for GDM in 1998.[3] Originally, its diagnostic criteria for GDM were adapted in 1991 from the WHO criteria for the 75-g OGTT.[28] There has been much debate whether universal or selective screening is more appropriate for GDM diagnosis in Australian women. ADIPS recommends that screening should be considered in all pregnant women, i.e., universal screening. However, if resources are limited, screening may be reserved for those at highest risk. In other words, they endorse both selective and universal screening. The screening test recommended is either a nonfasting 50-g or 75-g challenge test with thresholds to proceed for the OGTT of ≥7.8 or 8.0 mmol/L, respectively. The suggested diagnostic thresholds for GDM on the 75-g OGTT are ≥5.5 mmol/L and ≥ 8.0 mmol/L (either one/both) for fasting and 2-h glucose, respectively (Table 3.1).

The criteria of ADIPS are the most liberal of all the diagnostic benchmarks for GDM in that they classify more women as having GDM than any other criteria.[11] It has been suggested that one-third of women in Australia with type 2 diabetes could be identified earlier via a GDM pregnancy by the ADIPS diagnostic thresholds.[29] Thus, they may be the ideal criteria for prevention of future type 2 diabetes, since they detect more women with carbohydrate intolerance.

3.6 Evolution of New Zealand Society for the Study of Diabetes Criteria

In New Zealand, the 1998 consensus guidelines of the ADIPS[3] were accepted for the screening and diagnosis of GDM. However, by a majority decision of the New Zealand Society for the Study of Diabetes (NZSSD), the New Zealand criteria for GDM diagnosis were made more restrictive.[30,31] The 2-h cutoffs for the 75-g OGTT were raised to 9.0 mmol/L in New Zealand from the Australian 8.0 mmol/L threshold (Table 3.1) so that fewer women with GDM would be identified. The higher figure for the glucose threshold was also chosen "to reduce the worry and inconvenience for women of being given a false positive diagnosis and to reduce the strain on stretched specialist resources in many centers." Community-based studies have shown that this would reduce the number of women with GDM by half thereby giving respite to New Zealand's stretched resources.[31] Thus, standards were dictated by resource use concerns and cost. The NZSSD recommendation is a little different from the Australian approach but very unlike the American College of Obstetricians and Gynecologists (ACOG) approach.[32]

3.7 Evolution of Japan Diabetes Society Criteria

The Japan Diabetes Society (JDS) has been a leader in diabetes screening in Japan. Over the last four decades, the JDS has changed its criteria for the diagnosis of diabetes in 1970, 1982, and 1995 in order to keep pace with the changes made by major international bodies. However, regarding GDM, the JDS currently continues to endorse the approach to GDM established in the early 1980s.[33] These thresholds were established in 1984 by the Committee for Nutrition and Metabolism of the Japan Society of Obstetrics and Gynecology (JSOG). GDM is diagnosed when any two glucose values on the 75-g OGTT, exceeded 5.5, 10.0, and 8.3 mmol/L on the FPG, 1-h, and 2-h values respectively (Table 3.1). These cutoff values were initially selected from the mean value plus two standard deviations of healthy pregnancies. Later, their validity was also supported by greater frequency of abnormal perinatal outcomes in pregnant women. Subsequent studies have validated that these criteria as more predictive than the WHO criteria of pregnancy outcomes in Japanese women.[34]

After this initial report, some multicenter studies which investigated the screening of GDM in Japan became available. The accuracy and cost of various screening methods during the early and middle part of pregnancy were critically analyzed. In some of these reports, it was shown that in about 80% of Japanese women, GDM could be diagnosed during the first trimester of pregnancy. Further, it was also found that random blood glucose (threshold ≥5.5 mmol/L) and the glucose challenge test were valid screening methods.[33]

Thus, the JDS currently states that appropriate screening methods include a random blood glucose (cutoff : 5.3 mmol/L) in the first trimester and a glucose challenge test (cutoff: 7.8 mmol/L) in the second trimester. These recommendations differ from the findings of a study on screening tests for GDM in Japan.[35] Currently, a Committee on the Reassessment of Definition, Screening, and Diagnostic Criteria for Gestational Diabetes Mellitus has been established under the aegis of the JDS. Based on new information from the Hyperglycemia and Pregnancy Outcomes Study (HAPO), a chapter on which is included in this book, the criteria are scheduled to be updated.

3.8 Evolution of Brazilian Society of Diabetes Criteria

The Brazilian Society of Diabetes (BSD) is one of the unique organizations that recommends using the fasting venous plasma glucose (FPG) as a screening test for GDM.[36] An FPG of ≥4.7 mmol/L (at the first visit and at 24–28 weeks gestation) is used to decide if the diagnostic OGTT is needed. These recommendations are based on a study by the Brazilian Study of Gestational Diabetes (EBDG) Working Group published in 1998.[37] However, the value of the FPG as a screening test in this study has been controversial, as shown by a review about the utility of the FPG as a screening test for GDM.[38] The definitive diagnosis of GDM in Brazil is based on the criteria of the WHO-1999 for the 75-g OGTT (Table 3.1). The BSD submits that most of the current recommendations for GDM are based on consensus of specialists which should be replaced by recommendations based on evidence.[36]

3.9 International Diabetes Federation Guidelines

The International Diabetes Federation (IDF)[39] acknowledges that there are no randomized control trials testing the effectiveness of GDM screening. It also notes that there are many strategies available. Its 2005 recommendations are a hybrid of the ADA and WHO guidelines. Screening in low-risk women should be done by a plasma glucose (fasting, random, or postprandial not specified) at the time of the first antenatal visit or directly with a 75-g OGTT in women at high-risk for GDM (criteria not defined).

3.10 Regional Approaches to GDM

In this section, the actual screening practices in some selected countries and continents are outlined. In almost all countries without exception, there is a wide spectrum of practices for the screening and diagnosis of GDM.

3.10.1 Canada

In Canada, a decision not to screen, to screen all pregnant women, or to screen only women at "high-risk" would all be acceptable approaches based on the current recommendations. The two main associations that have published guidelines for GDM are the CDA[4] and the Society of the Obstetricians and Gynecologists of Canada (SOGC).[40] Both organizations have updated GDM guidelines over time based on available data. However, they differ considerably (Table 3.1). The SOGC-2002 recommends a scheme which is similar to that of the ADA i.e., selective screening with a 50-g GCT followed by a 100-g OGTT or 75-g OGTT, using the ADA criteria for diagnosis. However, the SOGC also agrees that not screening for GDM is also considered acceptable. The CDA prefers universal screening, due to the risk of missing cases with selective screening with a 50-g GCT.[4] However the diagnosis is based on the 75-g OGTT with much tighter thresholds than the ADA criteria; in fact the CDA criteria have some of the most stringent thresholds for the 75-g OGTT.[11]

The problem of a lack of consensus in Canada illustrates the challenges of GDM globally, if extended into a wider context. Consider a woman living in a Canadian province, who does not have GDM based on the 75-g OGTT by the CDA criteria. If she moves to another district in Canada, she will now have GDM if the SOGC recommendations are in vogue. A similar situation would also arise if she crosses the border into the USA, where the more liberal ADA criteria are used. The reverse would be true if she moved in the opposite direction. This lack of consensus is well summed up by the CDA: "In the year 2003, screening, diagnosis and management of GDM remain controversial and continue to be debated in the medical community.[4]"

3.10.2 United Kingdom

The National Institute for Health and Clinical Excellence (NICE) guidelines of March 2008 recommend that the random and fasting glucose, GCT, or urinalysis should not be used for screening of GDM. Rather, screening should be done using risk factors followed by a 75-g OGTT using the criteria of WHO-1999 for the diagnosis of GDM.[7]

The Scottish Intercollegiate Guidelines network (SIGN) advocates recommendations contrary to NICE for both the screening and diagnosis of GDM. Its latest guidelines (2001) propose the use of glucosouria and random venous glucose for screening, with the 75-g OGTT and the EASD criteria used for diagnosis.[41]

The CREST Working Group on Diabetes in Pregnancy guidelines were developed for Northern Ireland in 2001.[8] Guidelines recommend a diagnostic 75-g OGTT if (a) urine shows glycosuria, (b) fasting glucose or 2-h glucose levels after food exceed 5.5 mmol/L, or (c) plasma glucose within 2-h after food exceeds 7.0 mmol/L. They recommend diagnostic thresholds from the EASD-1991 study, i.e., either FPG ≥5.5 mmol/L or 2-h ≥9.0 mmol/L.

Not surprisingly, surveys in the U.K. have shown that there is wide variation in the practices for screening and diagnosis of GDM. In a recent mail-questionnaire study,[42] the screening practices among the respondents was variable and included glycosuria (40%), random venous glucose (28%), and FPG (6%). The confirmatory test was the 75-g OGTT, but the thresholds for diagnosis varied considerably. Two other studies have shown similar variation in the approach to GDM among the various caregivers/obstetric units in the U.K.[43,44]

3.10.3 Italy

The Italian Treatment Standards for Diabetes were drafted in 2007 by members from several Italian associations including the Italian scientific diabetes societies, Italian Society of Diabetology (SID), and the Italian Association of Diabetologists (AMD).[45] The guideline was formulated after considering all the major international recommendations for GDM, including the suggestions of the Italian Society of Obstetrics and Gynecology (SIGO). They have endorsed the latest approach of the ADA (the C&C thresholds for the 75-g OGTT) but are waiting for the results of the HAPO to make further recommendations.

A survey from Italy[46] has shown that only 50% of the laboratories performed the OGTT as per the protocols of their diabetes association. There was a wide variability in the OGTT used after a positive GCT. Some laboratories performed the 100-g OGTT, others the 75-g OGTT with 2–4 blood samples for diagnosis; many laboratories used only the 50-g GCT without confirmation by a follow-up OGTT. Some Italian laboratories used a variety of unique methods. A variable relationship between laboratories and diabetes organizations was detected, leading to the conclusion that there was a need for greater collaboration between the different regulatory bodies.

3.10.4 Australia

In Australia, despite the presence of ADIPS, an audit of 360 hospitals across the country[47] showed that the 50-g GCT was the most popular screening test, but 10% hospitals still used either a random glucose or a 75-g OGTT for screening. For the diagnosis for GDM, 30 (12%) hospitals used the obsolete 50-g OGTT, while 2% used the 100-g OGTT, which is not recommended by ADIPS.[3] Moreover, the number of glucose samples used to confirm a diagnosis varied from 1 to 3 values on the diagnostic OGTT.

3.10.5 Sweden

In Sweden, similar to many other countries, both the screening and diagnostic criteria for GDM have changed over time. In the early 1980s, screening for GDM was done by urine glucose. Subsequently, random blood glucose with a cutoff of 6.1 or 5.6 mmol/L for less or more than 2-h after a meal was used.[48] Later in 1985, repeated random blood glucose measurements became popular, with a cutoff of over 6.5 mmol/L as the threshold for proceeding to the OGTT.[49] In 1991, the popular Hemocue apparatus, which uses 5 μL of capillary whole blood (Hemocue AB, Angleholm, Sweden), was introduced into the Swedish market. Since then, most studies from Sweden have used capillary whole blood. In fact, even for the diagnostic OGTT, capillary whole blood is more likely to be used all over Sweden rather than plasma glucose. Currently, many large centers use 4–6 capillary glucose measurements as screening tests starting from the end of the first trimester with a value of ≥8.0 mmol/L as the threshold to proceed with the diagnostic OGTT.[50]

Regarding diagnosis, most Swedish units used the WHO-1985 diabetes criteria for capillary whole blood with either fasting ≥6.7 mmol/L or 2-h values ≥11.1 mmol/L after a 75-g OGTT. After the publication of the EASD study in 1991, a 2-h IGT value of 9.0–11.0 mmol/L was used for the diagnosis of GDM. With some exceptions, these criteria have been generally accepted in Sweden since the early 1990s, similar to many European countries. However, even as late as 2001 many counties (around Stockholm and Orebo) were using the WHO-1965 criteria for GDM, which did not consider "IGT in pregnancy"[51] as GDM. This was different from most of Sweden which included "IGT in pregnancy" as diagnostic for GDM. Thus in Sweden, there is heterogeneity in the diagnosis of GDM; additionally, using capillary whole blood extrapolated from values for plasma remains an additional complicating factor.[52]

3.10.6 Germany

There have been many discussions about the screening and diagnosis of GDM in Germany. In 2001, the guidelines were based on the suggestions of an expert panel of the German Society of Obstetrics and Gynecology (DGGG) and the German Diabetes Association (DDG). These were modified recommendations of the Fourth International Workshop-Conference on GDM. Women are screened on the basis of risk factors in the first trimester. Both the one-step (75-g OGTT alone) and the 2-step approach (50-g GCT followed by a 75-g OGTT) are accepted as valid methods for screening and diagnosis of GDM. The threshold for the GCT is a glucose value ≥ 7.8 mmol/L. Some of the diagnostic cutoffs for the 75-g OGTT have been retained from the original data of O'Sullivan and Mahan (1964), i.e., fasting ,1-h, and 2-h thresholds are 5.0, 10.0 and 8.6 mmol/L, respectively.[53] The possible reason is that in many parts of Germany, capillary whole blood was still being used for measuring glucose; formerly, the Hemocue was the only glucose meter approved by the German Diabetes Association for point-of-care testing.

3.10.7 China

In China, there is no consensus on which criteria are best suited for Chinese women; therefore, most hospitals have adopted one of the criteria of the various international organizations. In 1993, Dong Zhiguang suggested Chinese-specific criteria for the 75-g OGTT. They were lower than WHO criteria but similar to the criteria of the JDS. These criteria have been popular in China. However, it has also been shown that criteria of Carpenter and Couston as applied to the 100-g OGTT are suitable for Chinese women.[54] A chapter on diagnostic testing in China is included in this book.

3.10.8 South America, Africa, and Asia

There is a paucity of data about diabetes from many countries of these continents. Even lesser data is available about the practices regarding the screening and diagnosis of GDM. Hence, the methods used are harder to gauge in these regions. In South America, Brazil and Argentina are on the forefront of research on GDM.[37,55] Publications from Uruguay show that they follow the thresholds suggested by the NDDG. There is little information from Peru, Bolivia, Chile, and Venezuela. The African continent exhibits the same issues as South America, in that there is a lack of published data on OGTT reports. Studies from Ethiopia, Nigeria, Uganda, and South Africa show that the WHO criteria are popular.[56–59]

In some countries of Asia, like Korea,[60] Sri Lanka,[61] and Malaysia,[62] the WHO-1999 criteria appear to be used most frequently. However, other countries like Thailand[63] and Turkey[64] use the 50-g GCT followed by the 100-g OGTT as recommended by the ADA. In India[65,66] and the Middle-East,[11] both ADA and WHO criteria are frequently used. In Hong Kong, selective screening is popular[67]; additionally, the WHO criteria have been validated in pregnant Chinese women from Hong Kong.[68]

3.11 Conclusions

The evolution of the screening and diagnostic criteria for GDM worldwide have been in flux. As can be appreciated from this review, guidelines may lack updates and they often rely on expert opinion rather than evidence based data. We can best serve the interest of our pregnant patients by formulating unified universal guidelines for GDM[13,30,69]; this consistency is essential for GDM. In many other areas of medicine, such standardization in clinical research has been attained with fruitful results.[70] Consensus could be achieved due to the insight gained from the recent trials; an awareness of the shortcomings of the various global guidelines would help to avoid them in the future. With over four decades of hindsight, it is high time that we develop one clear-cut global guideline for GDM.

References

1. International Diabetes Federation. http://www.idf.org. Accessed 2.08.08.
2. American Diabetes Association Position Statement. Gestational diabetes mellitus. *Diabetes Care*. 2004;27(suppl 1):S88-S90.
3. The Australasian Diabetes in Pregnancy Society. Gestational diabetes mellitus guidelines. *Med J Aust*. 1998;169:93-97.

4. Canadian Diabetes Association Clinical Practice Guidelines Expert Committee. Canadian Diabetes Association 2003 Clinical Practice Guidelines for the Prevention and Management of Diabetes in Canada. *Can J Diabetes*. 2003;27(suppl 2):S99-S105.
5. Lind T, Philips PR. Influence of pregnancy on the 75-g OGTT: a prospective multicenter study. *Diabetes*. 1991;40(suppl 2):8-13.
6. World Health Organization. Definition, Diagnosis and Classification of Diabetes Mellitus and its Complications. Part 1: Diagnosis and Classification of Diabetes Mellitus. Report of a WHO Consultation. Geneva: World Health Organization; 1999.
7. National Institute for Health and Clinical Excellence (NICE). *Diabetes in pregnancy: management of diabetes and its complications from preconception to the postnatal period*. London: National Collaborating Centre for Women's and Children's Health; 2008.
8. Clinical Resource Efficiency Support Team, Belfast. Management of diabetes in pregnancy. http://www.crestni.org.uk;. 2001 Accessed 10.08.08.
9. Clark HD, Van Walraven C, Code C, et al. Did publication of a clinical practice guideline recommendation to screen for type 2 diabetes in women with gestational diabetes change practice? *Diabetes Care*. 2003;26:265-268.
10. Vogel N, Burnand B, Vial Y, et al. Screening for gestational diabetes: variation in guidelines. *Eur J Obstet Gynecol Reprod Biol*. 2000;91:29-36.
11. Agarwal MM, Dhatt GS, Punnose J, et al. Gestational diabetes: dilemma caused by multiple international diagnostic criteria. *Diabet Med*. 2005;22:1731-1736.
12. Hunt KJ, Schuller KL. The increasing prevalence of diabetes in pregnancy. *Obstet Gynecol Clin North Am*. 2007;34:173-199.
13. Cutchie WA, Cheung NW, Simmons D. Comparison of International and New Zealand Guidelines for the care of pregnant women with diabetes. *Diabet Med*. 2006;23:460-468.
14. Cheng LC, Salmon YM. Are the WHO (1980) criteria for the 75-g oral glucose tolerance test appropriate for pregnant women? *Br J Obstet Gynaecol*. 1993;100:645-648.
15. Schmidt MI, Duncan BB, Reichelt AJ, et al.; Brazilian Gestational Diabetes Study Group. Gestational diabetes mellitus diagnosed with a 2-h 75-g oral glucose tolerance test and adverse pregnancy outcomes. *Diabetes Care*. 2001;24:1151-1155.
16. Kim C, Newton KM, Knopp RH. Gestational diabetes and the incidence of type 2 diabetes. *Diabetes Care*. 2002;25:1862-1868.
17. O'Sullivan J, Mahan C. Criteria for the oral glucose tolerance test in pregnancy. *Diabetes*. 1964;13:278-285.
18. National Diabetes Data Group. Classification and diagnosis of diabetes mellitus and other categories of glucose intolerance. *Diabetes*. 1979;18:1039-1057.
19. Carpenter M, Coustan D. Criteria for screening tests for gestational diabetes. *Am J Obstet Gynecol*. 1982;144:768-773.
20. Sacks D, Abu-Fadil S, Greenspoon J, et al. Do the current standards for glucose tolerance testing in pregnancy represent a valid conversion of O'Sullivan's original criteria? *Am J Obstet Gynecol*. 1989;161:638-641.
21. Metzger B, Coustan D. Summary and recommendations of the Fourth International Workshop-Conference on Gestational Diabetes Mellitus: the Organizing Committee. *Diabetes Care*. 1998;21:B161-B167.
22. Mello G, Elena P, Ognibene A, et al. Lack of concordance between the 75-g and 100-g glucose load tests for the diagnosis of gestational diabetes mellitus. *Clin Chem*. 2006;52:1679-1684.
23. Brown CJ, Dawson A, Dodds R, et al. Report of the Pregnancy and Neonatal Care Group. *Diabet Med*. 1996;13:S43-S53.
24. Hanna FWF, Peters JR. Screening for gestational diabetes; past, present and future. *Diabet Med*. 2002;19:351-358.
25. Jensen DM, Damm P, Sorensen B, et al. Proposed diagnostic thresholds for gestational diabetes mellitus according to a 75-g oral glucose tolerance test. Maternal and perinatal outcomes in 3260 Danish women. *Diabet Med*. 2003;20:51-57.
26. Savona-Ventura C. Guidelines for the management of gestational diabetes in Malta. *J Malta College Family Doctors*. 2000;18:9-12.

27. Dungan K, Chapman J, Braithwaite SS, et al. Glucose measurement: confounding issues in setting targets for inpatient management. *Diabetes Care*. 2007;30:403-409.
28. Martin FIR. The diagnosis of gestational diabetes. *Med J Aust*. 1991;155:112.
29. Cheung NW, Byth K. Population health significance of gestational. diabetes. *Diabetes Care*. 2003;26:2005-2009.
30. Simmons D, Campbell N. Gestational diabetes mellitus in New Zealand Technical Report. www.ngamaia.co.nz. Accessed 12.08.2008.
31. Simmons D, Wolmarans L, Cutchie W, et al. Gestational diabetes mellitus: time for consensus on screening and diagnosis. *N Z Med J*. 2006;119(1228):U1807.
32. Simmons DS, Walters BN, Wein P, et al. Guidelines for the management of gestational diabetes mellitus revisited. *Med J Aust*. 2002;176:352.
33. Kuzuya T, Nakagawa S, Satoh J, et al. Committee of the Japan Diabetes Society on the diagnostic criteria of diabetes mellitus. Report of the Committee on the classification and diagnostic criteria of diabetes mellitu. *Diabetes Res Clin Pract*. 2002;55:65-85.
34. Sugaya A, Sugiyama T, Nagata M, et al. Comparison of the validity of the criteria for gestational diabetes mellitus by WHO and by the Japan Society of Obstetrics and Gynecology by the outcomes of pregnancy. *Diabetes Res Clin Pract*. 2000;50:57-63.
35. Maegawa Y, Sugiyama T, Kusaka H, et al. Screening tests for gestational diabetes in Japan in the 1st and 2nd trimester of pregnancy. *Diabetes Res Clin Pract*. 2003;62:47-53.
36. Gestational Diabetes Mellitus. Diagnosis, treatment and postgestational follow-up. *Int J Atherocsler*. 2007;2:91-150.
37. Reichelt AJ, Spichler ER, Branchtein L, et al. Fasting plasma glucose is a useful test for the detection of gestational diabetes. Brazilian Study of Gestational Diabetes (EBDG) Working Group. *Diabetes Care*. 1998;21:1246-1249.
38. Agarwal MM, Dhatt GS. Fasting plasma glucose as a screening test for gestational diabetes mellitus. *Arch Gynecol Obstet*. 2007;275:81-87.
39. International Diabetes Federation. Global guideline of Type 2 Diabetes. http://www.idf.org/Global_guideline. 2005. Accessed 9.05.10
40. Berger H, Crane J, Farine D, et al. Maternal-Fetal Medicine Committee; Executive and Council of the Society of Obstetricians and Gynaecologists of Canada. Screening for gestational diabetes mellitus. *J Obstet Gynaecol Can*. 2002;24:894-903.
41. Management of Diabetes. Scottish Intercollegiate Guidelines network. Scottish Intercollegiate Guidelines network. http://www.sign.ac.uk. Accessed 4.08.08.
42. Hanna FW, Peters JR, Harlow J, et al. Gestational diabetes screening and glycaemic management; National survey on behalf of the Association of British Clinical Diabetologists. *QJM*. 2008;101:777-784.
43. Nelson-Piercy C, Gale EA. Do we know how to screen for gestational diabetes? Current practice in one regional health authority. *Diabet Med*. 1994;11:493-498.
44. Mires GJ, Williams FL, Harper V. Screening practices for gestational diabetes mellitus in UK obstetric units. *Diabet Med*. 1999;16:138-141.
45. Italian Standards for Diabetes Mellitus. http://www.siditalia.it/documenti/AMD-SID_Italian%20standards%20for%20diabetes%20mellitus%20%202007.pdf. 2007 Accessed 3.09.08.
46. Federici MO, Mosca A, Testa R, et al. National survey on the execution of the oral glucose tolerance test (OGTT) in a representative cohort of Italian laboratories. *Clin Chem Lab Med*. 2006;44:568-573.
47. Rumbold AR, Crowther CA. Guideline use for gestational diabetes mellitus and current screening, diagnostic and management practices in Australian hospitals. *Aust N Z J Obstet Gynaecol*. 2001;41:86-90.
48. Lind T, Anderson J. Does random blood glucose sampling outdate testing for glycosuria in the detection of diabetes during pregnancy? *Br Med J (Clin Res Ed)*. 1984;289:1569-1571.
49. Ostlund I. *Aspects of Gestational Diabetes. Screening System, Maternal and Fetal Complications. Acta Universitatis Upsaliensis*. Comprehensive Summaries of Uppsala Dissertations from the Faculty of Medicine 1220; 2003:38 pp. Uppsala. ISBN 91-554-5511-5.

50. Fadl H, Ostlund I, Nilsson K, et al. Fasting capillary glucose as a screening test for gestational diabetes mellitus. *BJOG*. 2006;113:1067-1071.
51. Ostlund I, Hanson U, Björklund A, et al. Maternal and fetal outcomes if gestational impaired glucose tolerance is not treated. *Diabetes Care*. 2003;26:2107-2111.
52. Steffes MW, Sacks DB. Measurement of circulating glucose concentrations: the time is now for consistency among methods and types of samples. *Clin Chem*. 2005;51:1569-1570.
53. Schäfer-Graf UM. Management of pregnancies with gestational diabetes based solely on maternal glycemia versus glycemia plus fetal growth. http://edoc.hu-berlin.de/habilitationen/schaefer-graf-ute-m-2004-02-19/HTML/chapter1.html. 2004 Accessed 3.08.08.
54. Wu QK, Luo LM, Li P, et al. Gestational diabetes mellitus in Chinese women. *Int J Gyne Obs*. 2005;88:122-126.
55. de Sereday MS, Damiano MM, González CD, et al. Diagnostic criteria for gestational diabetes in relation to pregnancy outcome. *J Diabetes Complications*. 2003;17:115-119.
56. Seyoum B, Kiros K, Haileselase T, et al. Prevalence of gestational diabetes mellitus in rural pregnant mothers in northern Ethiopia. *Diabetes Res Clin Pract*. 1999;46:247-251.
57. Okonofua FE, Onwudiegwu U, Ugwu NC. An evaluation of the WHO criteria for abnormal glucose tolerance test during pregnancy in Nigerian women. *Afr J Med Med Sci*. 1995;24: 365-369.
58. Odar E, Wandabwa J, Kiondo P. Maternal and fetal outcome of gestational diabetes mellitus in Mulago Hospital, Uganda. *Afr Health Sci*. 2004;4:9-14.
59. Ranchod HA, Vaughan JE, Jarvis P. Incidence of gestational diabetes at Northdale Hospital, Pietermaritzburg. *S Afr Med J*. 1991;80:14-16.
60. Lee H, Jang HC, Park HK, et al. Prevalence of type 2 diabetes among women with a previous history of gestational diabetes mellitus. *Diabetes Res Clin Pract*. 2008;81:124-129.
61. Senanayake H, Seneviratne S, Ariyaratne H, et al. Screening for gestational diabetes mellitus in southern Asian women. *J Obstet Gynaecol Res*. 2006;32:286-291.
62. Tan PC, Ling LP, Omar SZ. Screening for gestational diabetes at antenatal booking in a Malaysian university hospital: the role of risk factors and threshold value for the 50-g glucose challenge test. *Aust N Z J Obstet Gynaecol*. 2007;47:191-197.
63. Boriboonhirunsarn D, Sunsaneevithayakul P. Abnormal results on a second testing and risk of gestational diabetes in women with normal baseline glucose levels. *Int J Gynaecol Obstet*. 2008;100:147-153.
64. Yalçin HR, Zorlu CG. Threshold value of glucose screening tests in pregnancy: could it be standardized for every population? *Am J Perinatol*. 1996;13:317-320.
65. Seshiah V, Das AK, Balaji V, et al. Diabetes in Pregnancy Study Group. Gestational diabetes mellitus–guidelines. *J Assoc Physicians India*. 2006;54:622-628.
66. Zargar AH, Sheikh MI, Bashir MI, et al. Prevalence of gestational diabetes mellitus in Kashmiri women from the Indian subcontinent. *Diabetes Res Clin Pract*. 2004;66:139-145.
67. Tan KCB. Impaired glucose tolerance in pregnancy. *Hong Kong Med J*. 1997;3:381-387.
68. Li DF, Wang ZQ, Wong VC, et al. Assessment of the glucose tolerance test in unselected pregnancy using 75 g glucose load. *Int J Gynaecol Obstet*. 1988;27:7-10.
69. Sacks DA, Greenspoon JS, Abu Fadil S, et al. Toward universal criteria for gestational diabetes: the 75-gram glucose tolerance test in pregnancy. *Am J Obstet Gynecol*. 1995;172: 607-614.
70. Gibler WB, Blomkalns AL. Achieving standardization in clinical research: changing cacophony into harmony. *Ann Emerg Med*. 2004;44:213-214.

Section II

Burden of GDM in US Populations

Prevalence of GDM

4

Jean M. Lawrence

4.1 Introduction

Recent studies have shown that the prevalence of gestational diabetes mellitus (GDM) has increased by 10–100% over the past 20 years, with greater increases observed among women from racial and ethnic minority groups.[1] Such an increase in GDM has important public health implications for these women as well as their offspring who are exposed to maternal hyperglycemia *in utero*. Women who develop GDM are at increased risk for GDM in subsequent pregnancies and are at increased risk for developing type 2 diabetes in the years after delivery.[2,3] Additionally, infants exposed to GDM *in utero* are at increased risk for obesity and future development of type 2 diabetes.[4,5] In this chapter, we describe the methodological challenges of conducting population-based studies of GDM and describe the trends in GDM prevalence over the past 20 years based on selected population-based studies from the United States, Canada, and Australia; chapter 6 provides an overview of the burden of GDM on developing countries.

4.2 Methodological Challenges in GDM Epidemiologic Research

Researchers designing epidemiologic studies to assess the trends in GDM face several methodological challenges, including how GDM is defined, the various blood glucose thresholds that are used to define women as having GDM, the proportion of the population screened for GDM during pregnancy, the sources of data that are available to identify women with GDM in population-based studies, and the terminology used (incidence vs. prevalence) when describing trends over time. Each of these challenges and how they affect the ability to compare study findings over time and across populations will be discussed in the sections that follow.

J.M. Lawrence
Department of Research and Evaluation, Kaiser Permanente Southern California, 100 South Los Robles, Pasadena, CA 91101, USA
e-mail: Jean.M.Lawrence@kp.org

C. Kim and A. Ferrara (eds.), *Gestational Diabetes During and After Pregnancy*, DOI: 10.1007/978-1-84882-120-0_4, © Springer-Verlag London Limited 2010

4.2.1 Definition of GDM

GDM is defined as carbohydrate intolerance of varying degrees of severity with onset *or* first recognition during pregnancy.[6,7] This definition applies regardless of treatment during pregnancy (insulin, glyburide, or dietary modification) and whether the condition persists after pregnancy. Based on this definition, women diagnosed with GDM include women with undiagnosed pregestational diabetes mellitus (PDM) as well as women with hyperglycemia induced by pregnancy. Women of childbearing age are not routinely screened for diabetes before pregnancy and large population-based studies of women screened for diabetes prior to pregnancy have not been undertaken. Additionally, screening for glucose intolerance that persists into the postpartum period among women with a history of GDM is variable, with few studies reporting postpartum testing with fasting plasma glucose or an oral glucose tolerance test in excess of 50% of women in recent periods.[8–14] In a recent review of 13 studies that reported glucose abnormalities after pregnancies complicated by GDM,[15] the prevalence of women with GDM who developed type 2 diabetes tested in periods ranging from 4 weeks to 1 year after delivery ranged from 2.5%[16] to 16.7%.[17] It is likely that some of these women had undiagnosed PDM that was identified during pregnancy.

4.2.2 Criteria Used to Define GDM

Various diagnostic criteria based on fasting and non-fasting blood glucose thresholds values are used to characterize women as having GDM (Table 4.1). These include definitions developed by the World Health Organization (WHO),[18] the National Diabetes Data Group (NDDG),[19] the American Diabetes Association (ADA),[20] the Canadian Diabetes Association (CDA),[21] the European Association for the Study of Diabetes (EASD),[22] and the Australasian Diabetes in Pregnancy Society (ADIPS).[23] Differences in defining thresholds that must be met or exceeded result in disparate estimates of GDM prevalence; prevalence estimates are particularly difficult to interpret when women with GDM are diagnosed based on different diagnostic criteria both within and between studies. A uniform approach to characterizing GDM, applied across multiple populations in the USA and other countries, would facilitate more direct comparisons of GDM prevalence within and between populations. Forthcoming results from the Hyperglycemia and Adverse Pregnancy Outcomes (HAPO) study may provide such a definition.[24,25] The HAPO study is discussed in detail in chapter 2.

4.2.3 Population-Based Screening for GDM

The estimate of the prevalence of GDM in any population is contingent upon screening for GDM in that population since the diagnosis of GDM requires screening for hyperglycemia during pregnancy. Studies that include both unscreened and screened women in the

Table 4.1 Various diagnostic criteria and authorities for gestational diabetes mellitus

Reference	Authority	Glucose load, g	GCT or OGTT	Number of results required for diagnosis ($n \geq$ mmol/L)	Blood glucose values (≥mmol/L)			
		f/nf			Fasting	1-h	2-h	3-h
Alberti and Zimmet[18]	WHO	75 f	OGTT	1	7.0		7.8	
Anonymous[19]	NDDG 1979	100 f	OGTT	2	5.8	10.5	9.2	8.0
Anonymous[20]	ADA	50 nf	GCT	1		7.8[a]		
Anonymous[20]	ADA	75 f	OGTT	2	5.3	10.0	8.6	
Anonymous[20]	ADA	100 f	OGTT	2	5.3	10.0	8.6	7.8
Meltzer et al[21]	CDA	50 nf	GCT	–		7.8		
Meltzer et al[21]	CDA	75 f	OGTT	2	5.3	10.6	8.9	
Brown et al[22]	EASD	75 f	OGTT	1	6.0		9.0	
Hoffman et al[23]	ADIPS	50 nf	GCT	–		7.8		
Hoffman et al[23]	ADIPS	75 nf	GCT	–		8.0		
Hoffman et al[23]	ADIPS Australia	75 f	OGTT	1	5.5		8.0	
Hoffman et al[23]	ADIPS New Zealand	75 f	OGTT	1	5.5		9.0	

f/nf Fasting/non-fasting; *GCT* Glucose challenge test; *OGTT* Oral glucose tolerance test

[a]If the result on the glucose challenge test (screening) is ≥10.3 mmol/L, GDM is diagnosed without further testing

denominator may draw a different conclusion than studies which are able to restrict their analysis to screened women and conduct sensitivity analysis to determine the impact of differential screening on the overall prevalence of GDM in their population. For example, studies of trends in GDM that have discussed screening in the populations under study have reported an increase in screening over time,[26] a consistently high rate of screening across the study period,[27, 28] and that screening was a component of usual care,[9] while other studies have not reported on the proportion of women screened for GDM in their populations under study.[29–32] In studies that do not limit their denominator to the population screened for GDM, some of the observed changes in the prevalence of GDM can be attributed to the increase in screening in the population over time, which would result in more complete case ascertainment over the years of the study. Studies that use hospital discharge diagnostic codes or infant birth certificates in the absence of information on prenatal screening for GDM include screened and unscreened women in their denominators when calculating trends in GDM. These studies are not able to make adjustments for inclusion of women who are not screened nor can they conduct sensitivity analysis to determine whether including women that are not screened has an impact on the results of their study. Keeping these limitations in mind, the results of these studies should be interpreted cautiously.

4.2.4 Sources of Information Used to Identify Persons with GDM

Population-based studies of GDM have used a variety of ways to identify women with GDM in their study samples. The information available to identify women as having GDM is often dependent on the populations under study. Studies from health plan-based populations,[9, 26–28] for example, may be based on blood glucose test results from oral glucose tolerance tests and glucose challenge tests conducted during pregnancy and as such they can apply a consistent criteria throughout the study period to identify women with GDM that is independent of hospital discharge diagnostic codes or infant birth certificates. Studies that must rely solely on information from infant birth certificates or hospital discharge data, as is the case for most studies from state, regional, or national populations, cannot determine if a uniform criteria was used to identify women as having GDM throughout the study period.[29–32] In their study of trends in the prevalence of GDM from 1989 through 2004 using data from the National Hospital Discharge Survey (NHDS), the authors note that the change in the criteria used to identify women as having GDM from the NDDG definition (19) to the Carpenter and Coustan criterion (20) during the period of the study, the latter of which had lower thresholds at which women were considered to have GDM, may have been the *most important* explanation for the increase in GDM prevalence in recent years in their study.[30]

Studies have identified women with GDM based on infants' birth certificates exclusively, infants' birth certificates or hospital discharge codes, hospital discharge diagnostic codes exclusively, hospital discharge code or laboratory test results, laboratory test results exclusively, local clinical databases, and medical record abstraction (Table 4.2). The ability of these sources of information to accurately identify women as having GDM is variable. The 1989 version of the US birth certificate did not differentiate between PDM and GDM, while the 2003 revision (the most recent national version of the US birth certificate)

Table 4.2 Selected studies of gestational diabetes mellitus in the USA, Canada, and Australia: 1985–2006

Population (geographic area)	Sample	N deliveries, race/ethnicity	Study period (years)[a]	GDM prevalence	Relative change[b] (%)	Criteria for GDM definition	Source of GDM information	Age adjusted
United States								
USA[30]	Country	58,922,266 Race distribution not reported for total sample	1989–2004	1.9% (1989–1990) to 4.2% (2003–2004)	122	Unknown	National Hospital Discharge Survey, ICD-9 code	Age-specific
Montana[38]	State	43,543 12% AI (below 88% White) 88% White;	2000–2003	White: AI 2.4–2.9% (below 2.0–2.2%) 2.0–2.2%	10 21	Unknown	Infant birth certificates	No
Minnesota[32]	State	130,671 77% NHW 4.2% Asian	1993, 2003	2.6–3.5% 2.5–3.2% 1.9–5.5%	35 28 189	Unknown	Infant birth certificates	Yes
Los Angeles County[31]	County	2,156,459 Race not reported	1991–2003	1.5–4.8%	220	Unknown	Hospital discharge data, ICD-9 code	Yes
New York City[39]	City	>1.5 million 43% Hispanic or Caribbean	1990, 2001	2.6–3.8%	46	Unknown	Infant birth certificates	Yes
New York City[29]	City	1,067,356 Many ethnic categories and sub-categories	1995–2003	5.0–5.4%	8	Unknown	Infant birth certificates and hospital discharge data	Yes

(*continued*)

Table 4.2 (continued)

Population (geographic area)	Sample	N deliveries, race/ethnicity	Study period (years)[a]	GDM prevalence	Relative change[b] (%)	Criteria for GDM definition	Source of GDM information	Age adjusted
Northern California[26]	MCO	267,051 45% NHW	1991–2000	3.7–6.6% 5.1–6.9%	78 35	2000 ADA	Laboratory test results Laboratory test results OR ICD-9 code	Yes
Colorado[27]	MCO	36,403 61% NHW	1994–2002	2.1–4.1%	95	NDDG	Clinical database	Yes
Southern California[28]	MCO	209,287 52% Hispanic, 26% NHW	1999–2005	7.5–7.4%	−1	2000 ADA	Laboratory test results	Yes
Oregon[9]	MCO	36,251 60% White	1999–2006	2.9–3.6%	24	NDDG	Laboratory test results OR ICD-9 code and pharmacy	No
Canada								
Manitoba[40]	Province	324,605 93.1% Not FN 6.9% FN	1985–2004	2.3–3.7% 1.8–3.0% 6.8–8.1%	61 67 19	Changed over time	Standard prenatal form	No
Ontario[37]	Province	659,164 Race not reported	1995–2002	3.2–3.6%	12	Unknown	Hospital Discharge data	No

James Bay, Ontario[41]	Region	1,298 FN (Cree)	1987–1995	8.5%	N/A	NDDG	Medical record review	N/A
James Bay, Quebec[47]	Region	579 FN (Cree)	1995–1996	12.8%	N/A	NDDG	Medical record review	N/A
Australia								
New South Wales[42]	State	370,703 51% Australian, 28% Asian	1998–2002	4.0–5.1%	27	(Primarily) ADIPS	Inpatient statistics (Hospital), midwives data collection, ICDM-10AM (Australian modification)	No
New South Wales[43]	State	956,738 75% Australia or New Zealand	1995–2005	3.0–4.4%	45	ADIPS	Midwives data collection	Yes
South Australia[45]	State	230,011	1988–1999			ADIPS or WHO	Laboratory test results	Yes
		98% Non-aboriginal		≈1.7–3.2%	88			
		2% Aboriginal		≈5.3–5.9%	11.3			

MCO managed care organization; *ADA* American Diabetes Association; *NDDG* National Diabetes Data Group; *WHO* World Health Organization; *OGTT* oral glucose tolerance test; *FPG* fasting plasma glucose; *ADIPS* Australasian Diabetes in Pregnancy Society; *NHW* non-Hispanic White; *AI* American Indian; *FN* First Nation

[a] For years with dashes between them (example, 1991–2000), data from all years were included in the study. For years with commas between them (example, 1993, 2003) only data from those 2 years are included in the study

[b] Relative change is calculated based on the prevalence in first and last year (or period) of the study

captures information on each of these conditions in separate categories.[33] The ability to exclude women with PDM from the denominator when studying trends in GDM is important as several recent studies have demonstrated that the prevalence of PDM in the populations giving birth is increasing.[28, 34] In a recent review paper, Devlin and colleagues reviewed 12 studies that evaluated the reliability of US birth certificates and hospital discharge diagnostic codes to identify births complicated by maternal diabetes.[35] Eight of these studies distinguished between PDM and GDM. Six studies conducted between 1989 and 2007 used infant birth certificates or hospital discharge to identify women with GDM and linked these data to other sources for validation. The sensitivities for the four studies that used birth certificates validated against a variety of sources to identify GDM ranged from 46 to 83%, while the sensitivities for the two studies that used hospital discharge data validated against medical records were 71% and 81%.[35] The identification of women with PDM using their infants' birth certificates performed less well, with sensitivities ranging from 47 to 52%. The sensitivities were 78 and 95% to identify women with PDM using hospital discharge diagnostic codes.

In a study conducted in New South Wales Australia, two population-based data sources; the Midwives Data Collection (birth data), which included information on maternal characteristics, pregnancy, labor, delivery, and infant outcomes and the Admitted Patient Data Collection (hospital data), a census of all public and private inpatient hospital discharges, were compared against the medical record for approximately 1,200 women. The sensitivities of birth data and hospital data to identify women with GDM were 63.3 and 68.6%, respectively, while the sensitivities of these data sources to identify women with PDM were 45.1 and 100%, respectively.[36] Thus, when the sensitivity of hospital discharge diagnostic codes were compared to the sensitivity of the birth certificate to identify women with PDM and GDM, hospital discharge codes were more likely to correctly identify women as having PDM and GDM than was information on the birth certificates. The differences in the sensitivity between the two sources of data were greater when identifying women with PDM than when identifying women with GDM.

4.2.5 Terminology – Incidence vs. Prevalence

Studies that describe trends in GDM have used the terms "prevalence" and "incidence" somewhat interchangeably, although the term prevalence has been more commonly used. Incidence is the number of cases of a disease or illness *newly identified* in a specific population in a specified period of time. Prevalence is the total number of persons *having* a disease or condition in a specific population during a specific period of time. To be characterized as having the condition in the period under study, a person may either *develop the condition before the beginning of the study period* or be *newly diagnosed* with the condition during the study period. In either case, to be included in the denominator the person with the condition must be part of the population under study during the specified period. Prevalence can be further categorized as point prevalence (a specific point in time), period prevalence (at any time during a specific period), and annual prevalence (at any time during the year).

Most studies of GDM examine the number of women giving birth after a specific point in the pregnancy (i.e., 20 weeks gestation) or whose pregnancies result in live birth during a specific period, often one calendar year, who develop GDM during that pregnancy. Given that the duration of pregnancy is, on average, 40 weeks and GDM is most often identified between 24 and 28 weeks, GDM may develop during the calendar year in which the delivery occurs or the previous calendar year, as would be the case for women who give birth early in the year. Ferrara distinguished between cumulative incidence and prevalence of GDM based on the composition of the denominator. Studies which limit the denominator to women with screened pregnancies, regardless of whether they resulted in a live birth, yield cumulative incidence rates while studies including only women with live births yield prevalence estimates.[1] The composition of the denominator will vary based on the source of information used to identify women at risk for the outcome who are to be included in the denominator. Studies based on infant birth certificate data cannot include women who were pregnant but did not have a live birth, studies using hospital discharge diagnoses codes may include women who had late second trimester or third trimester fetal losses resulting in hospitalization, while clinical databases may include women with fetal losses beyond a specific time in pregnancy. Thus, when comparing trends in GDM across studies, it is important to take into account the composition of the sample that comprise both the numerator (women with GDM) and the denominator (the population at risk for GDM) to determine the comparability of finding across studies instead of solely relying on the terminology (incidence or prevalence) used to describe the methodological approach in any given study.

4.2.6 Other Methodological Issues Affecting Studies of GDM

4.2.6.1 Maternal Race and Ethnicity

A variety of other factors may impact our ability to compare trends in GDM across studies and to adjust for key risk factors that may impact these trends. The availability of accurate information to categorize maternal race/ethnicity is important as it impacts on the studies' ability to reliably provide race/ethnicity-specific prevalence or incidence estimates and to adjust for changes in the racial/ethnic composition of the population when doing trend analyses. One large study conducted over a 7-year period in the province of Ontario in Canada which focused on the risk of developing diabetes after a GDM-affected pregnancy did not provide race/ethnicity specific GDM estimates since this study was conducted using administrative data which did not include this information.[37] While this study provides information on the trend in the prevalence of GDM in Ontario, it does not provide information on how these trends may be differentially affected by women from the various racial and ethnic groups in that province over time. Studies that must rely on data from administrative sources to categorize the race/ethnicity of the women in the population have a significant amount of missing data and may define their categories less precisely than studies that include maternal race/ethnicity from infant birth certificates. For example, in an analyses of data from the NHDS, the authors reported that data on race was missing for up to 20% of births from 1995 to 2001 and up to 29% of births from 2002 to 2004. Additionally, Hispanic ethnicity was not included as a separate category from white or black race, and women of Asian or Pacific Islander race were excluded from the analyses due to a small number of annual births in this racial group.[30] Thus, while this was the only study identified that provided national estimates of GDM prevalence by US geographic region and maternal age category, its race/ethnicity specific conclusions must be interpreted cautiously as the racial/ethnic group with the highest GDM prevalence, Asian and Pacific Islanders, was excluded from the analysis and women of Hispanic ethnicity, another group with a high GDM prevalence could not be analyzed separately, but were combined into the two main race categories, White and Black, most likely increasing GDM prevalence in these groups due to the proportion of women who were both Hispanic and white or black. Other studies have derived information on maternal race/ethnicity from infant birth certificates,[9, 28, 29, 32, 38, 39] hospital records,[26] self-reported First Nation status,[40] band number to identify native American status,[41] and country and region of maternal birth.[42, 43]

4.2.6.2
Maternal Prepregnancy Weight and Body Mass Index

Prepregnancy body mass index (BMI) is a risk factor for GDM, with overweight and obese women having a higher risk of GDM than women of healthy weight.[44] Based on data from 75,403 women from 26 states and New York City who self-reported prepregnancy weight and height on the Pregnancy Risk Assessment Monitoring System (PRAMS) survey from 2004 and 2005, 23% of women giving birth were overweight and 19% were obese in 2004 and 2005.[45] Maternal BMI has rarely been included in population-based studies of GDM given the limited availability of maternal height and weight in these study samples. In the study of trends in GDM prevalence in New York City, prepregnancy weight but not height was used as an adjustment factor in models presenting trends in GDM from 1995 to 2003 but was not discussed in the paper.[29] In a study from a managed health care plan in Oregon, prepregnancy BMI was included based on information from the medical records, although BMI was discussed in the context of postpartum screening (the primary aim of the study) and not in relation to trends in GDM.[9]

As of 2007, 24 states and Puerto Rico included prepregnancy height and weight on their birth certificates (*personal communication, Joyce Martin, National Center for Health Statistics*). However, published reports which evaluate the validity of prepregnancy height and weight on the birth certificate compared to a gold standard such as a clinical database are lacking and the results would most likely be variable by location within states as well as between states. Electronic medical records, which are being implemented across the country in a variety of health plans and practices, may ultimately provide additional information on BMI for women giving birth. The availability of these data may increase our understanding of the contribution of maternal prepregnancy BMI as well as weight gain during pregnancy in the development of GDM, particularly as it may differ by racial or ethnic group. Another chapter in this book includes a more comprehensive discussion of the role of obesity in GDM.

4.3 Trends in Prevalence of GDM

Despite the methodological challenges in studying the epidemiology of GDM, we must rely on these population-based studies to further our understanding of the trends in GDM prevalence over time. We must consider the strengths and limitations of each study when comparing and contrasting estimates across studies. There are often significant trade-offs between the size and diversity of the populations available for study in terms of geographic diversity (counties, states, regions, and countries), insurance status (insured women only vs. all women regardless of insurance status), and the amount of detailed information available to identify women with GDM and characterize these trends in population-based studies. In the selected studies over the past 20 years, summarized in Table 4.2, almost all studies reported an increase in the prevalence of pregnancies affected by GDM, although the magnitude of the increase varied significantly by the populations studied and the methods use to undertake these studies.

4.3.1 Comparison of Trends Across Studies

The change in prevalence for the studies reviewed from the USA, Canada, and Australia varied significantly by region, data source, racial/ethnic composition of the population giving birth, and years included in the study but almost all demonstrated increases in GDM over the course of the period under study with one exception[28] (Table 4.2). The greatest increase in prevalence of GDM was reported in a study of Los Angeles County births, which observed a 220% increase based on hospital discharge diagnostic codes from 1991 to 2003[31] while there was no significant change observed in a managed health care population in Southern California (a 6-county area which included Los Angeles County) based on laboratory-identified cases of GDM from 1999 to 2005.[28] The prevalence reported by the Los Angeles County study from 1999 through 2003, the period during which these two studies overlap, ranged from approximately 4.2 to 4.5%[31] based on hospital discharge diagnostic codes. This estimate was significantly lower than the prevalence reported by the managed health care population study for these same years, which ranged from 7.5 to 8.2% using laboratory test results.[28] Differences in the results between the two studies may be based on several factors which include the difference in the composition of the denominator (screened plus unscreened women in the Los Angeles County study vs. screened women only in the health plan study) and the way that cases were identified (hospital discharge diagnostic codes in the Los Angeles County study vs. a consistent cut-point applied to blood glucose test results from the laboratory database in the health plan study).

When results were compared within one large managed health care plan across four different regions of the USA (northern and southern California [two studies], Oregon, and Colorado),[9, 26–28] the study from the southern California region exhibited the highest prevalence of GDM based on laboratory-identified cases but no significant change in prevalence from 1999 to 2005 while the other studies reported an increase in prevalence, with a doubling reported in Colorado from 1994 to 2002, a 25% increase in Oregon from 1999 to 2006, and an increase of 35 or 78% depending on the case definition used in northern California from 1991 to 2000. The two California studies were the most comparable, as they both restricted their denominator to women with documented screening for GDM during pregnancy, and used a consistent laboratory cut-point to identify women with GDM throughout the study period. Southern California presented their results based solely on laboratory-identified cases while northern California reported results using this same laboratory-defined case definition in addition to a second case definition that included laboratory defined cases and cases identified using hospital discharge diagnostic codes.[26, 28] Both California studies reported a higher prevalence or cumulative incidence of GDM than did the studies in the other regions. Non-Hispanic white women, who are at lower risk for GDM than women from other racial/ethnic groups, comprised about 60% of the populations giving birth in the samples from Oregon and Colorado but comprised only about one-quarter of women in southern California and less than half of the women in northern California. The Oregon and Colorado studies relied on the NDDG criteria to establish GDM clinically while the California studies used the ADA criteria, which require a lower blood glucose level to characterize the women as having GDM.

The single study that included the entire US population (almost 59 million births over 16 years) was based on results from the NHDS and reported a 122% increase in GDM from 1989–1990 to 2003–2004.[30] As previously noted, the results of this study could be affected by the differences in diagnostic criteria used during the study period, inclusion of Hispanic women in the specific race categories, and inclusion of unscreened women in the denominator. Among white women, the prevalence of GDM increased by 80% while a 172% increase was observed among Black women. Increases in GDM were observed in all geographic regions of the country.[30] Studies using birth certificate data from Montana[38] and Minnesota[32] reported an increase of 10% over 3 years and a 28% increase over 10 years, respectively, among white women. The increase among American Indian women in Montana was 21%, about twice that of white women, while the increase among Asian women in Minnesota was 189%, or almost seven times the increase observed among white women in the same period. The two studies from New York City reported quite different prevalence estimates of GDM. In the study based exclusively on birth certificates, a 46% increase was observed in the year 2001 as compared to the prevalence of the year 1990[39] while in the study which used both birth certificates and hospital discharge data, an 8% increase was observed in the year 2003 when compared with the prevalence of the year 1995.[29] However, as expected, the prevalence of GDM was higher in the study using birth certificates and hospital discharge data combined than in the study that used birth certificate data only.

In the two studies conducted in Canada which reported trends in prevalence of GDM, a 12% increase in the prevalence was reported in the province of Ontario from 1995 to 2002,[37] while a 61% increase was observed among women in the province of Manitoba from 1985 to 2004.[40] As we previously mentioned, the study conducted for the province of Ontario was not able to examine the differences in prevalence of GDM by race/ethnicity as this information was not included in their administrative data.[37] However, in the study conducted in the province of Manitoba, the overall increase in prevalence was 61%, with a smaller increase observed among First Nation women (19%) compared to 67% among non-First Nation women.[40] However, while the absolute increase was lower, the prevalence of GDM was much higher in First Nation women (8.1%) as compared to non-First Nation women (3.0%) in 2004, the last year of their study.

In the two studies conducted in the state of New South Wales, Australia, a 27% increase in the prevalence of GDM was reported from 1998 to 2002 based on hospital information, midwives data collection, and hospital discharge codes combined[42] whereas a 45% increase was observed in the same state from 1995 through 2005, from a prevalence of 3.0% in 1995 to 4.4% in 2005.[43] In the state of South Australia, the prevalence of GDM increased by 88% among non-Aboriginal women and 11.3% in Aboriginal women from 1988 to 1999 based on laboratory test results only.[46] Studies that examined trends in GDM within European countries could not be identified for inclusion in this review.

4.3.2 Comparison of Prevalence by Racial and Ethnic Group

Studies of GDM conducted in the US have consistently demonstrated that women of Native American, Hispanic, and Asian race/ethnicity are at greater risk for developing GDM than are non-Hispanic white women,[26–28, 30, 31] while GDM prevalence for African American women has been reported as being about the same[26, 28, 30, 31] or higher[29, 32] than non-Hispanic white women, depending on the study reviewed. In several studies that had significant diversity in the racial and ethnic composition of their populations under study and sample sizes that were sufficient to produce stable estimates of prevalence,[26, 28, 29, 31] women of Asian and Pacific Islander race/ethnicity have the highest prevalence of GDM. Ferrara et al[26] reported that the cumulative incidence of GDM was 10.9% in 2000, the last year of their study; while Lawrence et al[28] reported a prevalence of 11.8% among Asian/Pacific Islander women (the majority of whom were Asian) in 2005. Hispanic women had the next highest burden of GDM during pregnancy, reporting estimates of 7.6 and 8.5%, respectively, in these two studies. Non-Hispanic white and African American women had a similar burden of GDM in each study.

Few studies have had sufficient sample size to report on the prevalence of GDM among Native American women. Two studies describing the trends in the prevalence of GDM among First Nation Cree women in the provinces of Ontario and Northern Quebec in Canada reported that 8.5% (1987–1995) and 12.8% (1995–1996) of the women in their study samples, respectively, developed GDM during their pregnancies.[41, 47] In Manitoba Canada, the prevalence of GDM rose from 6.8% (1985–1989) to 8.1% (2000–2004) among First Nation women.[40] During the same period, the prevalence rose from 1.8 to 3.0% among non-First Nation women. GDM prevalence in American Indian women in Montana in 2004 was 2.9% compared to 2.2% in White women based on information on infant birth certificates.[38]

Within racial/ethnic groups that are often combined when reporting results from US studies, there are significant differences in the prevalence of GDM by subgroups of women included in these categories. Several studies have compared the prevalence of GDM across women from Asian groups using consistent methodologies for the comparison. Savitz et al reported a risk of GDM of 6.6% for East Asian women, ranging from 3.0% for Japanese women and 3.3% for Korean women to 7.7% for Taiwanese women and 9.9% for women from Hong Kong among women living in New York City.[29] Among South Central Asian women, the risk was 14.3%, ranging from 4.6% for Iranian women to 16.2% for Pakistani women and 21.2% for Bangladeshi women. In this study, the only groups of Asian women that did not have a higher risk for GDM than non-Hispanic white women after adjustment for age, education, prepregnancy weight, parity, and smoking status were Japanese and Iranian women. Lawrence et al reported a similar difference in prevalence of GDM among Asian American women in southern California, with Japanese and Korean women having a prevalence of 6.8 and 7.8%, respectively, while Indian (12.7%), Filipina (12.6%), Vietnamese (12.2%), and Southeast Asian women (9.9%) all had a high prevalence of GDM.[48] Rao et al found a significant difference in GDM prevalence among Japanese, Chinese and Filipina women, with a prevalence of GDM of 3.4, 6.5, and 6.1% respectively.[49] In a study of GDM prevalence in Australia, women born in Northeast and Southeast Asia as well as South Asia had a prevalence of GDM of 9.4 and 10.5%, respectively, in comparison with 2.7% among women born in Australia and New Zealand.[43]

In the New York City study,[29] women that would traditionally be grouped as black or African American in other studies, including women defined as African, from Sub-Saharan Africa, and non-Hispanic Caribbean women had risks of GDM of 4.3, 5.9, and 6.9%, respectively.[29] Within these groups, subgroup differences were also observed, with the risk for Sub-Saharan African women ranging from 4.1 to 6.9% depending on their country of birth, although samples sizes in these groups became quite small. None of the other studies reported provided subgroup information on women in the group that were described as Black or African American.

4.3.3 Demographic Changes that may Affect Trends in GDM

Shifts in the demographics of the population giving birth can increase the overall prevalence of GDM in the population. Two such trends in the USA are the increasing maternal age at birth and the increase in proportion of births to women from minority populations, both of which are associated with the risk of GDM. The birth rate for women aged 35–39 years has increased each year since 1978 (19.0), rising by almost 50% since 1990 (31.7) to 47.3 births per 1,000 women in 2006. The birth rate for women age 40–44 years (9.4) increased each year since 2000, and has more than doubled since 1981 (3.8) while the birth rate for women aged 45–49 years increased to 0.6 births per 1,000 women in 2006; this rate more than doubled between 1990 (0.2) and 2000 (0.5), but was stable until 2005.[50] The racial/ethnic composition of the population giving birth in the USA has also changed over time. In 2006, 54.1% of the 4,265,555 women giving birth were non-Hispanic white, compared to 64.7% of the 3,903,012 women giving birth in 1989, a decrease of about 20% in the proportion of women giving birth who were non-Hispanic white. In 2006, 24% of the women giving birth in the USA were Hispanic, while about 5.6% were Asian or Pacific Islander.[49] For women in age categories 30–34, 35–39, and 40–44 years, the age-specific birth rates are consistently higher for Hispanic women and Asian or Pacific Islander women than non-Hispanic white women.[33] The convergence of these two demographic trends may also contribute to the increasing prevalence of GDM over time.

4.4 Conclusions and Future Research

The increasing prevalence of GDM signals an impending surge in the number of women that will be affected by diabetes in the coming years. Both women who develop GDM during their pregnancies and their offspring who are exposed to the environmental influence of GDM *in utero* are at increased risk of developing diabetes in the future. In order to better characterize these populations and to evaluate future trends in GDM and PDM, the methodological challenges described in this chapter must be addressed. A more uniform case definition for GDM, better quality data to identify women as having GDM or PDM in large population-based samples, information on maternal height as well as maternal weight both prepregnancy and at the time of delivery and information to characterize their race/ethnicity in more precise and self-defined categories are needed.

References

1. Ferrara A. Increasing prevalence of gestational diabetes mellitus: a public health perspective. *Diabetes Care*. 2007;30(suppl 2):S141-S146.
2. Kim C, Newton KM, Knopp RH. Gestational diabetes and the incidence of type 2 diabetes: a systematic review. *Diabetes Care*. 2002;25:1862-1868.
3. Kim C, Berger DK, Chamany S. Recurrence of gestational diabetes mellitus: a systematic review. *Diabetes Care*. 2007;30:1314-1319.
4. Hillier TA, Pedula KL, Schmidt MM, Mullen JA, Charles MA, Pettitt DJ. Childhood obesity and metabolic imprinting: the ongoing effects of maternal hyperglycemia. *Diabetes Care*. 2007;30:2287-2292.
5. Dabelea D, Mayer-Davis EJ, Lamichhane AP, et al. Association of intrauterine exposure to maternal diabetes and obesity with type 2 diabetes in youth: the SEARCH Case-Control Study. *Diabetes Care*. 2008;31:1422-1426.
6. Metzger BE, Buchanan TA, Coustan DR, et al. Summary and recommendations of the Fifth International Workshop-Conference on Gestational Diabetes Mellitus. *Diabetes Care*. 2007;30(suppl 2):S251-S260.
7. Metzger BE, Coustan DR. Summary and recommendations of the Fourth International Workshop-Conference on Gestational Diabetes Mellitus. The Organizing Committee. *Diabetes Care*. 1998;21(suppl 2):B161-B167.
8. Almario CV, Ecker T, Moroz LA, Bucovetsky L, Berghella V, Baxter JK. Obstetricians seldom provide postpartum diabetes screening for women with gestational diabetes. *Am J Obstet Gynecol*. 2008;198(528):e1-e5.
9. Dietz PM, Vesco KK, Callaghan WM, et al. Postpartum screening for diabetes after a gestational diabetes mellitus-affected pregnancy. *Obstet Gynecol*. 2008;112:868-874.
10. Ferrara A, Peng T, Kim C. Trends in postpartum diabetes screening and subsequent diabetes and impaired fasting glucose among women with histories of gestational diabetes mellitus. A report from the Translating Research Into Action for Diabetes (TRIAD) Study. *Diabetes Care*. 2009;32:269-274.
11. Hunt KJ, Conway DL. Who returns for postpartum glucose screening following gestational diabetes mellitus? *Am J Obstet Gynecol*. 2008;198:404-406.

12. Russell MA, Phipps MG, Olson CL, Welch HG, Carpenter MW. Rates of postpartum glucose testing after gestational diabetes mellitus. *Obstet Gynecol.* 2006;108:1456-1462.
13. Smirnakis KV, Chasan-Taber L, Wolf M, Markenson G, Ecker JL, Thadhani R. Postpartum diabetes screening in women with a history of gestational diabetes. *Obstet Gynecol.* 2005;106:1297-1303.
14. Lawrence JM, Hsu JW, Chen W, Black MH, Sacks DA. Prevalence and timing of postpartum glucose testing and sustained glucose dysregulation after gestational diabetes mellitus. *Diabetes Care.* 2010;33:569-576.
15. Kitzmiller JL, Dang-Kilduff L, Taslimi MM. Gestational diabetes after delivery. Short-term management and long-term risks. *Diabetes Care.* 2007;30(suppl 2):S225-S235.
16. Costa A, Carmona F, Martinez-Roman S, Quinto L, Levy I, Conget I. Post-partum reclassification of glucose tolerance in women previously diagnosed with gestational diabetes mellitus. *Diabet Med.* 2000;17:595-598.
17. Jang HC, Yim CH, Han KO, et al. Gestational diabetes mellitus in Korea: prevalence and prediction of glucose intolerance at early postpartum. *Diabetes Res Clin Pract.* 2003;61: 117-124.
18. Alberti KG, Zimmet PZ. Definition, diagnosis and classification of diabetes mellitus and its complications. Part 1: diagnosis and classification of diabetes mellitus provisional report of a WHO consultation. *Diabet Med.* 1998;15:539-553.
19. Anonymous. Classification and diagnosis of diabetes mellitus and other categories of glucose intolerance. National Diabetes Data Group. *Diabetes.* 1979;28:1039-1057.
20. Anonymous. Gestational diabetes mellitus. *Diabetes Care.* 2004;27(suppl 1):S88-S90.
21. Meltzer S, Leiter L, Daneman D, et al. 1998 clinical practice guidelines for the management of diabetes in Canada. Canadian Diabetes Association. *CMAJ.* 1998;159(suppl 8):S1-S29.
22. Brown CJ, Dawson A, Dodds R, et al. Report of the Pregnancy and Neonatal Care Group. *Diabet Med.* 1996;13:S43-S53.
23. Hoffman L, Nolan C, Wilson JD, Oats JJ, Simmons D. Gestational diabetes mellitus–management guidelines. The Australasian Diabetes in Pregnancy Society. *Med J Aust.* 1998;169: 93-97.
24. Anonymous. The hyperglycemia and adverse pregnancy outcome (HAPO) study. *Int J Gynaecol Obstet.* 2002;78:69-77.
25. Trujillo AL, Jovanovic L. Waiting for HAPO. *Diabetes Metab Res Rev.* 2008;24(suppl 2): S1-S2.
26. Ferrara A, Kahn HS, Quesenberry CP, Riley C, Hedderson MM. An increase in the incidence of gestational diabetes mellitus: Northern California, 1991-2000. *Obstet Gynecol.* 2004;103:526-533.
27. Dabelea D, Snell-Bergeon JK, Hartsfield CL, Bischoff KJ, Hamman RF, McDuffie RS. Increasing prevalence of gestational diabetes mellitus (GDM) over time and by birth cohort: Kaiser Permanente of Colorado GDM Screening Program. *Diabetes Care.* 2005;28:579-584.
28. Lawrence JM, Contreras R, Chen W, Sacks DA. Trends in the prevalence of preexisting diabetes and gestational diabetes mellitus among a racially/ethnically diverse population of pregnant women, 1999-2005. *Diabetes Care.* 2008;31:899-904.
29. Savitz DA, Janevic TM, Engel SM, Kaufman JS, Herring AH. Ethnicity and gestational diabetes in New York City, 1995-2003. *BJOG.* 2008;115:969-978.
30. Getahun D, Nath C, Ananth CV, Chavez MR, Smulian JC. Gestational diabetes in the United States: temporal trends 1989 through 2004. *Am J Obstet Gynecol.* 2008;198(525):e1-e5.
31. Baraban E, McCoy L, Simon P. Increasing prevalence of gestational diabetes and pregnancy-related hypertension in Los Angeles County, California, 1991-2003. *Prev Chronic Dis.* 2008; 5:A77.
32. Devlin HM, Desai J, Holzman GS, Gilbertson DT. Trends and disparities among diabetes-complicated births in Minnesota, 1993-2003. *Am J Public Health.* 2008;98:59-62.

33. Martin JA, Kung HC, Mathews TJ, et al. Annual summary of vital statistics: 2006. *Pediatrics*. 2008;121:788-801.
34. Feig DS, Razzaq A, Sykora K, Hux JE, Anderson GM. Trends in deliveries, prenatal care, and obstetrical complications in women with pregestational diabetes: a population-based study in Ontario, Canada, 1996-2001. *Diabetes Care*. 2006;29:232-235.
35. Devlin HM, Desai J, Walaszek A. Reviewing performance of birth certificate and hospital discharge data to identify births complicated by maternal diabetes. *Matern Child Health J*. 2009;13(5):660-666. epub ahead of print.
36. Bell JC, Ford JB, Cameron CA, Roberts CL. The accuracy of population health data for monitoring trends and outcomes among women with diabetes in pregnancy. *Diabetes Res Clin Pract*. 2008;81:105-109.
37. Feig DS, Zinman B, Wang X, Hux JE. Risk of development of diabetes mellitus after diagnosis of gestational diabetes. *CMAJ*. 2008;179:229-234.
38. Montana Department of Public Health and Human Services Chronic Disease Prevention and Health Promotion Program (2009) Trends in diabetes in pregnancy among American Indian and White mothers in Montana 1989-2003: An update. 1-7
39. Thorpe LE, Berger D, Ellis JA, et al. Trends and racial/ethnic disparities in gestational diabetes among pregnant women in New York City, 1990-2001. *Am J Public Health*. 2005;95: 1536-1539.
40. Aljohani N, Rempel BM, Ludwig S, et al. Gestational diabetes in Manitoba during a twenty-year period. *Clin Invest Med*. 2008;31:E131-E137.
41. Godwin M, Muirhead M, Huynh J, Helt B, Grimmer J. Prevalence of gestational diabetes mellitus among Swampy Cree women in Moose Factory, James Bay. *CMAJ*. 1999;160: 1299-1302.
42. Shand AW, Bell JC, McElduff A, Morris J, Roberts CL. Outcomes of pregnancies in women with pre-gestational diabetes mellitus and gestational diabetes mellitus; a population-based study in New South Wales, Australia, 1998-2002. *Diabet Med*. 2008;25:708-715.
43. Anna V, van der Ploeg HP, Cheung NW, Huxley RR, Bauman AE. Sociodemographic correlates of the increasing trend in prevalence of gestational diabetes mellitus in a large population of women between 1995 and 2005. *Diabetes Care*. 2008;31:2288-2293.
44. Chu SY, Callaghan WM, Kim SY, et al. Maternal obesity and risk of gestational diabetes mellitus. *Diabetes Care*. 2007;30:2070-2076.
45. Chu SY, Kim SY, Bish CL. Prepregnancy Obesity Prevalence in the United States, 2004-2005. *Am J Obstet Gynecol*. 2008;200(271):e1-e7.
46. Ishak M, Petocz P. Gestational diabetes among Aboriginal Australians: prevalence, time trend, and comparisons with non-Aboriginal Australians. *Ethn Dis*. 2003;13:55-60.
47. Rodrigues S, Robinson E, Gray-Donald K. Prevalence of gestational diabetes mellitus among James Bay Cree women in northern Quebec. *CMAJ*. 1999;160:1293-1297.
48. Lawrence JM, Contrera R. Prevalence of pre-gestational and gestational diabetes mellitus (GDM) among Asian American Women by Ethnic Subgroup, 1999-2005. *Diabetologia*. 2007;50:S54.
49. Rao AK, Cheng YW, Caughey AB. Perinatal complications among different Asian-American subgroups. *Am J Obstet Gynecol*. 2006;194:e39-e41.
50. Martin JA, Hamilton BE, Sutton PD, et al. Births: final data for 2006. *Natl Vital Stat Rep*. 2009;57:1-104.

Risk Factors for Gestational Diabetes: from an Epidemiological Standpoint

5

Cuilin Zhang

5.1 Introduction

5.1.1 Public Health and Clinical Implications of Risk Factors for GDM

Gestational diabetes mellitus (GDM) complicates approximately 1–14% of all pregnancies. With more than 200,000 cases diagnosed annually in U.S., it continues to be a significant public health and clinical problem.[1] Importantly, this number is increasing with the increasing prevalence of obesity among women of reproductive age.[2] GDM has been related to substantial short-term and long-term adverse health outcomes for both mothers and offspring. Women with GDM have increased risk for perinatal morbidity and a considerably elevated risk for impaired glucose tolerance and type 2 diabetes mellitus in the years following pregnancy.[1, 3–6] Children of women with GDM are more likely to be obese and have impaired glucose tolerance and diabetes in childhood and early adulthood.[1] Moreover, accumulating evidence from in vivo and animal studies demonstrate that maternal hyperglycemia impairs embryogenesis as early as the pre-implantation stages of development.[7, 8] Collectively, these data highlight the importance of understanding risk factors for GDM and preventing GDM among high risk populations. Ongoing research and public health goals are to understand and short-circuit the vicious cycle involving GDM, childhood obesity and metabolic disorders, and adulthood obesity and diabetes.

5.1.2 Risk Factors Both Before and During Pregnancy are Relevant

Normal pregnancy, especially the third trimester, is characterized by profound metabolic stresses on maternal lipid and glucose homeostasis, including marked insulin resistance and hyperinsulinemia.[9–11] Although the underlying mechanisms are yet to be precisely identified,

C. Zhang
Division of Epidemiology, Statistics and Prevention Research,
Eunice Kennedy Shriver National Institute of Child Health and Human Development,
National Institutes of Health, Rockville, MD, USA
e-mail: zhangcu@mail.nih.gov

C. Kim and A. Ferrara (eds.), *Gestational Diabetes During and After Pregnancy*,
DOI: 10.1007/978-1-84882-120-0_5, © Springer-Verlag London Limited 2010

insulin resistance and inadequate insulin secretion to compensate for it play a central role in the pathophysiology of GDM.[9] Women who develop GDM are thought to have a compromised capacity to adapt to the increased insulin resistance characteristic of late pregnancy, primarily during the 3rd trimester.[9] Pregnancy-related metabolic challenges unmask a predisposition to glucose metabolic disorders in some women.[9, 12, 13] The majority of women with GDM have β-cell dysfunction against a background of chronic insulin resistance to which the insulin resistance of pregnancy is partially additive.[9] Factors that contribute to insulin resistance or relative insulin deficiency both before and during pregnancy may have a deleterious effect during pregnancy and may be risk factors for GDM. Less attention has been paid to pregravid risk factors for GDM. This chapter reviews major risk factors not only during, but also before pregnancy. Particular attention will be paid to emerging modifiable factors as these likely have substantial implications for the prevention of GDM.

5.2 Risk Factors

5.2.1 Overview of Risk Factors of GDM: Evidence from Epidemiologic Studies

Relatively few epidemiological studies have been conducted to identify risk factors of GDM.[14, 15] As discussed in earlier chapters, the diagnostic criteria and screening strategy for GDM and the measurements of risk factors vary significantly across study periods and study populations, which makes it difficult to compare findings across studies. Moreover, substantial heterogeneity exists in the approach analyzing the association between risk factors and GDM risk. The majority of earlier studies on risk factors of GDM failed to address bias due to potential confounding by other risk factors. Further, the actual number of GDM cases in the majority of studies is rather low, hampering solid conclusions. Despite these methodological concerns, several GDM risk factors consistently emerge.

Excessive adiposity, advanced maternal age, a family history of type 2 diabetes, and a prior history of GDM are well recognized risk factors of GDM.[14–18] Among them, excessive adiposity is the most important modifiable risk factor, especially in view of the escalating burden of obesity among women of reproductive age across different race/ethnicity populations in the past decade.[19] The risk of GDM increases significantly and progressively in overweight, obese, and morbidly obese women.[20–22] Women with a family history of type 2 diabetes (particularly maternal history), as compared with women without such a history, experience a 1.4–2-fold increase in the risk of GDM.[14–18, 23] Cigarette smoking has not been consistently identified as a risk factor of GDM.[14, 16, 18, 24–28] Available data suggest that the magnitude of possible association between maternal smoking (before and during pregnancy) and GDM may be modest. Asian, Hispanic, and Native American women, as compared with Caucasian women, have an increased risk of GDM.[14, 16, 18, 29] African American women have been reported to have an increased risk of GDM, as compared with Caucasians, by some,[18, 30] although not all[16, 29] investigators. A very small, but emerging literature also suggests that short maternal stature may be associated with an increased risk of GDM.[31–35] For instance, results from one study of Greek women demonstrated that the mean height of GDM patients was significantly shorter than normoglycemic controls (158 cm vs. 161 cm; p-value <0.05). This average reduction in height was independent of maternal prepregnancy obesity, age, and socio-economic status.[32] Studies among women of other race/ethnicity also provided evidence suggestive of an increased risk of GDM associated with short maternal stature.[31, 33–35] Other reported risk factors include, but are not limited to, polycystic ovary syndrome, previous stillbirth, high blood pressure during pregnancy, and multiple pregnancies.[14]

5.2.2 Modifiable Risk Factors

In the past decade, increasing efforts were made to identify risk factors for GDM, in part due to the escalating prevalence of diabetes and obesity worldwide. Subsequently, several potentially novel risk factors for GDM have been identified. A series of studies have linked physical activity before and/or during pregnancy with a reduced risk of GDM.[36–43] This effect seems to increase with increasing intensity of and time spent on the physical activity. Moreover, a few studies provided some suggestive evidence of dietary factors both before and during pregnancy acting as potentially modifiable contributors to GDM risk.[44–52] For instance, findings from some studies,[46, 47] (although not all),[46, 47, 53] suggested that polyunsaturated fat intake may be protective against glucose intolerance in pregnancy, and high intake of saturated fat may be detrimental.[48] Prepregnancy overall dietary patterns, in particular, a diet characterized by high intake of red meat, processed meat, refined grain products, sweets, French fries, and pizza was associated with an increased risk of developing GDM.[50]

5.2.3 Nonmodifiable (Genetic) Risk Factors

Available data suggests that genetic factors may also play a role in the etiology of GDM, as discussed in greater detail in a separate chapter in this book. For instance, GDM is clustered in families and displays a familial tendency.[17, 54] Moreover, GDM recurred in at least 30% (range 30–91%) of women with a history of GDM[14,52, 54–56] suggesting that there is a subgroup of women who may be genetically predisposed to developing this complication of pregnancy. Furthermore, defects in both insulin secretion and insulin activity are crucial in the pathogenesis of GDM. A recent study has shown major genetic components in both traits; more than 75% of the variations in insulin secretion trait can be explained by genetic component and at least 53% by peripheral insulin sensitivity.[57] Very few studies have been conducted to identify susceptibility genes for GDM.[58, 59] Inference from limited studies was hindered by small sample size, retrospective design, lack of systematic analysis of common variants of the candidate gene, and lack of consideration of the effect of nongenetic factors.

The remainder of this chapter concerns emerging modifiable risk factors that may contribute to the early prevention of GDM, which may help to dissect the vicious circle involving GDM, childhood obesity and metabolic disorders, and adulthood obesity and diabetes.

5.3 Modifiable Factors and GDM Risk

5.3.1 Physical Activity

Accumulating evidence from epidemiological and clinical studies among nonpregnant individuals support the thesis that physical activity can influence glucose homeostasis through its direct or indirect impact on insulin sensitivity and secretion. By increasing insulin sensitivity and improving glucose tolerance via several mechanisms, physical activity has a beneficial effect on many aspects of insulin resistance syndromes.[60–62] After an episode of physical activity, insulin sensitivity was improved for up to 48 h by increasing cellular sensitivity to circulating insulin.[63] In addition to this acute effect, longer-term, even relatively modest, increases in habitual physical activity induce adaptations that can profoundly affect glucose tolerance[61] and potentially reduce GDM risk. Long-term improvement in glucose tolerance and increased insulin sensitivity may also result from physical activity-induced reductions in fat mass and increases in lean muscle mass.[64, 65]

Recently emerging studies on the impact of physical activity on pregnant women are limited. The definitions used to classify intensity, amount, and type of physical activity varied considerably, making comparisons between studies difficult. Furthermore, the actual number of GDM cases in the majority of studies is rather low, hampering solid conclusions. Despite these limitations, several studies have linked physical activity before and/or during pregnancy to a reduced risk of GDM.[36–43] This effect seems to increase with increasing intensity of and time spent on the physical activity. For instance, in a prospective study of 21,765 women who reported at least one singleton pregnancy in the Nurses' Health Study II, women in the highest quintile of habitual recreational physical activity before pregnancy (specifically vigorous activity, which is equivalent to approximately 30 min a day of brisk walking) had a ~20% risk reduction for the development of GDM.[43] Similarly, Oken et al observed that physical activity before pregnancy (particularly vigorous activity) was associated with a reduced risk of either GDM or any antepartum glucose intolerance (risk reductions of 44 and 24%, respectively).[41] In both a prospective study and a case-control study, Dempsey et al found that leisure-time physical activity (i.e., nonoccupational activity) in the year prior to pregnancy was correlated with a significantly lower risk of GDM.[37, 38]

Evidence of the effects of physical activity *during* pregnancy on GDM risk is suggestive but inconclusive. One study reported a significant protective effect,[37] while others found an association,[36, 38, 39, 41, 66] albeit at statistically insignificant levels. In a case-control study, Dempsey et al found that participating in any recreational activities during the first 20 weeks of pregnancy reduced GDM risk by 48%.[37] Both Dempsey et al and Oken et al[38, 41] in prospective cohort studies reported that physical activity during early pregnancy appeared to be associated with lower risk of developing GDM; however, the findings were not statistically significant. Dye et al observed that women who exercised weekly for at least 30 min, at some time during pregnancy, had lower risk of GDM, although this result was found only for morbidly obese women (body mass index (BMI) >33 kg/m^2).[39] Using data that were nationally representative of women with live births, Liu et al found considerable evidence that those who began physical activity during pregnancy had less risk of developing GDM than those who were inactive.[40] Women with activity levels above the median had 67% lower odds of developing GDM.

5.3.2 Dietary Factors

Substantial evidence indicates that diet is linked to the development of glucose intolerance. An extensive body of literature has reported both protective and risk-enhancing associations between particular dietary factors and type 2 diabetes in adult men and nonpregnant women. These studies suggest that total carbohydrate and fat intake are not related to type 2 diabetes risk, but specific types of carbohydrates may be protective, e.g., whole grains,[67–70] and specific types of fats (e.g., *trans* and n-3 polyunsaturated fats)[71–75] may be risk-enhancing.[76, 77] Dietary treatment/counseling has long been recommended for women who developed GDM. However, studies of the association of dietary factors with the risk of development of GDM have just emerged recently.

A limited number of studies have examined diet before and/or during pregnancy as a potentially modifiable contributor to the development of GDM.[44–52] Earlier studies on the effect of diet during pregnancy, many of which were cross-sectional or retrospective in design, suggested that macronutrient components of the diet in mid-pregnancy may predict incidence[46, 48, 49] or recurrence[52] of GDM. For instance, findings from some studies,[46, 47] although not all,[46, 47, 53] suggested that polyunsaturated fat intake may be protective against glucose intolerance in pregnancy and high intake of saturated fat may be detrimental.[48] Of note, these analyses did not adjust for or consider the impact from other types of fat, which is important as intake of different fat subtypes tends to be correlated and may have opposing effects.[76] A recent prospective study, considering the correlation of nutrients, showed that higher intake of fat and lower intake of carbohydrates may be associated with increased risk of GDM and IGT.[49] The number of GDM cases in the majority of studies is rather low. Thus far, no concrete conclusion can be drawn as to the role of dietary factors during pregnancy in the development of GDM.

Emerging data,[45,50] primarily from the Nurses' Health Study II, suggested that pregravid diet is associated with the risk for glucose intolerance during pregnancy. In this large prospective study, strong associations were observed between the Western diet, on one hand, and prudent dietary patterns on the other, and GDM risk.[50] The prudent pattern was characterized by a high intake of fruits, green leafy vegetables, poultry, and fish, whereas the Western pattern was characterized by high intake of red meat, processed meat, refined grain products, sweets, French fries, and pizza. The association with the Western pattern was largely explained by intake of red and processed meat products. Pregravid intake of red and processed meats were both significantly and positively associated with GDM risk, independent of known risk factors for type 2 diabetes and GDM. For instance, compared with those women who consumed less than two servings of red meat per week, those who consumed more than six servings of red meat per week had a 1.74-fold increased risk of GDM (relative risk (RR), 95% confidence interval (CI) 1.74 (1.35, 2.26)). In addition, pregravid consumption of dietary total fiber and cereal and fruit fiber were significantly and inversely associated with GDM risk.[45] In contrast, dietary glycemic load was positively associated with GDM risk. The glycemic index is a relative measure of the glycemic impact of carbohydrates in different foods.[78] Total glycemic load was calculated by first multiplying the carbohydrate content of each food by its glycemic index value, then by multiplying this value by the frequency of consumption and summing the values from all food. Dietary glycemic load thus represents the quality and quantity of carbohydrate intake and the interaction between the two. Each 10-g/day increment in total fiber intake was associated with a 26% (95% CI 9–49) reduction in risk; each 5-g/day increment in cereal or fruit fiber was associated with a 23%[9–36] or 26%[5–42] reduction, respectively. The combination of high glycemic load and low cereal fiber diet was associated with 2.15-fold (95% CI 1.04–4.29) increased risk of GDM compared with the reciprocal diet. Although the observational design of the study does not prove causality, these findings suggested that pregravid diet was associated with women's susceptibility to GDM. Future clinical and metabolic studies are warranted to confirm these findings.

5.3.3 Cigarette Smoking

Cigarette smoking has been associated with increased insulin resistance and increased risk for developing type 2 diabetes among men and nonpregnant women.[79] Despite some evidence for heterogeneity, the association was overall robust and consistent across a range and variety of smoking patterns, demographics, and study characteristics.[80, 81]

Cigarette smoking is still common among pregnant women although an 8% reduction in the number of women who smoke during pregnancy was observed in the past decade.[82] Cigarette smoking has not been repeatedly identified as a risk factor for GDM.[14, 16, 18, 24–28] Available data suggest that the magnitude of possible association is modest, with limited studies reported an elevated risk associated smoking.[24, 25] Some of the variation between studies can be attributed to variations in study design, characteristics of study population, ascertainment of the dose of cigarette smoking, the content of cigarettes such as nicotine and additives, and the degree of adjustment for confounding effects. Although many women who smoke before pregnancy stop smoking or reduce the number of cigarettes smoked once they are pregnant, in the Nurses' Health Study II, habitual smokers had a 1.43-fold increased risk for GDM in subsequent pregnancies (RR (95% CI): 1.43 (1.14, 1.80)) after the adjustment of potential confounders, including BMI.[18]

5.3.4 Weight Characteristics

Excessive adiposity is the major well-characterized modifiable risk factor for GDM. Numerous studies across diverse populations have reported an increased risk of GDM among women who are overweight or obese compared with lean or normal-weight women.[1, 15, 18, 20–22] In a recent meta-analyses[20] of 20 relevant studies published between 1980 and 2006, the risk of developing GDM is approximately 2, 3, and 6 times higher among overweight, obese, and severely obese women, respectively, as compared with normal-weight pregnant women; the adjusted odds ratios (95% CI) of GDM were 1.86 (1.22–2.78), 3.34 (2.43–4.55), and 5.77 (3.60–9.39), respectively. Moreover, the meta-analysis found no evidence that these estimates were substantially affected by selected study characteristics (publication date, study location, parity, study design (prospective vs. retrospective), and the prevalence of GDM among normal-weight women).

In addition to prepregnancy adiposity, emerging evidence suggests that weight change, specifically excessive weight gain during various periods of adult life before pregnancy, is associated with increased risk of GDM. In two prospective studies,[18, 22] self-reported weight gain of 10.0 kg or more from 18 years to shortly before pregnancy was associated with more than a twofold increased risk for GDM as compared with relatively stable weight. Weight gain 2.3–10.0 kg within 5 years before pregnancy was related to a significantly increased risk of GDM in a recent nested case-control study.[21] Taken together, all these data suggest that efforts to prevent obesity and weight gain among young women may help to reduce GDM risk.

5.4 Conclusions and Research Agenda

The escalating prevalence of obesity and diabetes worldwide, the substantial increase in the incidence of GDM during recent years, and the short-term and long-term adverse health outcomes for both women and offspring associated with GDM, highlight the significance of preventing GDM among women at high risk. Emerging evidence from observational studies suggest that several modifiable factors, in particular, pregravid excessive adiposity, recreational physical activity before and during pregnancy, and pregravid western dietary patterns may be related to elevated GDM risk. Pregnant women, or women planning pregnancy, are generally highly motivated to follow advice to improve the outcome of pregnancy, and hence pregnancy represents an ideal time in life to advocate a healthy lifestyle.

At present, there are no large-scale systematic lifestyle intervention studies of GDM for women at high risk. Before initiating such studies, adequately powered dose response studies are needed to evaluate the efficiency and efficacy of interventions and to define optimal interventions. Such interventions must also be evaluated in the context of neonatal outcomes and offspring's long-term health outcomes.

References

1. Anonymous. Gestational diabetes mellitus. *Diabetes Care*. 2004;27(suppl 1):88-90.
2. Dabelea D, Snell-Bergeon JK, Hartsfield CL, Bischoff KJ, Hamman RF, McDuffie RS. Increasing prevalence of gestational diabetes mellitus (GDM) over time and by birth cohort: Kaiser Permanente of Colorado GDM Screening Program. *Diabetes Care*. 2005;28:579-584.
3. Coustan DR, Carpenter MW, O'Sullivan PS, Carr SR. Gestational diabetes: predictors of subsequent disordered glucose metabolism. *Am J Obstet Gynecol*. 1993;168:1139-1144.
4. Kjos SL, Peters RK, Xiang A, Henry OA, Montoro M, Buchanan TA. Predicting future diabetes in Latino women with gestational diabetes. Utility of early postpartum glucose tolerance testing. *Diabetes*. 1995;44:586-591.
5. Metzger BE, Cho NH, Roston SM, Radvany R. Prepregnancy weight and antepartum insulin secretion predict glucose tolerance five years after gestational diabetes mellitus. *Diabetes Care*. 1993;16:1598-1605.
6. Kim C, Newton KM, Knopp RH. Gestational diabetes and the incidence of type 2 diabetes: a systematic review. *Diabetes Care*. 2002;25:1862-1868.

7. Moley KH. Diabetes and preimplantation events of embryogenesis. *Semin Reprod Endocrinol.* 1999;17:137-151.
8. Fraser RB, Waite SL, Wood KA, Martin KL. Impact of hyperglycemia on early embryo development and embryopathy: in vitro experiments using a mouse model. *Hum Reprod.* 2007; 22:3059-3068.
9. Buchanan TA, Xiang AH. Gestational diabetes mellitus. *J Clin Invest.* 2005;115:485-491.
10. Catalano PM, Tyzbir ED, Wolfe RR, et al. Carbohydrate metabolism during pregnancy in control subjects and women with gestational diabetes. *Am J Physiol.* 1993;264:E60-E67.
11. Catalano PM, Tyzbir ED, Roman NM, Amini SB, Sims EA. Longitudinal changes in insulin release and insulin resistance in nonobese pregnant women. *Am J Obstet Gynecol.* 1991; 165:1667-1672.
12. Knopp RH, Bergelin RO, Wahl PW, Walden CE, Chapman M, Irvine S. Population-based lipoprotein lipid reference values for pregnant women compared to nonpregnant women classified by sex hormone usage. *Am J Obstet Gynecol.* 1982;143:626-637.
13. Knopp RH, Warth MR, Charles D, et al. Lipoprotein metabolism in pregnancy, fat transport to the fetus, and the effects of diabetes. *Biol Neonate.* 1986;50:297-317.
14. Ben-Haroush A, Yogev Y, Hod M. Epidemiology of gestational diabetes mellitus and its association with Type 2 diabetes. *Diabet Med.* 2004;21:103-113.
15. Metzger BE, Buchanan TA, Coustan DR, et al. Summary and recommendations of the Fifth International Workshop-Conference on Gestational Diabetes Mellitus. *Diabetes Care.* 2007; 30(suppl 2):S251-S260.
16. Berkowitz GS, Lapinski RH, Wein R, Lee D. Race/ethnicity and other risk factors for gestational diabetes. *Am J Epidemiol.* 1992;135:965-973.
17. Martin AO, Simpson JL, Ober C, Freinkel N. Frequency of diabetes mellitus in mothers of probands with gestational diabetes: possible maternal influence on the predisposition to gestational diabetes. *Am J Obstet Gynecol.* 1985;151:471-475.
18. Solomon CG, Willett WC, Carey VJ, et al. A prospective study of pregravid determinants of gestational diabetes mellitus. *JAMA.* 1997;278:1078-1083.
19. Okosun IS, Chandra KM, Boev A, et al. Abdominal adiposity in U.S. adults: prevalence and trends, 1960-2000. *Prev Med.* 2004;39:197-206.
20. Chu SY, Callaghan WM, Kim SY, et al. Maternal obesity and risk of gestational diabetes mellitus. *Diabetes Care.* 2007;30:2070-2076.
21. Hedderson MM, Williams MA, Holt VL, Weiss NS, Ferrara A. Body mass index and weight gain prior to pregnancy and risk of gestational diabetes mellitus. *Am J Obstet Gynecol.* 2007;198(4):409.e1-409.e7.
22. Rudra CB, Sorensen TK, Leisenring WM, Dashow E, Williams MA. Weight characteristics and height in relation to risk of gestational diabetes mellitus. *Am J Epidemiol.* 2007;165: 302-308.
23. Williams MA, Qiu C, Dempsey JC, Luthy DA. Familial aggregation of type 2 diabetes and chronic hypertension in women with gestational diabetes mellitus. *J Reprod Med.* 2003;48: 955-962.
24. England LJ, Levine RJ, Qian C, et al. Glucose tolerance and risk of gestational diabetes mellitus in nulliparous women who smoke during pregnancy. *Am J Epidemiol.* 2004;160: 1205-1213.
25. Joffe GM, Esterlitz JR, Levine RJ, et al. The relationship between abnormal glucose tolerance and hypertensive disorders of pregnancy in healthy nulliparous women. Calcium for Preeclampsia Prevention (CPEP) Study Group. *Am J Obstet Gynecol.* 1998;179:1032-1037.
26. Rodrigues S, Robinson E, Gray-Donald K. Prevalence of gestational diabetes mellitus among James Bay Cree women in northern Quebec. *CMAJ.* 1999;160:1293-1297.
27. Rodrigues S, Robinson EJ, Ghezzo H, Gray-Donald K. Interaction of body weight and ethnicity on risk of gestational diabetes mellitus. *Am J Clin Nutr.* 1999;70:1083-1089.

28. Terry PD, Weiderpass E, Ostenson CG, Cnattingius S. Cigarette smoking and the risk of gestational and pregestational diabetes in two consecutive pregnancies. *Diabetes Care*. 2003; 26:2994-2998.
29. Savitz DA, Janevic TM, Engel SM, Kaufman JS, Herring AH. Ethnicity and gestational diabetes in New York City, 1995-2003. *BJOG*. 2008;115:969-978.
30. Dooley SL, Metzger BE, Cho N, Liu K. The influence of demographic and phenotypic heterogeneity on the prevalence of gestational diabetes mellitus. *Int J Gynaecol Obstet*. 1991;35:13-18.
31. Meza E, Barraza L, Martinez G, et al. Gestational diabetes in a Mexican-U.S. border population: prevalence and epidemiology. Rev. *Invest Clin*. 1995;47:433-438.
32. Anastasiou E, Alevizaki M, Grigorakis SJ, Philippou G, Kyprianou M, Souvatzoglou A. Decreased stature in gestational diabetes mellitus. *Diabetologia*. 1998;41:997-1001.
33. Branchtein L, Schmidt MI, Matos MC, Yamashita T, Pousada JM, Duncan BB. Short stature and gestational diabetes in Brazil. Brazilian Gestational Diabetes Study Group. *Diabetologia*. 2000;43:848-851.
34. Yang X, Hsu-Hage B, Zhang H, et al. Gestational diabetes mellitus in women of single gravidity in Tianjin City, China. *Diabetes Care*. 2002;25:847-851.
35. Jang HC, Min HK, Lee HK, Cho NH, Metzger BE. Short stature in Korean women: a contribution to the multifactorial predisposition to gestational diabetes mellitus. *Diabetologia*. 1998;41:778-783.
36. Chasan-Taber L, Schmidt MD, Pekow P, et al. Physical activity and gestational diabetes mellitus among Hispanic women. *J Womens Health (Larchmt)*. 2008;17:999-1008.
37. Dempsey JC, Butler CL, Sorensen TK, et al. A case-control study of maternal recreational physical activity and risk of gestational diabetes mellitus. *Diabetes Res Clin Pract*. 2004; 66:203-215.
38. Dempsey JC, Sorensen TK, Williams MA, et al. Prospective study of gestational diabetes mellitus risk in relation to maternal recreational physical activity before and during pregnancy. *Am J Epidemiol*. 2004;159:663-670.
39. Dye TD, Knox KL, Artal R, Aubry RH, Wojtowycz MA. Physical activity, obesity, and diabetes in pregnancy. *Am J Epidemiol*. 1997;146:961-965.
40. Liu J, Laditka JN, Mayer-Davis EJ, Pate RR. Does physical activity during pregnancy reduce the risk of gestational diabetes among previously inactive women? *Birth*. 2008;35:188-195.
41. Oken E, Ning Y, Rifas-Shiman SL, Radesky JS, Rich-Edwards JW, Gillman MW. Associations of physical activity and inactivity before and during pregnancy with glucose tolerance. *Obstet Gynecol*. 2006;108:1200-1207.
42. Retnakaran R, Qi Y, Sermer M, Connelly PW, Zinman B, Hanley AJ. Pre-gravid physical activity and reduced risk of glucose intolerance in pregnancy: the role of insulin sensitivity. *Clin Endocrinol (Oxf)*. 2008;70(4):615-622.
43. Zhang C, Solomon CG, Manson JE, Hu FB. A prospective study of pregravid physical activity and sedentary behaviors in relation to the risk for gestational diabetes mellitus. *Arch Intern Med*. 2006;166:543-548.
44. Zhang C, Williams MA, Sorensen TK, et al. Maternal plasma ascorbic Acid (vitamin C) and risk of gestational diabetes mellitus. *Epidemiology*. 2004;15:597-604.
45. Zhang C, Liu S, Solomon CG, Hu FB. Dietary fiber intake, dietary glycemic load, and the risk for gestational diabetes mellitus. *Diabetes Care*. 2006;29:2223-2230.
46. Wang Y, Storlien LH, Jenkins AB, et al. Dietary variables and glucose tolerance in pregnancy. *Diabetes Care*. 2000;23:460-464.
47. Wijendran V, Bendel RB, Couch SC, et al. Maternal plasma phospholipid polyunsaturated fatty acids in pregnancy with and without gestational diabetes mellitus: relations with maternal factors. *Am J Clin Nutr*. 1999;70:53-61.
48. Bo S, Menato G, Lezo A, et al. Dietary fat and gestational hyperglycaemia. *Diabetologia*. 2001;44:972-978.

49. Saldana TM, Siega-Riz AM, Adair LS. Effect of macronutrient intake on the development of glucose intolerance during pregnancy. *Am J Clin Nutr*. 2004;79:479-486.
50. Zhang C, Schulze MB, Solomon CG, Hu FB. A prospective study of dietary patterns, meat intake and the risk of gestational diabetes mellitus. *Diabetologia*. 2006;49:2604-2613.
51. Zhang C, Williams MA, Frederick IO, et al. Vitamin C and the risk of gestational diabetes mellitus: a case-control study. *J Reprod Med*. 2004;49:257-266.
52. Moses RG. The recurrence rate of gestational diabetes in subsequent pregnancies. *Diabetes Care*. 1996;19:1348-1350.
53. Radesky JS, Oken E, Rifas-Shiman SL, Kleinman KP, Rich-Edwards JW, Gillman MW. Diet during early pregnancy and development of gestational diabetes. *Paediatr Perinat Epidemiol*. 2008;22:47-59.
54. Egeland GM, Skjaerven R, Irgens LM. Birth characteristics of women who develop gestational diabetes: population based study. *BMJ*. 2000;321:546-547.
55. Kim C, Berger DK, Chamany S. Recurrence of gestational diabetes mellitus: a systematic review. *Diabetes Care*. 2007;30:1314-1319.
56. Nohira T, Kim S, Nakai H, Okabe K, Nohira T, Yoneyama K. Recurrence of gestational diabetes mellitus: rates and risk factors from initial GDM and one abnormal GTT value. *Diabetes Res Clin Pract*. 2006;71:75-81.
57. Poulsen P, Levin K, Petersen I, Christensen K, Beck-Nielsen H, Vaag A. Heritability of insulin secretion, peripheral and hepatic insulin action, and intracellular glucose partitioning in young and old Danish twins. *Diabetes*. 2005;54:275-283.
58. Watanabe RM, Black MH, Xiang AH, Allayee H, Lawrence JM, Buchanan TA. Genetics of gestational diabetes mellitus and type 2 diabetes. *Diabetes Care*. 2007;30(suppl 2):S134-S140.
59. Shaat N, Groop L. Genetics of gestational diabetes mellitus. *Curr Med Chem*. 2007;14: 569-583.
60. Sato Y, Iguchi A, Sakamoto N. Biochemical determination of training effects using insulin clamp technique. *Horm Metab Res*. 1984;16:483-486.
61. Regensteiner JG, Mayer EJ, Shetterly SM, et al. Relationship between habitual physical activity and insulin levels among nondiabetic men and women. San Luis Valley Diabetes Study. *Diabetes Care*. 1991;14:1066-1074.
62. Helmrich SP, Ragland DR, Leung RW, Paffenbarger RS Jr. Physical activity and reduced occurrence of non-insulin-dependent diabetes mellitus. *N Engl J Med*. 1991;325:147-152.
63. Holloszy JO. Exercise-induced increase in muscle insulin sensitivity. *J Appl Physiol*. 2005;99:338-343.
64. Yki-Jarvinen H, Koivisto VA. Effects of body composition on insulin sensitivity. *Diabetes*. 1983;32:965-969.
65. Shulman GI, Rothman DL, Jue T, Stein P, DeFronzo RA, Shulman RG. Quantitation of muscle glycogen synthesis in normal subjects and subjects with non-insulin-dependent diabetes by 13C nuclear magnetic resonance spectroscopy. *N Engl J Med*. 1990;322:223-228.
66. Chasan-Taber L, Erickson JB, Nasca PC, Chasan-Taber S, Freedson PS. Validity and reproducibility of a physical activity questionnaire in women. *Med Sci Sports Exerc*. 2002;34: 987-992.
67. Meyer KA, Kushi LH, Jacobs DR Jr, Slavin J, Sellers TA, Folsom AR. Carbohydrates, dietary fiber, and incident type 2 diabetes in older women. *Am J Clin Nutr*. 2000;71:921-930.
68. Montonen J, Knekt P, Jarvinen R, Aromaa A, Reunanen A. Whole-grain and fiber intake and the incidence of type 2 diabetes. *Am J Clin Nutr*. 2003;77:622-629.
69. Liu S, Manson JE, Stampfer MJ, et al. A prospective study of whole-grain intake and risk of type 2 diabetes mellitus in US women. *Am J Public Health*. 2000;90:1409-1415.
70. Fung TT, Hu FB, Pereira MA, et al. Whole-grain intake and the risk of type 2 diabetes: a prospective study in men. *Am J Clin Nutr*. 2002;76:535-540.

71. Salmeron J, Hu FB, Manson JE, et al. Dietary fat intake and risk of type 2 diabetes in women. *Am J Clin Nutr*. 2001;73:1019-1026.
72. Feskens EJ, Bowles CH, Kromhout D. Inverse association between fish intake and risk of glucose intolerance in normoglycemic elderly men and women. *Diabetes Care*. 1991;14: 935-941.
73. Adler AI, Boyko EJ, Schraer CD, Murphy NJ. Lower prevalence of impaired glucose tolerance and diabetes associated with daily seal oil or salmon consumption among Alaska Natives. *Diabetes Care*. 1994;17:1498-1501.
74. Meyer KA, Kushi LH, Jacobs DR Jr, Folsom AR. Dietary fat and incidence of type 2 diabetes in older Iowa women. *Diabetes Care*. 2001;24:1528-1535.
75. van Dam RM, Willett WC, Rimm EB, Stampfer MJ, Hu FB. Dietary fat and meat intake in relation to risk of type 2 diabetes in men. *Diabetes Care*. 2002;25:417-424.
76. Hu FB, van Dam RM, Liu S. Diet and risk of Type II diabetes: the role of types of fat and carbohydrate. *Diabetologia*. 2001;44:805-817.
77. Schulze MB, Hu FB. Primary prevention of diabetes: what can be done and how much can be prevented? *Annu Rev Public Health*. 2005;26:445-467.
78. Wolever TM, Jenkins DJ, Jenkins AL, Josse RG. The glycemic index: methodology and clinical implications. *Am J Clin Nutr*. 1991;54:846-854.
79. Rimm EB, Manson JE, Stampfer MJ, et al. Cigarette smoking and the risk of diabetes in women. *Am J Public Health*. 1993;83:211-214.
80. Ding EL, Hu FB. Smoking and type 2 diabetes: underrecognized risks and disease burden. *JAMA*. 2007;298:2675-2676.
81. Willi C, Bodenmann P, Ghali WA, Faris PD, Cornuz J. Active smoking and the risk of type 2 diabetes: a systematic review and meta-analysis. *JAMA*. 2007;298:2654-2664.
82. Anonymous. Smoking during pregnancy–United States, 1990-2002. *MMWR Morb Mortal Wkly Rep*. 2004;53:911-915.

Section III

Burden of GDM in Developing Countries

Burden of GDM in Developing Countries

6

Chong Shou and Huixia Yang

6.1 Epidemiological Studies

Diabetes is rapidly emerging as a global health care problem that threatens to reach pandemic levels by 2030; the number of people with diabetes worldwide is projected to increase from 171 million in 2000 to 366 million by 2030. According to the World Health Organization (WHO), Southeast Asia and the Western Pacific region are at the forefront of the current diabetes epidemic, with India and China facing the greatest challenges.[1] These increases are driven by decreased physical activity and over-consumption of cheap, energy-dense food. The subsequent obesity also contributes to greater risk for gestational diabetes mellitus (GDM).

While screening for GDM is common in China, there is significant variation between geographical regions due to differing lifestyle behaviors as well as varying diagnostic criteria. Xu et al[2] reported the prevalence of GDM was 2.9%, using American Diabetes Association (ADA) criteria. Yang et al[3] reported the total incidence of gestational abnormal glucose metabolism was 7.3%, and had increased gradually between 1995 and 2004 based on National Diabetes Diagnostic Group (NDDG) criteria. Between January 1995 and December 1999, there was a gradual increase in GDM incidence [4.3% (376/8,739)]. Between January 2000 and December 2001, there was a more rapid rise with an average incidence of 10.8% (445/4,133). Between January 2002 and December 2004, GDM incidence was stable at 8.9% (678/7,640). In the largest Chinese GDM surveillance study, Yang et al[4] showed that the prevalence of GDM in Tianjing City is 2.3% by WHO criteria, much lower than that of Chinese women in western countries using the same diagnostic criteria. A 75-g-2h oral glucose tolerance tests (OGTT) was performed in 4000 gravidas who were 28–30 weeks pregnant. Women were recruited from Kunming City in southwestern China and were less likely to be Han Chinese and more likely to be of southeast Asian racial/ethnic origin. GDM prevalence was much higher, 11.6% as opposed to the 2.3% prevalence rate found by Yang et al.[4]

H. Yang (✉)
Department of Obstetrics and Gynecology,
Peking University First Hospital, Beijing, P.R. China
e-mail: yanghuixia688@sina.com

C. Kim and A. Ferrara (eds.), *Gestational Diabetes During and After Pregnancy*,
DOI: 10.1007/978-1-84882-120-0_6, © Springer-Verlag London Limited 2010

Established risk factors for GDM include advanced maternal age, obesity, and family history of diabetes. The trends for a greater proportion of mothers who are older and obese, along with the adoption of modern lifestyles in developing countries, may all contribute to an increase in the prevalence of GDM. We have evaluated the risk factors for GDM and gestational impaired glucose tolerance (GIGT) at Peking University First Hospital. In 2004, we performed a prospective case–control study in 85 women with GDM, 63 cases with GIGT, and 125 controls. Results showed that[1] mean age and body mass index (BMI) before pregnancy and larger maternal weight gains during pregnancy were significantly different between GDM/GIGT and control groups[2] ($p<0.05$). Greater intake of fruits and carbohydrates per day was associated with increased incidence of GDM and GIGT ($p<0.05$),[3] and there was a higher proportion of women with a family history of diabetes among the GDM (42.2%) and GIGT groups (36.5%) compared with the control group (19.2%, $p<0.05$).[5] In the GDM and GIGT groups, irregular menses (16.5, 23.8%) and polycystic ovary syndrome (PCOS) (5.9, 3.2%) were more prevalent compared with controls (6.4%, 0).[5] Multivariate logistic regression showed that age, irregular menses, BMI before pregnancy, history of spontaneous abortion, and educational level all were independent factors for GDM or GIGT.[5]

Data on changes in incidence over time are generally not available from other countries, but cross-sectional data suggest that risk factors are similar to western and Chinese populations. In Iran, Hossein et al[6] reported that the prevalence of GDM was 4.7%. Women with GDM had significantly higher parity and BMI than did nondiabetic women. Women with GDM were also more likely to have a family history of diabetes and a history of poor obstetric outcome. Keshavarz et al[7] reported similar risk factors for GDM in Iran and also included maternal age >30 years, previous macrosomia, and glycosuria. In India, Zargar et al[8] reported that the prevalence of GDM among Kashmiri women was 3.8%. GDM prevalence steadily increased with age (from 1.7% in women below 25 years to 18% in women 35 years or older). GDM occurred more frequently in women who were residing in urban areas, had borne three or more children, had history of abortion(s) or GDM during previous pregnancies, had given birth to a macrosomic baby, or had a family history of diabetes. Women with obesity, hypertension, osmotic symptoms, proteinuria, or hydramnios also had a higher prevalence of GDM. In South Africa, Mamabolo et al[9] reported that the prevalence of GIGT and GDM was 8.8% (7.3% GIGT; 1.5% GDM). The prevalence of GDM in this region is high as compared to other parts of Africa, which could have lower GDM prevalence due to chronic malnutrition precipitated by famine, drought, and war, as well as racial/ethnic differences. In Ethiopia, Seyoum et al[10] reported that the prevalence of GDM was as low as 3.7%.

6.2 Screening and Diagnostic Criteria in Developing Countries

As discussed in the chapters on screening, screening for GDM consists of a 1- or 2-step approach. The initial screening test occurs between 24 and 28 weeks and consists of plasma glucose 1-h after 50-g oral glucose load (glucose challenge test or GCT). A 1-h value

>140 mg/dL identifies 80% of women with GDM. Lowering the threshold to 130 mg/dL increases the sensitivity to 90% but at the cost of false positivity. The ADA and American College of Obstetricians and Gynecology (ACOG) recognize both thresholds.[11] Confirmation of GDM is based on a second step, the subsequent 3-h OGTT. The WHO has proposed different diagnostic criteria, based on a 75-g OGTT with GDM defined as either the fasting plasma glucose (FPG) ≥126 mg/dL or 2-h plasma glucose ≥140 mg/dL. Both algorithms are valid options for the diagnosis of GDM and the prediction of adverse pregnancy outcomes.[12]

In the last decade, the 50-g GCT and management of gestational impaired glucose metabolism has become standard in most hospitals in China. Between 1995 and 2001, at Peking University First Hospital, we examined GCT values from pregnant women to determine the optimal GDM screening value.[13] The 1-h average plasma glucose level of the GCT was 6.8 ± 1.7 mmol/L. The abnormal rate of GCT was 25.2% using 7.8 mmol/L as the cutoff, which missed 5.3% of women (17/321) with GDM by OGTT. When the cutoff was lowered to 7.2 mmol/L, the abnormal GCT rate was increased to 36.5%, and only 2.8% (9/321) of women with GDM by the OGTT were missed. With a value of 8.3 mmol/L as a threshold, 15.9% (51/321) women with GDM by OGTT were missed. When the glucose after the GCT is ≥11.2 mmol/L, the incidence of GDM is 55.8% (92/165).[13] Among these women, 62.0% (57/92) GDM could be diagnosed according to the FPG alone. When the GCT glucose level is ≥11.2 mmol/L, FPG could be done first to diagnose GDM, without the OGTT.[13]

We have also investigated the effects of setting different OGTT thresholds. We examined OGTT data from 647 women with GDM and 233 women with GIGT diagnosed between 1 January 1989 and 31 December 2002.[14] Among GDM women, 535 cases were diagnosed by the 75-g OGTT and 112 cases of GDM diagnosed by the FPG alone. Of 535 cases of GDM diagnosed by OGTT, 49.2% (263/535) women had an FPG value >5.8 mmol/L; 90.1% (482/535) women had 1-h glucose values >10.6 mmol/L; 64.7% (359/535) had 2-h glucose levels >9.2 mmol/L.

In this particular series, women also had a 3-h glucose level done despite the fact that only a 75-g challenge was given. There were only 114 cases (21.3%) with abnormal 3-h plasma glucose levels among the 535 women with OGTT. Among those with abnormal 3-h level, 49.1% (56/114) had abnormal glucose values at the other three points of OGTT, and 34.2% (39/114) with two other abnormal values of OGTT. Our study showed that omission of the 3-h PG of OGTT only missed 19 cases of GDM and these women would be diagnosed as having GIGT. Among the 233 women with GIGT, only four cases had abnormal 3-h PG. Thus, omission of the 3-h glucose value of OGTT only resulted in failure to diagnose 3.6% (19/535) women with GDM, which means 2.9% (19/647) of all the GDM and 1.7% (4/233) of GIGT in this cohort. A glucose level >11.2 mmol/L following a 50-g GCT was highly associated with GDM necessitating insulin therapy (75.4%). An elevated FPG level was also associated with insulin therapy (59.7%).[14]

A diagnosis of GDM in China now is based on a fasting glucose level ≥5.8 mmol/L (105 mg/dL) on more than two occasions, or two or more abnormal values on the 3-h OGTT, with cut-off values of 5.8 mmol/L (105 mg/dL), 10.6 mmol/L (190 mg/dL), 9.2 mmol/L (165 mg/dL), and 8.1 mmol/L (145 mg/dL) at fasting, 1-, 2-, and 3-h, respectively. GIGT is diagnosed when there is only one abnormal value during the OGTT.

In Iran, Shirazian et al[15] also evaluated the effects of various criteria on GDM prevalence. They reported that among 670 pregnant women, GDM was diagnosed in 41 (6.1%), 81 (12.1%), and 126 (18.8%) on the basis of ADA, WHO, and Australian Diabetes in Pregnancy Society (ADIPS) criteria, respectively. The kappa value was 0.38 ($p<0.0001$) for the agreement between ADA and WHO criteria, 0.41 ($p<0.0001$) for agreement between ADA and ADIPS criteria, and 0.64 ($p<0.0001$) for agreement between WHO and ADIPS criteria.

We also evaluated the effect of gestational age on glucose tolerance. We found no difference in the abnormal GCT rates when GCT was administered between 24 and 36 weeks of gestation.[13] Among 4,151 Indian women who underwent sequential OGTTs,[16] 741 were diagnosed with GDM by WHO criteria. Of these women, 16% were identified within the first 16 weeks of gestation, 22% were identified between 17 and 23 weeks gestation, and 61% were identified after the 24th week of gestation. In summary, glucose intolerance occurred early in gestation, leading the investigators to suggest earlier OGTT testing in their population.

6.3 Adverse Pregnancy Outcomes

6.3.1 Maternal Adverse Outcomes

Adverse maternal short-term outcomes can be categorized as exacerbation of GDM and other complications that impact on maternal morbidity and mortality such as hydramnios, hypertension, preeclampsia, and increased risk of cesarean section.

Yang et al[17] reported that the incidence of preeclampsia was 12.6% in 1,202 pregnant women at Peking University First Hospital with abnormal glucose metabolism. The incidence of preeclampsia in diabetic women, women with glucose intolerance preceding pregnancy (IGT), and GIGT pregnant women was 34.9, 11.8 and 6.9%, respectively. Incidence of preeclampsia in women with diabetes and GDM women was higher than glucose tolerant women (8.1%, 3,634/44,899). Yang et al[18] also found women with GDM were more likely to develop pregnancy-induced hypertension (14.7 vs. 7.9%) and macrosomia (13.8 vs. 7.54%) than glucose tolerant women. However, there were no significant differences in pregnancy outcomes between GDM women and women with GIGT.

Recently, we investigated risk factors for preeclampsia in pregnant Chinese women with abnormal glucose metabolism ($n=1{,}499$) in a retrospective cohort study.[19] Subjects were women who delivered between January 1995 and December 2004. The prevalence of preeclampsia in women diagnosed with diabetes mellitus prior to pregnancy was higher than that in women with GDM or GIGT (29.1 vs. 8.7 vs. 7.8%, $p<0.01$). Prepregnancy BMI was significantly higher in women with preeclampsia than in those without. A higher rate of preeclampsia was found in women with chronic hypertension and those with poor glucose control. The independent risk factors for preeclampsia were chronic hypertension and elevated prepregnancy BMI. Our study indicated that the type of diabetes, chronic hypertension, and elevated prepregnancy BMI are risk factors for preeclampsia in pregnant women with abnormal glucose metabolism.

Long-term maternal adverse effects are mainly due to increased risk of developing diabetes later in life with the magnitude of the risk ranging from 20 to 80%.[20] We are still lacking evidence of long-term adverse maternal outcomes of GDM in China, although such studies are ongoing. In other developing countries, the risk of diabetes after delivery is similar to that observed in western countries. Krishnaveni et al[21] found that 37% of women with GDM developed type 2 diabetes within 5 years, with greater insulin levels, waist-to-hip ratios, BMIs, and 30 min insulin levels associated with greater incidence of diabetes.

6.3.2 Adverse Fetal Outcomes

The infants of GDM women are at an increased risk of stillbirth and aberrant fetal growth (macrosomia and growth restriction) as well as metabolic (e.g., hypoglycemia and hypocalcemia), hematological (e.g., hyperbilirubinemia and polycythemia) and respiratory complications that increase neonatal intensive care unit admission rates and birth trauma (e.g., shoulder dystocia).[22]

In China, the incidence of macrosomia is 2.2–13%.[23] We have investigated the impact of GDM and an abnormal GCT on macrosomia.[24] We examined the prenatal and delivery records of 8,656 pregnant women who delivered in Peking University First Hospital from January 1995 to March 2001. The incidence of macrosomia was 8.1% (700/8,656). The incidence of infants with macrosomia in GDM or IGT women was 12.5% (69/552), which was significantly higher than that of infants of women with normal glucose levels (7.8% or 631/8,104, $p<0.01$). The macrosomia rate in women with GDM Class A2 (13.8%) was significantly higher than that of women with GDM Class A1 (6.0%, $p<0.01$). The macrosomia rate among the women under age 25 years (5.9%) was lower than that of the women over 35 years (9.9%, $p<0.01$). The macrosomia rate of infants of mothers with GDM or IGT (18.2%) was higher than that of those whose mothers did not have these conditions. The average BMI of the women between 26 and 28 gestational weeks was 24.9 ± 2.9 kg/m^2. The women with BMI ≥27.8 kg/m^2 had infants with a macrosomia rate of 16.2%, which was higher than that of women with lesser BMIs (6.3%, $p<0.01$). The obese women without GDM or IGT had infants with a similar rate of macrosomia (15.9%) to women with GDM (18.3%). Women with GIGT or GDM have a higher rate of infants with macrosomia than do women with normal glucose tolerance, despite good glycemic control, especially in GDM type A2. Among Indian women, optimal glycemic control during a GDM pregnancy, as assessed by hemoglobin A1c, was associated with birthweights similar to birthweights of infants of mothers with normal glucose tolerance.[25]

We also analyzed fetal lung maturity in 1,198 women with abnormal glucose metabolism and tested amniotic fluid lamellar body counts (LBC) in 42 women with abnormal glucose metabolism and 42 normal pregnant women.[26] The incidence of respiratory distress among infants of women with abnormal glucose metabolism was 0.67%. LBC from women with abnormal glucose metabolism was $10{,}013\pm6{,}318\times10/3$ μL vs. $84.2\pm52.2\times10/\mu$L in the control group, a nonsignificant difference ($p=0.21$). In other words, under strict glucose control, fetal lung maturity is not delayed in mothers with abnormal glucose metabolism, and if the gestational age exceeded 37 weeks, the fetal lung maturity should not be detected before delivery.

In order to understand neonatal outcomes after standard management, we conducted a retrospective study of neonatal outcomes in 1,490 pregnant women who were diagnosed and treated for abnormal glucose metabolism and delivered in the Peking University First Hospital from January 1995 to December 2004.[3] The selected cases consisted of 79 women with diabetes mellitus, 777 women with GDM, including 355 cases of Class A1 GDM, 316 with Class A2 GDM, 106 women whose glucose tolerant status was not known, and 634 women with GIGT. Fetal outcomes were analyzed in comparison with 19,013 pregnant women with normal glucose metabolism who delivered during the same period. We found that the perinatal mortality rate of the abnormal glucose metabolism group was 1.2% (18/1,513) which was significantly higher in the diabetes group (4.93%) than the GDM (1.1%) and GIGT groups (0.78%, $p<0.01$). The incidence of neonatal asphyxia, hypoglycemia, malformation, and admission to the neonatal intensive care unit in the diabetes group were all higher than in the GDM and GIGT groups ($p<0.01$). Neonatal respiratory distress syndrome (NRDS) was found in nine cases among 1,505 neonates (0.6%) and all were delivered preterm. Our results indicated that macrosomia and preterm birth remain the two most common complications, even after standardized glycemic management, but neonatal complications (other than macrosomia) are reduced in the GIGT group. Women in the DM group had a higher rate of neonatal complications than those in GDM and GIGT groups, so management in these patients should be intensified. NRDS is no longer a primary neonatal complication provided proper management is performed.[3]

Kashavarz et al[7] reported that women with GDM had a higher rate of stillbirth ($p<0.001$; odds ratio 17.1, 95% CI=4.5–65.5), hydramnios ($p<0.001$; odds ratio 15.5, 95% CI=4.8–50.5), gestational hypertension ($p<0.001$; odds ratio 6, 95% CI=2.3–15.3), macrosomia ($p<0.05$; odds ratio 3.2, 95% CI=1.2–8.6), and cesarean section ($p<0.001$) than women with normal glucose tolerance.

Since Barker's primary epidemiologic studies in 1989 showing an inverse relationship between birthweight and mortality due to adult ischemic heart disease,[27] it has become increasingly clear that fetal stress may lead to fetal programming and an alteration of normal developmental gene expression. Research indicates that the child of a diabetic mother remains at increased risk for a variety of developmental disturbances including obesity, IGT or diabetes, and diminished neurobehavioral capacities.[28] In developing countries such as China, it has not yet been demonstrated that the fetal distress that causes all the short-term neonatal complications in infants of GDM mothers may also be associated with the above long-term risks.

In India, children whose mothers were tested for glucose tolerance during pregnancy had detailed anthropometry performed at birth and annually thereafter.[29] While infants of GDM mothers were larger than controls, at 1 year these differences were not significantly large. However, at 5 years, the female offspring of diabetic mothers had a greater percentage of body fat and higher insulin levels at 30 and 120 min than control children, leading the authors to conclude that GDM *in utero* was associated with greater offspring adiposity and glucose and insulin concentrations.

6.4
Focus of GDM Research in China

Our group at Peking University First Hospital has done some basic research on pathophysiology of GDM. Our results have shown that women with GDM have the highest values of tumor necrosis factor alpha (TNFα) and leptin and the lowest value of adiponectin compared to women with GIGT and healthy controls ($p<0.01$) at 14–20 weeks of gestation. These differences persisted at 24–32 weeks gestation. These results indicate that the concentrations of TNFα, leptin, and adiponectin may change before the appearance of the abnormal glucose level during pregnancy.[30] In addition, we investigated the relationship between the polymorphism of site rs228648 in the urotensin II gene and the genetic susceptibility to GDM in northern Chinese women. Genotyping was conducted to investigate the polymorphism of site rs228648 (G-A) in urotensin II gene among 70 unrelated GDM subjects and 70 normal controls.[31] We found that the distribution of genotype frequencies of site rs228648 was in accord with Hardy–Weinberg's equation law, being colony representative. The frequency of G allele of site rs228648 was 70.7% in GDM group, significantly higher than that in the control group (57.9%, $p<0.05$), and the frequency of A allele of site rs228648 was 29.3% in the GDM group, significantly lower than that of the control group (42.1%, $p<0.05$). There was no significant difference in the frequency of G/G genotype between the GDM group and control group (52.9 vs. 41.4%, $p>0.05$). Women in the control group were more likely to be homozygous for the allele A of site rs228648 than were women with GDM. The frequency of A/A genotype of rs228648 was negatively correlated with the GDM group. After adjustment for age and gestational weeks, the association was still significant (odds ratio 0.312, $p=0.031$).

Literature searches of English-language databases may not capture the extent of GDM research performed in other countries, particularly China. We searched the Chinese full-text literature database for all original and experimental research articles on GDM published in Chinese. We notice that the quantity of publications has increased yearly since 1981: 10 in 1999, 51 in 2003 and 133 in 2006. The focus of these studies were: etiology and pathogenesis (71 articles, 54.2%), the mechanism of influence on pregnancy outcome (21, 16.0%), and laboratory results reports (19, 14.5%). The main themes of the clinical studies were on maternal-fetal outcome (196, 51.0%), analysis of maternal-fetal outcome after clinical treatment (88, 22.9%), screening and diagnosis of GDM (56, 14.6%), risk factors for GDM (25, 6.5%) and long-term follow up after a GDM delivery (9, 2.3%). Five papers in all were multi-centered research reports from Beijing, Tianjin, and Shanghai, respectively. Therefore, while the study of GDM has drawn remarkable attention during the past 30 years, the number of basic mechanism studies lags behind the clinical studies. Moreover, clinical studies are focused on clinical outcome reports and there is a lack of prospective multi-centered reports and clinical trials.[32]

Type 2 diabetes is presently thought to affect 246 million people, representing 5.9% of the global adult population, with the vast majority of diabetes affected subjects living in developing countries.[33] The number is expected to reach some 380 million by 2025, representing 7.1% of the adult population. For developing countries, there will be a projected increase of 170% of cases. Thus, diagnosis and management of GDM are necessary to decrease short-term adverse complications during pregnancy as well as to identify the group of women and offspring at increased risk for the development of later diabetes and possibly atherosclerotic cardiovascular disease. Resource allocation for research on GDM in developing countries, particularly for countries with high annual birth rates such as China, is needed.

References

1. Hossain P, Kawar B, El Nahas M. Obesity and diabetes in the developing world – a growing challenge. *N Engl J Med*. 2007;356(3):213-215.
2. Xu XM, Jiang ML, Dong YY. Study on the necessity for low- risk pregnant women to be screened for gestational diabetes mellitus. *Curr Adv Obstet Gynecol*. 2001;1:34-36 [Chinese].
3. Sun WJ, Yang HX. Maternal and fetal outcomes in pregnant women with abnormal glucose metabolism. *Zhonghua Fu Chan Ke Za Zhi*. 2007;42(6):374-376 [Chinese].
4. Yang X, Hsu-Hage B, Zhang H, et al. Gestational diabetes mellitus in women of single gravidity in Tianjin city, China. *Diabetes Care*. 2002;25(5):847-851.
5. Yang HX, Zhang MH, Sun WJ, Zhao Y. A prospective study of risk factors in pregnant women with abnormal glucose metabolism. *Zhonghua Fu Chan Ke Za Zhi*.2005;40(11):725-728 [Chinese].
6. Hossein-Nezhad A, Maghbooli Z, Vassigh AR, Larijani B. Prevalence of gestational diabetes mellitus and pregnancy outcomes in Iranian women. *Taiwan J Obstet Gynecol*. 2007;46(3):236-241.
7. Keshavarz M, Cheung NW, Babaee GR, Moqhadam HK, Ajami ME, Shariati M. Gestational diabetes in Iran: incidence, risk factors and pregnancy outcomes. *Diabetes Res Clin Pract*. 2005;69(3):279-286.
8. Zargar AH, Sheikh MI, Bashir MI, et al. Prevalence of gestational diabetes mellitus in Kashmiri women from the Indian subcontinent. *Diabetes Res Clin Pract*. 2004;66(2):139-145.
9. Mamabolo RL, Alberts M, Levitt NS, Delemarre-van de Waal HA, Steyn NP. Prevalence of gestational diabetes mellitus and the effect of weight on measures of insulin secretion and insulin resistance in third-trimester pregnant rural women residing in the Central Region of Limpopo Province, South Africa. *Diabet Med*. 2007;24(3):233-239.
10. Seyoum B, Kiros K, Haileselase T, Leole A. Prevalence of gestational diabetes mellitus in rural pregnant mothers in northern Ethiopia. *Diabetes Res Clin Pract*. 1999;46(3):247-251.
11. Carpenter MW, Coustan DR. Criteria for screening tests for gestational diabetes. *Am J Obstet Gynecol* 1982;144:768-773.
12. Schmidt MI, Duncan BB, Reichelt AJ, et al.; Brazilian Gestational Diabetes Study Group. Gestational diabetes mellitus diagnosed with a 2-h 75-g oral glucose tolerance test and adverse pregnancy outcomes. *Diabetes Care*. 2001;24(7):1151-1155.
13. Shi CY, Yang HX, Dong Y, et al. Study of 8665 cases of the 50 g oral glucose challenge test to screen the gestational diabetes mellitus. *Zhonghua Fu Chan Ke Za Zhi*. 2003;38(3):136-139 [Chinese].
14. Yang HX, Gao XL, Dong Y, Shi CY. Analysis of oral glucose tolerance test in pregnant women with abnormal glucose metabolism. *Chin Med J (Engl)*. 2005;118(12):995-999.
15. Shirazian N, Mahboubi M, Emdadi R, et al. Comparison of different diagnostic criteria for gestational diabetes mellitus based on the 75-g oral glucose tolerance test: a cohort study. *Endocr Pract*. 2008;14(3):312-317.
16. Seshiah V, Balaji V, Balaji MS, et al. Gestational diabetes mellitus manifests in all trimesters of pregnancy. *Diabetes Res Clin Pract*. 2007;77(3):482-484.
17. Yang HX, Zhong MH, Sun WJ, Dong Y. Associated factors of pre-eclampsia complicated in pregnant women with abnormal glucose metabolism. *Zhonghua Fu Chan Ke Za Zhi*. 2005; 40(9):577-580 [Chinese].

18. Yang HX, Zhao Y, Duan XH, Wu BS. A controlled study for pregnant outcomes in women with abnormal glucose tolerance. *Chinese General Practice*. 2004;7(14):1044-1045 [Chinese].
19. Sun Y, Yang HX, Sun WJ. Risk factors for pre-eclampsia in pregnant Chinese women with abnormal glucose metabolism. *Int J Gynaecol Obstet*. 2008;101:74-76.
20. Kim C, Newton KM, Knopp RH. Gestational diabetes and the incidence of type 2 diabetes: a systematic review. *Diabetes Care*. 2002;25(10):1862-1868.
21. Krishnaveni GV, Hill JC, Veena SR, et al. Gestational diabetes and the incidence of diabetes in the 5 years following the index pregnancy in South Indian women. *Diabetes Res Clin Pract*. 2007;78(3):398-404.
22. Langer O, Yogev Y, Most O, Xenakis MJ. Gestational diabetes: the consequences of not treating. *AmJ Obstet Gynecol*. 2005;192:989-997.
23. Jin HZ, Huang DM, Guan XJ. *Practical Neonatology*. 2nd ed. Beijing: People`s Medical; 1997:350-355.
24. Shi CY, Yang HX, Xie CY, Dong Y. Influences of abnormal carbohydrate metabolism during pregnency. *Zhonghua Wei Chan Yi Xue Za Zhi*. 2005;8(1):9-12 [Chinese].
25. Seshiah V, Cynthia A, Balaji V, et al. Detection and care of women with gestational diabetes mellitus from early weeks of pregnancy results in birth weight of newborn babies appropriate for gestational age. *Diabetes Res Clin Pract*. 2008;80(2):199-202.
26. Sun WJ, Yang HX. Effect of pregnancies with abnormal glucose metabolism on fetal lung maturity. *CGP Zhong Guo Quan Ke Yi Xue*. 2005;8(3):191-195 [Chinese].
27. Barker DJ, Osmond C, Golding J, Kuh D, Wadsworth ME. Growth in utero, blood pressure in childhood and adult life, and mortality from cardiovascular disease. *BMJ*. 1989;298(6673): 564-567.
28. Pettitt DJ, Lawrence JM, Beyer J, et al. Association between maternal diabetes in utero and age at offspring's diagnosis of type 2 diabetes. *Diabetes Care*. 2008;31(11):2126-2130.
29. Krishnaveni GV, Hill JC, Leary SD, et al. Anthropometry, glucose tolerance, and insulin concentrations in Indian children: relationships to maternal glucose and insulin concentrations during pregnancy. *Diabetes Care*. 2005;28(12):2919-2925.
30. Gao XL, Yang HX, Zhao Y. Variations of tumor necrosis factor-alpha, leptin and adiponectin in mid-trimester of gestational diabetes mellitus. *Chin Med J (Engl)*. 2008;121(8):701-705.
31. Tan YJ, Fan ZT, Yang HX. Role of urotensin II gene in the genetic susceptibility to gestational diabetes mellitus in northern Chinese women. *Zhonghua Fu Chan Ke Za Zhi*. 2006;41(11):732-725 [Chinese].
32. Gao XL, Yang HX. Current situation of the studies on gestational diabetes mellitus in China. *Zhong Guo Quan Ke Yi Xue*. 2008;11:547-550 [Chinese].
33. King H, Aubert RE, Herman WH. Global burden of diabetes, 1995-2025: prevalence, numerical estimates, and projections. *Diabetes Care*. 1998;21(9):1414-1431.

Section IV

Pathophysiology and Genetics of GDM

Insulin and the Placenta in GDM 7

Ursula Hiden and G. Desoye

7.1 Introduction

The placenta is a fetal organ with widespread functions located at the interface between mother and fetus. It transports maternal nutrients to sustain fetal growth, synthesizes hormones and growth factors to facilitate maternal adaptation to pregnancy, represents an immunologic barrier, and dissipates thermic energy resulting from fetal metabolism. Proper function of the placenta is essential to pregnancy outcome. Because of its position between the maternal and fetal compartment, the placenta is susceptible to regulation by hormones, growth factors, and metabolites present in both circulations. These factors, along with their binding proteins and receptors, form a complex network allowing tight control of placental development and function. Any disturbance of this network e.g., by concentration changes in one or several components may also compromise placental functioning.

GDM is associated with alterations in concentrations of a wide range of hormones, growth factors, cytokines, and metabolites in the maternal circulation. Available evidence, though limited, also shows changes in the fetal blood and in the placenta. These include cytokines secreted by adipose tissue, called adipocytokines, insulin, and glucose levels. As a consequence, placentas from GDM pregnancies display various changes in both morphology and function. These changes may represent adaptive responses to the altered maternal and fetal milieu.

In this chapter, the effect of GDM-associated maternal and fetal hyperinsulinemia on the placenta will be discussed. The impact of diabetes and GDM, obesity and diabetes therapies on the placental insulin receptor and its signaling molecules will be elucidated.

G. Desoye (✉)
Department of Obstetrics and Gynecology, Medical University of Graz, Graz, Austria
e-mail: gernot.desoye@meduni-graz.at

C. Kim and A. Ferrara (eds.), *Gestational Diabetes During and After Pregnancy*,
DOI: 10.1007/978-1-84882-120-0_7, © Springer-Verlag London Limited 2010

7.2 The Human Placenta

The human placenta has a tree-like, villous structure. The terminally differentiated syncytiotrophoblast, a syncytium that is formed from fusion of subjacent, mitotically-active cytotrophoblast cells, covers the surface of all villi. It thus represents the outermost interface of the placenta that is in contact with the maternal circulation. Some villi are physically anchored in the maternal uterus, whereas others freely float in the intervillous space that is filled with maternal blood. The establishment of a proper maternal blood stream into the intervillous space is an important step early in placental development. It depends on the invasion of trophoblast cells into the maternal uterus, followed by remodeling and opening of the maternal uterine spiral arterioles.

Inside the villous core, tissue-resident macrophages, fibroblasts, and placental blood vessels are surrounded by extracellular matrix. The big vessels from the umbilical cord ramify into smaller vessels and capillaries at the tips of the villi and merge again to form the vein of the umbilical cord. Thus, the maternal and the fetal compartments are in contact with different surfaces of the placenta: the microvillous membrane of the syncytiotrophoblast is in contact with the maternal blood, whereas the endothelium of the placental vasculature is in contact with the fetal blood.

The remodeling of the uterine arteries by trophoblasts is completed in the second trimester and, thus, will likely not be affected by GDM that clinically manifests at midgestation. However, placental vascularization as well as placental growth continue up to term of gestation and may be affected by the diabetic environment of GDM.

7.3 Insulin Therapy and Antidiabetic Drugs

When dietary management fails to achieve adequate glucose control, the therapeutic use of insulin has been regarded as the most physiological and safe way to treat hyperglycemia in GDM. This is because free insulin cannot cross the placenta.[1] However, insulin complexed to anti-insulin antibodies has been detected in cord blood suggesting transplacental transport of insulin bound to maternal antibodies via placental Fc-receptors.[2] By this route insulin escapes degradation by placental insulinases.[3]

Most diabetic pregnant women treated with porcine insulin are reported to have anti-insulin antibodies. Their prevalence depends on duration of the disease and on the kind of insulin administered.[4] Thus, in patients with insulin-treated pregestational diabetes, anti-insulin antibodies will occur, although even GDM women treated with insulin produce anti-insulin IgG.[5] Higher levels of insulin antibodies have been found when animal insulin is used for therapy as compared with human insulin.[6] The biological effect of the maternally-derived insulin in the fetal circulation is unclear. The presence of maternal anti-insulin antibody levels does not correlate with birth weight or fetal metabolic disorders.[5]

In recent years, insulin analogs such as insulin lispro[7] and insulin aspart[8] are often used. They do not increase insulin antibody levels. Hence, they do not utilize the transplacental transport mechanism via Fc-receptors and are not detectable in the fetal circulation.

The use of glucose-lowering oral agents in pregnancy has raised discussion and concern because of limited data on their short- and long-term risk for the fetus and neonate, respectively. The suitability of several classes of antidiabetic agents for treatment of diabetes in pregnancy has been determined in ex vivo perfusion of human placentas. The PPAR-gamma agonists thiazolidinediones (rosiglitazone, pioglitazone), alpha-glucosidase inhibitors (acarbose) and biguanides (metformin) readily cross the placental barrier.[9] Nevertheless, metformin and acarbose have been used increasingly for GDM therapy. Various studies showed no consistent evidence for an increase in adverse maternal or neonatal consequences.[10] However, the use of compounds crossing the placenta has to be considered very critically.

Exenatide, a synthetic exendin-4 with incretin effect stimulating insulin secretion is transported across the placenta in negligible amounts, resulting in insignificant exposure to the fetus.[11] The sulfonylureas glipizide and glyburide block ATP-sensitive potassium channels in β-cells and thus stimulate insulin secretion. Both show little or no transport across the placenta.[12] Although the potential transport of these drugs across the placenta has been studied, almost no information is available on potential effects of these drugs on the placenta itself. It is conceivable that some cellular processes and placental functions are modified by drugs in the maternal circulation. In the single study to examine this question, glipizide induced a dose-dependent upregulation of placental insulin receptors (IR) in vitro[13] (Fig. 7.1), and may alter placental function. Glyburide is safe and has been used for the treatment of GDM.[12]

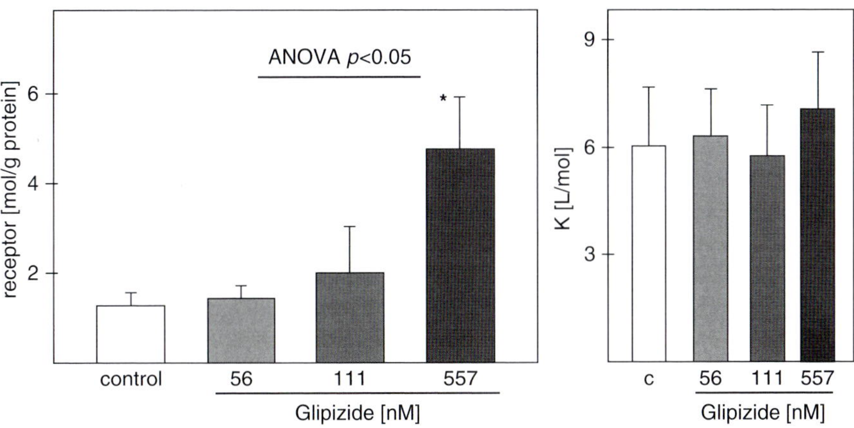

Fig. 7.1 Amount of insulin receptors (IR) on isolated placental trophoblasts after 48 h treatment with glipizide shows a dose-dependent increase (**a**). The affinity of receptors towards insulin remains stable upon glipizide treatment (**b**). Data taken from[13]

7.4
Hyperglycemia, Hyperinsulinemia and Proinflammatory Cytokines

Hyperglycemia in the fetal circulation produces hyperinsulinemia in the fetal compartment. In GDM women treated with insulin, maternal plasma insulin levels are also elevated.[14] The elevated insulin levels in the maternal and fetal circulation will particularly affect placental development, because of the high expression of IR[15] on both placental surfaces.[16]

Adipocytokines, biologically active peptides, profoundly influence insulin sensitivity, contribute to insulin resistance, and produce a proinflammatory state. They appear to be involved in the development of obesity-mediated adverse effects on glucose and lipid metabolism[17] and may represent a molecular link between increased adiposity and impaired insulin sensitivity.

Several adipocytokines display altered levels in the maternal or fetal circulation in GDM pregnancies. Tumor necrosis factor alpha (TNF-α) has elevated and reduced levels in the maternal and fetal circulation, respectively,[18] whereas, plasma leptin is increased in mother[19] and fetus[20] and placental leptin production is increased GDM.[20] Furthermore, decreased plasma levels of maternal adiponectin in GDM have been reported.[21] Resistin levels are lower in infants born to mothers with GDM.[22] Thus, adiposity may further influence and promote insulin resistance in pregnancy in general and in GDM in particular, ultimately leading to maternal and, hence, fetal hyperglycemia.

7.5
Morphological Alteration of the Placenta in GDM

The placenta in GDM is characterized by a variety of morphological and functional changes reviewed in detail elsewhere.[23,24]

GDM first appears in the second half of gestation when fundamental steps in placental development such as placentation and opening of the uterine spiral arteries have been completed. However, central placental functions and processes such as nutrient transport, synthesis of hormones and growth factors, as well as placental growth and vascularization may still be influenced by metabolic derangements in both circulations. Ultimately, these lead to changes in placental morphology observed at term of gestation.

A well known placental alteration in GDM is the increase in placental weight.[25] This is paralleled by an increase in fetal weight, resulting from excessive fat accumulation.[26] The reason for the elevated weight of placenta and fetus are unclear, although changes in transplacental transport may be implicated.

In addition to augmented growth, gross placental structure may be altered in GDM predominantly as a result of an enlargement of placental surface and exchange areas; i.e., the syncytiotrophoblast and the placental endothelium as a result of hyperproliferation and hypervascularization.[27] Their underlying mechanisms are not clear, but maternal hyperinsulinemia early in gestation is a candidate for increased trophoblast proliferation[28] and for inducing structural modifications.[29] However, other maternal growth factors are likely to contribute.

The greater placental capillary surfaces may result from feto-placental counter regulatory mechanisms to fetal hypoxia. Presence of fetal hypoxia can be deduced from the elevated fetal erythropoietin levels often observed in the fetuses of diabetic women[30] and may result from changes in GDM. The low oxygen levels may have profound consequences for fetus and placenta and upregulate expression of proangiogenic factors such as VEGF and FGF-2 in the feto-placental compartment hence stimulating placental vascularization.[31,32] Hypervascularization resulting from stimulated vascular branching is a common feature of the placenta in GDM.[33]

7.6 Functional Alteration of the Placenta in GDM

7.6.1 Gene Expression

Comparison of gene expression of placentas from obese women with insulin-treated GDM with those from healthy controls, revealed 435 genes differentially expressed. Most of these were related to inflammatory pathways, which may reflect the obesity of these mothers.[34] A more recent study measured gene expression in total placental tissue from normal and nonobese GDM subjects. Among 22,215 genes surveyed, the expression of 66 genes was altered. Their functions were predominantly related to immune response, and development and regulation of cell death.[35] These differences in gene expression arise from the interaction of the maternal and fetal diabetic milieu with the placenta, including altered levels of hormones, growth factors, and metabolites. For instance, insulin in a concentration similar to that present in fetal cord plasma in GDM alters the expression of 146 genes on primary placental endothelial cells.[36] These gene expression studies will help reveal biological processes that are most affected by GDM and thus will contribute to improving our understanding for the mechanisms underlying changes in placental phenotype associated with GDM.

7.6.2 Placental Transport

The transporting epithelium in the human placenta is the syncytiotrophoblast with its microvillous plasma membrane bathing in the maternal blood in the intervillous space. At specialized sites, the syncytiotrophoblast basal membrane is in contact with the endothelial cells lining the fetal capillary. These sites are the key structures across which all nutrients such as glucose, amino acids, and lipids destined for the fetus have to be transported.

The increased transplacental glucose flux underlying fetal hyperglycemia is not accounted for by changes in glucose transporter expression because perfusion experiments demonstrate an unaltered or even reduced glucose transfer across the placenta in diet- and insulin-treated GDM, respectively.[37,38] This suggests the steeper maternal-fetal glucose gradient as the driving force for the enhanced glucose fluxes across the placenta in GDM.

The unchanged concentration differences of glucose between umbilical arteries and vein in GDM[39] support this notion.

Conflicting data exist on amino acid transport systems in GDM. Upregulation of the placental syncytiotrophoblast system A amino-acid transporter, which transports alanine, serine, proline, and glutamine, has been observed[40] although not uniformly.[41, 42] As amino acid transport systems are complex and several transporter systems exist with overlapping specificity, conclusions from one transport system may not apply to general amino acid transport. Future studies measuring amino acid transport in placental perfusion using GDM placentas would allow better identification of potential GDM-associated changes in the transport and help to elucidate the role of amino acid transport in fetal adiposity.

Almost all fatty acids circulate in esterified form in triglycerides, phospholipids, and cholesterol esters. Together with apolipoproteins and lipid-soluble vitamins they are complexed in lipoproteins. GDM does not significantly alter maternal cholesterol levels, but maternal as well as fetal hypertriglyceridemia, particularly in the VLDL and HDL fraction, has been a well known feature of GDM.[43, 44] At present the mechanism of fatty acid transport across the placental barrier is still not fully understood. The lipoproteins have to bind to LDL, HDL, and VLDL receptors on the syncytiotrophoblast surface. Subsequently, they are either endocytosed (LDL[45]) or depleted of cholesterol (HDL[46]). In addition, endothelial lipase alone[47] or in concert with other yet unidentified lipases, hydrolyzes maternal triglycerides. The released free fatty acids will then be taken up by and transferred across the trophoblast, a complex process involving several fatty acids transport molecules and binding proteins.[48, 49] Cellular membranes of GDM placentas contain a higher proportion of these fatty acids. Several scenarios may be involved: selective uptake and intermediate storage of these fatty acids into the placenta, their increased placental synthesis, their reduced conversion into eicosanoids and/or their decreased release into the fetal circulation.[50] The fetal concentrations of arachidonic acid and docosahexaenoic acid are reduced in GDM,[51] whereas those in the mothers are unchanged.[52] A more detailed analysis found these changes only in the arterial, but not in the venous, cord plasma coming from the placenta. This indicates that altered fetal metabolism of long-chain fatty acids rather than altered placental transport account for alteration of fatty acids in the fetal circulation in GDM.[53]

7.6.3 Oxygen Delivery in Diabetes

Several utero-placental alterations in GDM are unfavorable for oxygen delivery to the fetus. A higher proportion of glycosylated hemoglobin,[54] which has a stronger binding affinity for oxygen than nonglycosylated hemoglobin, will impair oxygen delivery to the placenta. This may be further augmented by a reduced utero-placental blood flow, especially without tight glycemic control of the mothers.[55] In the placenta, thickening of the trophoblast basement membrane is frequently found. It mainly results from increased amounts of collagen.[56, 57] Collectively, these changes may lead to reduced oxygen delivery to the fetus. In addition, fetal demand for oxygen may be increased, because of hyperinsulinemia- and hyperglycemia-induced stimulation of the fetal aerobic metabolism. In the situation of imbalanced fetal oxygen demand and maternal supply, fetal hypoxia may ensue. Elevated fetal plasma erythropoietin levels in GDM pregnancies may reflect such imbalance.[30]

7.7 Insulin Effects in the Human Placenta

The placenta is a rich source of IR and has served as the tissue of origin for isolation of the receptor protein. The IR distribution pattern in the placenta is complex and varies with gestational age. In the first trimester IRs are mainly expressed on the trophoblasts and are thus in contact with the maternal circulation, whereas at term most IRs are located at the placental endothelium and are directed toward the fetal blood. At this stage of gestation the trophoblast contains only a modest IR amount, located at the microvillous membrane. This change in IR location during gestation may reflect a change in control of insulin-dependent processes in the placenta from the mother early in gestation to the fetus later in gestation. For obvious reasons, IR expression in placentas from uncomplicated pregnancies at mid-gestation has not been investigated, leaving unresolved the question of which distinct time period in gestation this change in location occurs. Hence, insulin target cells at the time period of the clinical manifestation of GDM and for the initial effects of hyperinsulinemia on placental processes is unknown.

Although IR expression in the trophoblast decreases toward term of gestation, several insulin effects have been reported in isolated term trophoblasts, mainly relating to transport function and hormone synthesis. Insulin stimulates the uptake of the amino-acid analog α-aminoisobutyric acid, a synthetic substrate for the system A amino acid transporter.[58, 59] This is an isolated finding and a general conclusion on GDM-associated alterations in transplacental amino acid transport remains to be established.

Insulin's endocrine activity affects the synthesis and secretion of placental hormones. Trophoblast estradiol-β secretion is downregulated[60, 61] paralleled by the inhibition of aromatase (CYP19A1), the enzyme that catalyzes the last step in estrogen biosynthesis.[62] The effect of GDM on maternal estrogen levels is controversial. Couch et al[44] found elevated levels of β-estradiol in plasma of women with diet-treated GDM, while others reported reduced levels, when women were insulin-treated,[63] or no change.[64, 65]

Moreover, insulin upregulates placental lactogen (hPL) secretion from isolated trophoblasts.[60, 61] Since more than 99% of hPL is released into the maternal circulation, higher maternal hPL concentrations in insulin-treated GDM women would be expected. However, plasma levels are rather reduced at term,[63] suggesting additional regulators of circulating hPL levels beyond insulin, and IGF-I may be a candidate. Insulin also reduces the expression of placental growth hormone in choriocarcinoma cells used as trophoblast models.[66] This is an interesting finding because placental growth hormone can induce insulin resistance.[67]

In line with its lipogenic effects in other tissues the combination of insulin and fatty acids upregulate adipophilin expression in trophoblasts.[68] Adipophilin is a protein implicated in cellular fatty acid uptake and storage of neutral lipids in adipocytes. Hence, elevated adipophilin levels along with the lipogenic activity of insulin may contribute to elevated storage of triglycerides in GDM placentas.[69]

Despite the high amounts of IR on placental endothelial cells at term of gestation,[15] no distinct insulin effects on these cells have been identified so far, apart from a general regulation of gene expression.[36] Interestingly, the IRs are particularly expressed at branching sites of placental capillaries with high proliferative activity.[70] This suggests that the general insulin effect on vascular endothelium such as the activation of endothelial NO synthase (eNOS) and subsequent expression of proangiogenic factors such as VEGFA,[71] ultimately promoting angiogenesis and vascularization, may also be operative in the placenta.[70]

The GDM-associated elevation of insulin levels in the fetal and – if insulin treated – also in the maternal circulation[14] may contribute to placental changes observed in GDM in vivo. The insulin-induced increase in amino acid transport may sustain fetal overgrowth in GDM. The upregulated VEGFA expression in the endothelial cells may contribute to the diabetes-associated placental hypervascularization (cf. above).

7.8 Placental Insulin Receptor Expression in Normal and Diabetic Pregnancy

The amount of IR can be regulated by ambient insulin concentrations. Hence, it comes as no surprise that in GDM IR protein is also changed in total placental tissue and on trophoblast membranes.[14,23] The alterations depend on the type of diabetes and on the treatment modality and, obviously on maternal obesity. Whereas mild forms of GDM treated with a restriction in nutrient uptake down-regulate trophoblast IRs, severe insulin-treated cases show an upregulation of IRs on trophoblast membranes similar to Type 1 diabetes[14] (Fig. 7.2). In GDM, IR expression in total placental tissue depends on the metabolic control. Whereas well controlled insulin-treated GDM reveals no change,[72] in poorly controlled or even untreated GDM, insulin receptor expression is down-regulated.[73,74]

The mechanisms accounting for the changes in IR in diabetes are unknown. Among several scenarios these may be the result of the different maternal insulin levels in diet- vs. insulin-treated GDM cases[14] or of elevated glucocorticoid levels[75,76] which, similar to other tissues,[77] may up-regulate IR expression in the more severe cases of GDM and in T1DM.

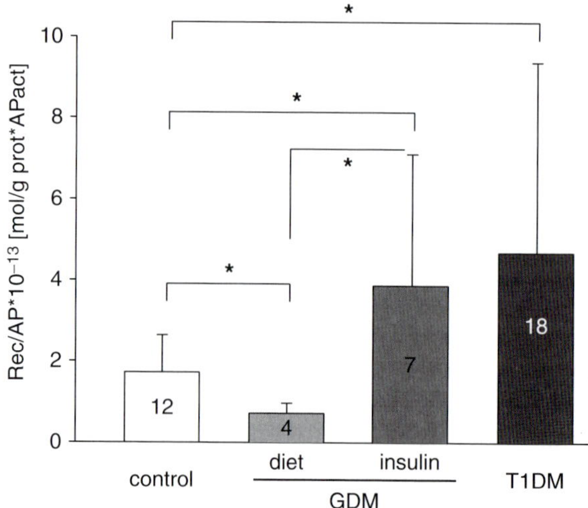

Fig. 7.2 Diabetes alters the number of IR on trophoblast plasma membranes. Diet-treated GDM reduces insulin receptor numbers, whereas insulin-treated GDM and Type 1 diabetes increase the amount of trophoblast IR. Data taken from[13]

7.9
Insulin Resistance in GDM

Insulin resistance is a common phenomenon in the second half of normal pregnancy resulting from the insulin-antagonizing action of various pregnancy-related hormones. In GDM, insulin resistance cannot be sufficiently compensated for by maternal insulin production and as a consequence hyperglycemia arises. Insulin resistance emerges from elevated levels of cytokines and hormones counter-acting IR signaling and from altered expression levels of components of the insulin signaling cascade.[78] Both will result in reduced insulin action. In GDM, maternal levels of the cytokine TNFα are increased.[18] Plasma levels of leptin are elevated in the maternal[19, 79] and the fetal[20] circulation. Both interfere with IR signal transduction. TNFα impairs IR signaling by inhibition of IR substrate 1 (IRS1) activity, whereas hyperleptinemia leads to insulin resistance by activation of SOCS (suppressor of cytokine signaling) proteins, which, ultimately, attenuate leptin and IR signaling.[80]

The placenta expresses TNFα and leptin receptors and hence, may also be a target of the weakening effects of TNFα and leptin on insulin signaling. The role of the pregnancy-related hormones such as estrogen, progesterone, prolactin, and human placental lactogen in the development of the accentuated insulin resistance of GDM is unclear as they do not significantly correlate with insulin resistance.[81]

In addition to factors counteracting insulin signaling, altered activation or expression of components of the IR signaling cascade in the insulin target cells may contribute to insulin resistance. Also in GDM, alterations in activation, phosphorylation or expression of proteins related to insulin signaling in classical insulin target tissues (adipose tissue[78, 82]; skeletal muscle[78, 83]) have been shown. In the placenta, only limited data about insulin resistance or alteration in insulin signaling resulting from GDM are available.[72, 84] However, these are restricted to measurements of total IR-protein phosphorylation and do not include information on activation or inhibition of site-specific insulin signaling by i.e., phosphorylation of tyrosine or serine residues, respectively. This information is important because signaling may be induced or inhibited depending on the phosphorylation site.

7.10
GDM Alters Placental Insulin Receptor Signaling Components

Basically, insulin activates two main signaling pathways: the phosphatidylinositol 3-kinase/protein kinase B (PI3K/PKB) and the mitogen-activated protein kinase (MAPK) pathway. The PI3K/PKB pathway induces the metabolic effects of insulin such as translocation of GLUT4 glucose transporters, glycogen and protein synthesis. The PI3K is composed of a regulatory 85-kDa subunit and a catalytic 110-kDa subunit. The MAPK pathway stimulates proliferation, migration and angiogenesis.[85] Gene knock out experiments in mice and isolated cells *in vitro* strongly suggest that MAPK signaling is mainly activated via insulin receptor substrate 1 (IRS1) whereas insulin receptor substrate 2 (IRS2) plays a key role in the regulation of carbohydrate metabolism.[86] Thus, expression changes of any insulin signaling component may affect insulin receptor signal transduction and, ultimately, insulin effects.

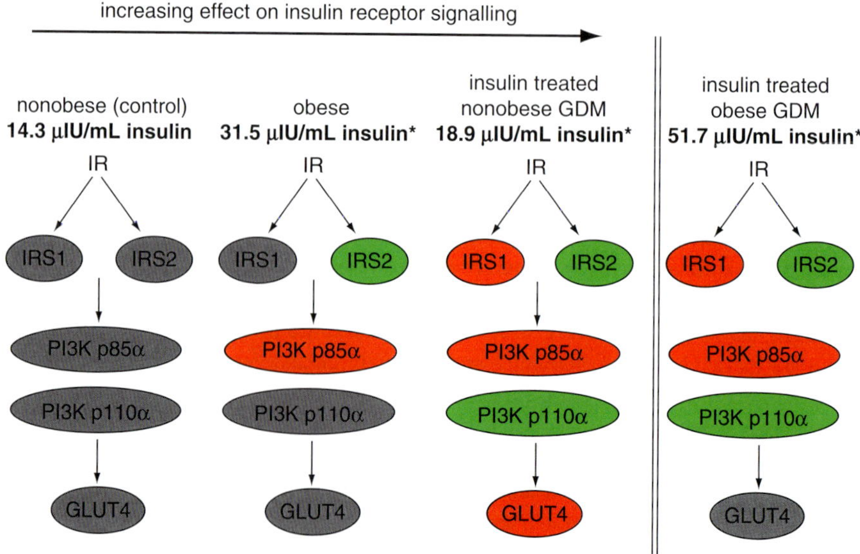

Fig. 7.3 Altered expression of placental insulin signaling components in nonobese and obese women without or with insulin-treated GDM. The pathway illustrated is one of several insulin signaling cascades resulting in GLUT4 translocation to the plasma membrane. Obesity alone alters the expression of IRS2 and PI3K p85α (second pathway) vs. healthy, nonobese controls (first pathway). Placentas from insulin-treated non obese women with GDM showed additional changes in IRS1, PI3K p85α and GLUT4 (third pathway). Similar changes to those found in insulin-treated nonobese GDM were found in obese insulin-treated GDM. Insulin concentrations refer to those measured in the late third trimester; *indicates significant difference from controls. The red and green color indicates upregulation and downregulation vs. control, respectively. According to data from[72]

Obesity and GDM are associated with altered expression of several downstream components of the insulin signaling pathway in the placenta (Fig. 7.3). When obesity is associated with GDM, or *vice versa,* the changes are more pronounced. A reduction of IRS1 expression is a common feature in skeletal muscle and adipose tissue in women with GDM.[78] The obese, nondiabetic women have higher plasma insulin levels than the nonobese group, whereas the glucose levels are normal. This indicates that the elevated insulin levels in obesity with normal glucose tolerance may already induce changes in the placental insulin signaling pathway similar to but less severe than those observed in insulin-treated GDM. Alternatively, or in addition, the inflammation associated with obesity and GDM may contribute as well.

7.11 Conclusion

Because of the presence of IR on the maternal and fetal surface the placenta is a target tissue of insulin in both circulations. Whereas various effects of insulin have been identified in isolated placental cells, their relevance remains to be shown in vivo. GDM is a condition associated with exacerbated maternal insulin resistance. To date, presence and character of insulin resistance in the placenta in GDM has not been determined, and the few existing studies present conflicting data on insulin receptor autophosphorylation. Elevated levels of TNFα and leptin in the maternal and/or fetal circulation may impair insulin signaling and alter levels of insulin signaling molecules. This then may modify insulin effects in GDM and produce changes observed in placentas obtained from GDM women.

Only few studies exist that define treatment modality or even distinguish between diet-treated and insulin-treated GDM cases, and between placentas from obese and nonobese women. Over the years , it has become clear that these represent different groups with different degrees of metabolic derangement. Furthermore, obesity, even with normal glucose tolerance, is associated with a change in the levels of insulin signaling components in the placenta, which resembles changes observed in insulin-treated GDM and, therefore, may represent a modest form of inflammatory response of the placenta. Placental alterations associated with maternal obesity might represent a stage preceding placental alterations in GDM. In order to understand the effect of GDM on the placenta, it appears of central importance to define and distinguish between these groups. A detailed analysis of the placental response to the diabetic environment is still pending.

References

1. Kalhan SC, Schwartz R, Adam PA. Placental barrier to human insulin-I125 in insulin-dependent diabetic mothers. *J Clin Endocrinol Metab*. 1975;40(1):139-142.
2. Menon RK et al. Transplacental passage of insulin in pregnant women with insulin-dependent diabetes mellitus. Its role in fetal macrosomia. *N Engl J Med*. 1990;323(5):309-315.
3. Weirich G et al. Immunohistochemical evidence of ubiquitous distribution of the metalloendoprotease insulin-degrading enzyme (IDE; insulysin) in human non-malignant tissues and tumor cell lines. *Biol Chem*. 2008;389(11):1441-1445.
4. Martikainen A et al. Disease-associated antibodies in offspring of mothers with IDDM. *Diabetes*. 1996;45(12):1706-1710.
5. Weiss PA et al. Anti-insulin antibodies and birth weight in pregnancies complicated by diabetes. *Early Hum Dev*. 1998;53(2):145-154.
6. Velcovsky HG, Federlin KF. Insulin-specific IgG and IgE antibody response in type I diabetic subjects exclusively treated with human insulin (recombinant DNA). *Diabetes Care*. 1982; 5(suppl 2):126-128.
7. Jovanovic L et al. Metabolic and immunologic effects of insulin lispro in gestational diabetes. *Diabetes Care*. 1999;22(9):1422-1427.
8. McCance DR et al. Evaluation of insulin antibodies and placental transfer of insulin aspart in pregnant women with type 1 diabetes mellitus. *Diabetologia*. 2008;51(11):2141-2143.
9. Nanovskaya TN et al. Transfer of metformin across the dually perfused human placental lobule. *Am J Obstet Gynecol*. 2006;195(4):1081-1085.
10. Nicholson W et al. Benefits and risks of oral diabetes agents compared with insulin in women with gestational diabetes: a systematic review. *Obstet Gynecol*. 2009;113(1):193-205.
11. Hiles RA, Bawdon RE, Petrella EM. Ex vivo human placental transfer of the peptides pramlintide and exenatide (synthetic exendin-4). *Hum Exp Toxicol*. 2003;22(12):623-628.
12. Feig DS, Briggs GG, Koren G. Oral antidiabetic agents in pregnancy and lactation: a paradigm shift? *Ann Pharmacother*. 2007;41(7):1174-1180.

13. Desoye G, Barnea ER, Shurz-Swirsky R. Increase in insulin binding and inhibition of the decrease in the phospholipid content of human term placental homogenates in culture by the sulfonylurea glipizide. *Biochem Pharmacol.* 1993;46(9):1585-1590.
14. Desoye G, Hofmann HH, Weiss PA. Insulin binding to trophoblast plasma membranes and placental glycogen content in well-controlled gestational diabetic women treated with diet or insulin, in well-controlled overt diabetic patients and in healthy control subjects. *Diabetologia.* 1992;35(1):45-55.
15. Desoye G et al. Insulin receptors in syncytiotrophoblast and fetal endothelium of human placenta. Immunohistochemical evidence for developmental changes in distribution pattern. *Histochemistry.* 1994;101(4):277-285.
16. Hiden U, et al. Insulin and the IGF system in the human placenta of normal and diabetic pregnancies. *J Anat.* 2009;215:60-68.
17. Matsuzawa Y, Funahashi T, Nakamura T. Molecular mechanism of metabolic syndrome X: contribution of adipocytokines adipocyte-derived bioactive substances. *Ann N Y Acad Sci.* 1999;892:146-154.
18. Ategbo JM et al. Modulation of adipokines and cytokines in gestational diabetes and macrosomia. *J Clin Endocrinol Metab.* 2006;91(10):4137-4143.
19. Vitoratos N et al. Maternal plasma leptin levels and their relationship to insulin and glucose in gestational-onset diabetes. *Gynecol Obstet Invest.* 2001;51(1):17-21.
20. Lea RG et al. Placental leptin in normal, diabetic and fetal growth-retarded pregnancies. *Mol Hum Reprod.* 2000;6(8):763-769.
21. Worda C et al. Decreased plasma adiponectin concentrations in women with gestational diabetes mellitus. *Am J Obstet Gynecol.* 2004;191(6):2120-2124.
22. Ng PC et al. Plasma ghrelin and resistin concentrations are suppressed in infants of insulin-dependent diabetic mothers. *J Clin Endocrinol Metab.* 2004;89(11):5563-5568.
23. Desoye G, Shafrir E. The human placenta in diabetic pregnancy. *Diabetes Rev.* 1996;4: 70-89.
24. Desoye G, Kaufmann P. The human placenta in diabetes. In: Porta M, Matschinsky FM, eds. *Diabetology of Pregnancy.* Basel:Karger; 2006:94-109.
25. Taricco E et al. Foetal and placental weights in relation to maternal characteristics in gestational diabetes. *Placenta.* 2003;24(4):343-347.
26. Durnwald C et al. Evaluation of body composition of large-for-gestational-age infants of women with gestational diabetes mellitus compared with women with normal glucose tolerance levels. *Am J Obstet Gynecol.* 2004;191(3):804-808.
27. Mayhew TM et al. Growth and maturation of villi in placentae from well-controlled diabetic women. *Placenta.* 1994;15(1):57-65.
28. Mandl M et al. Serum-dependent effects of IGF-I and insulin on proliferation and invasion of human first trimester trophoblast cell models. *Histochem Cell Biol.* 2002;117(5):391-399.
29. Hiden U et al. MT1-MMP expression in first-trimester placental tissue is upregulated in type 1 diabetes as a result of elevated insulin and tumor necrosis factor-alpha levels. *Diabetes.* 2008;57(1):150-157.
30. Madazli R et al. The incidence of placental abnormalities, maternal and cord plasma malondialdehyde and vascular endothelial growth factor levels in women with gestational diabetes mellitus and nondiabetic controls. *Gynecol Obstet Invest.* 2008;65(4):227-232.
31. Black SM, Devol JM, Wedgwood S. Regulation of fibroblast growth factor-2 expression in pulmonary arterial smooth muscle cells involves increased reactive oxygen species generation. *Am J Physiol Cell Physiol.* 2008;294(1):C345-C354.
32. Josko J, Mazurek M. Transcription factors having impact on vascular endothelial growth factor (VEGF) gene expression in angiogenesis. *Med Sci Monit.* 2004;10(4): RA89-RA98.
33. Jirkovska M et al. Topological properties and spatial organization of villous capillaries in normal and diabetic placentas. *J Vasc Res.* 2002;39(3):268-278.

34. Radaelli T et al. Gestational diabetes induces placental genes for chronic stress and inflammatory pathways. *Diabetes*. 2003;52(12):2951-2958.
35. Enquobahrie DA, et al. Global placental gene expression in gestational diabetes mellitus. *Am J Obstet Gynecol*. 2009;200(2):206 e1-e13.
36. Hiden U et al. Insulin control of placental gene expression shifts from mother to foetus over the course of pregnancy. *Diabetologia*. 2006;49(1):123-131.
37. Osmond DT et al. Placental glucose transport and utilisation is altered at term in insulin-treated, gestational-diabetic patients. *Diabetologia*. 2001;44(9):1133-1139.
38. Osmond DT et al. Effects of gestational diabetes on human placental glucose uptake, transfer, and utilisation. *Diabetologia*. 2000;43(5):576-582.
39. Radaelli T, et al. Oxygenation, acid-base-balance and glucose levels in fetuses from gestational diabetic pregnancies. *J Soc Gynecol Invest*. 2005;2(suppl):221A.
40. Jansson T et al. Alterations in the activity of placental amino acid transporters in pregnancies complicated by diabetes. *Diabetes*. 2002;51(7):2214-2219.
41. Dicke JM, Henderson GI. Placental amino acid uptake in normal and complicated pregnancies. *Am J Med Sci*. 1988;295(3):223-227.
42. Kuruvilla AG et al. Altered activity of the system A amino acid transporter in microvillous membrane vesicles from placentas of macrosomic babies born to diabetic women. *J Clin Invest*. 1994;94(2):689-695.
43. Merzouk H et al. Changes in serum lipid and lipoprotein concentrations and compositions at birth and after 1 month of life in macrosomic infants of insulin-dependent diabetic mothers. *Eur J Pediatr*. 1999;158(9):750-756.
44. Couch SC et al. Elevated lipoprotein lipids and gestational hormones in women with diet-treated gestational diabetes mellitus compared to healthy pregnant controls. *J Diabetes Complications*. 1998;12(1):1-9.
45. Malassine A et al. Acetylated low density lipoprotein endocytosis by human syncytiotrophoblast in culture. *Placenta*. 1990;11(2):191-204.
46. Wadsack C et al. Selective cholesteryl ester uptake from high density lipoprotein by human first trimester and term villous trophoblast cells. *Placenta*. 2003;24(2–3):131-143.
47. Gauster M et al. Dysregulation of placental endothelial lipase and lipoprotein lipase in intrauterine growth-restricted pregnancies. *J Clin Endocrinol Metab*. 2007;92(6):2256-2263.
48. Cunningham P, McDermott L. Long chain PUFA transport in human term placenta. *J Nutr*. 2009;139(4):636-639.
49. Herrera E et al. Maternal lipid metabolism and placental lipid transfer. *Horm Res*. 2006;65 (suppl 3):59-64.
50. Bitsanis D et al. Gestational diabetes mellitus enhances arachidonic and docosahexaenoic acids in placental phospholipids. *Lipids*. 2006;41(4):341-346.
51. Thomas B et al. Plasma AA and DHA levels are not compromised in newly diagnosed gestational diabetic women. *Eur J Clin Nutr*. 2004;58(11):1492-1497.
52. Thomas BA et al. Plasma fatty acids of neonates born to mothers with and without gestational diabetes. *Prostaglandins Leukot Essent Fatty Acids*. 2005;72(5):335-341.
53. Ortega-Senovilla H et al. Gestational diabetes mellitus upsets the proportion of fatty acids in umbilical arterial but not venous plasma. *Diabetes Care*. 2009;32(1):120-122.
54. Madsen H, Ditzel J. Red cell 2, 3-diphosphoglycerate and hemoglobin-oxygen affinity during diabetic pregnancy. *Acta Obstet Gynecol Scand*. 1984;63(5):403-406.
55. Nylund L et al. Uteroplacental blood flow in diabetic pregnancy: measurements with indium 113m and a computer-linked gamma camera. *Am J Obstet Gynecol*. 1982;144(3):298-302.
56. al-Okail MS, al-Attas OS. Histological changes in placental syncytiotrophoblasts of poorly controlled gestational diabetic patients. *Endocr J*. 1994;41(4):355-360.
57. Leushner JR et al. Analysis of the collagens of diabetic placental villi. *Cell Mol Biol*. 1986;32(1):27-35.

58. Guyda HJ. Metabolic effects of growth factors and polycyclic aromatic hydrocarbons on cultured human placental cells of early and late gestation. *J Clin Endocrinol Metab*. 1991; 72(3):718-723.
59. Karl PI, Alpy KL, Fisher SE. Amino acid transport by the cultured human placental trophoblast: effect of insulin on AIB transport. *Am J Physiol*. 1992;262(4 pt 1):C834-C839.
60. Hochberg Z et al. Insulin regulates placental lactogen and estradiol secretion by cultured human term trophoblast. *J Clin Endocrinol Metab*. 1983;57(6):1311-1313.
61. Perlman R et al. The effect of inhibitors on insulin regulation of hormone secretion by cultured human trophoblast. *Mol Cell Endocrinol*. 1985;43(1):77-82.
62. Nestler JE et al. Insulin mediators are the signal transduction system responsible for insulin's actions on human placental steroidogenesis. *Endocrinology*. 1991;129(6):2951-2956.
63. Olszewski J, Szczurowicz A, Wojcikowski C. Changes in levels of human placenta lactogen (hPL), progesterone, and estriol in blood serum and estrogens in urine during gestational diabetes mellitus. *Ginekol Pol*. 1995;66(3):145-150.
64. Grigorakis SI et al. Hormonal parameters in gestational diabetes mellitus during the third trimester: high glucagon levels. *Gynecol Obstet Invest*. 2000;49(2):106-109.
65. Montelongo A et al. Longitudinal study of plasma lipoproteins and hormones during pregnancy in normal and diabetic women. *Diabetes*. 1992;41(12):1651-1659.
66. Zeck W et al. Regulation of placental growth hormone secretion in a human trophoblast model–the effects of hormones and adipokines. *Pediatr Res*. 2008;63(4):353-357.
67. Barbour LA et al. Human placental growth hormone causes severe insulin resistance in transgenic mice. *Am J Obstet Gynecol*. 2002;186(3):512-517.
68. Elchalal U et al. Insulin and fatty acids regulate the expression of the fat droplet-associated protein adipophilin in primary human trophoblasts. *Am J Obstet Gynecol*. 2005;193(5):1716-1723.
69. Shafrir E, Barash V. Placental function in maternal-fetal fat transport in diabetes. *Biol Neonate*. 1987;51(2):102-112.
70. Hiden U, et al. Insulin action on the human placental endothelium in normal and diabetic pregnancy. *Curr Vasc Pharmacol*. 2009;7:460-466.
71. Jiang ZY et al. Characterization of multiple signaling pathways of insulin in the regulation of vascular endothelial growth factor expression in vascular cells and angiogenesis. *J Biol Chem*. 2003;278(34):31964-31971.
72. Colomiere M et al. Defective insulin signaling in placenta from pregnancies complicated by gestational diabetes mellitus. *Eur J Endocrinol*. 2009;160(4):567-578.
73. Duran-Garcia S, Nieto JG, Cabello AM. Effect of gestational diabetes on insulin receptors in human placenta. *Diabetologia*. 1979;16(2):87-91.
74. al-Attas OS, al-Okail MS. Features of insulin receptor interaction in placenta from normal, overt and poorly controlled gestational diabetic patients. *Mol Cell Biochem*. 1993;126(2):135-142.
75. Roy MS et al. The ovine corticotropin-releasing hormone-stimulation test in type I diabetic patients and controls: suggestion of mild chronic hypercortisolism. *Metabolism*. 1993; 42(6):696-700.
76. Tomlinson JW et al. Impaired glucose tolerance and insulin resistance are associated with increased adipose 11beta-hydroxysteroid dehydrogenase type 1 expression and elevated hepatic 5alpha-reductase activity. *Diabetes*. 2008;57(10):2652-2660.
77. Mamula PW et al. Regulating insulin-receptor-gene expression by differentiation and hormones. *Diabetes Care*. 1990;13(3):288-301.
78. Barbour LA, et al. Cellular mechanisms for insulin resistance in normal pregnancy and gestational diabetes. *Diabetes Care*. 2007;30(suppl 2):S112-S119.
79. Kautzky-Willer A et al. Increased plasma leptin in gestational diabetes. *Diabetologia*. 2001;44(2):164-172.
80. Howard JK, Flier JS. Attenuation of leptin and insulin signaling by SOCS proteins. *Trends Endocrinol Metab*. 2006;17(9):365-371.

81. Kirwan JP et al. TNF-alpha is a predictor of insulin resistance in human pregnancy. *Diabetes*. 2002;51(7):2207-2213.
82. Tomazic M et al. Comparison of alterations in insulin signalling pathway in adipocytes from Type II diabetic pregnant women and women with gestational diabetes mellitus. *Diabetologia*. 2002;45(4):502-508.
83. Shao J et al. Decreased insulin receptor tyrosine kinase activity and plasma cell membrane glycoprotein-1 overexpression in skeletal muscle from obese women with gestational diabetes mellitus (GDM): evidence for increased serine/threonine phosphorylation in pregnancy and GDM. *Diabetes*. 2000;49(4):603-610.
84. Alonso A et al. Effects of gestational diabetes mellitus on proteins implicated in insulin signaling in human placenta. *Gynecol Endocrinol*. 2006;22(9):526-535.
85. Van Obberghen E et al. Surfing the insulin signaling web. *Eur J Clin Invest*. 2001;31(11):966-977.
86. Withers DJ et al. Disruption of IRS-2 causes type 2 diabetes in mice. *Nature*. 1998; 391(6670):900-904.

What Causes Gestational Diabetes? 8

Thomas A. Buchanan and Anny H. Xiang

8.1 Introduction

Gestational diabetes mellitus (GDM) is hyperglycemia that is first detected during pregnancy. Like other forms of hyperglycemia, GDM is characterized by an insulin supply that is insufficient to meet the body's insulin needs. The causes of an insufficient insulin supply reflect the causes of hyperglycemia in general, including autoimmune disease, monogenic causes, and insulin resistance. The hyperglycemia that characterizes GDM is often, although not always less severe than the hyperglycemia that defines diabetes outside of pregnancy. Thus, GDM often represents an early manifestation of diabetes in evolution. As such, GDM provides an opportunity to study diabetes in evolution to develop and test strategies for diabetes prevention.

8.2 Detection: Population Screening for Glucose Intolerance

The clinical detection of GDM is generally accomplished by applying one or more of the following procedures: (a) clinical risk assessment, (b) glucose tolerance screening, and (c) formal glucose tolerance testing. The procedures are applied to pregnant women not already known to have diabetes. Criteria used to make the diagnosis vary from region to region, but may soon be standardized as a result of the Hyperglycemia and Adverse Pregnancy Outcomes (HAPO) study,[1] a chapter on which appears in this book. Importantly, GDM screening is one of the very few times when glucose intolerance is assessed in a

T.A. Buchanan (✉)
Departments of Medicine, Obstetrics and Gynecology, and Physiology and Biophysics, Keck School of Medicine, University of Southern California, 1500 San Pablo Street, Los Angeles, CA 90033, USA
e-mail: buchanan@usc.edu

C. Kim and A. Ferrara (eds.), *Gestational Diabetes During and After Pregnancy*, DOI: 10.1007/978-1-84882-120-0_8, © Springer-Verlag London Limited 2010

large number of otherwise healthy individuals. Screening identifies relatively young individuals whose glucose levels are in the upper end of the population distribution during pregnancy. A few of those women have glucose levels that would be diagnostic of diabetes outside of pregnancy. The remainder have lower glucose levels, but are nonetheless at high risk for developing worsening hyperglycemia and diabetes after pregnancy.

8.3 Glucose Regulation in Pregnancy and GDM

Pregnancy is normally attended by progressive insulin resistance. It begins near mid-pregnancy and progresses through the third trimester to levels that approximate the insulin resistance seen in type 2 diabetes. The insulin resistance of pregnancy may result from a combination of increased maternal adiposity and the insulin-desensitizing effects of placental products such as human placental lactogen,[2] placental growth hormone,[3,4] and tumor necrosis factor alpha.[5] Studies by Friedman et al[6] indicate that, at the cellular level in skeletal muscle, the insulin resistance of pregnancy results from multiple changes in the insulin signaling pathway starting with impaired activation of the insulin receptor by insulin. Women with GDM have additional changes (e.g., serine phosphorylation of insulin receptor substrate-1) that downregulate insulin signaling in a manner typically seen in obesity.

Pancreatic β-cells normally increase their insulin secretion to compensate for the insulin resistance of pregnancy. As a result, changes in circulating glucose levels over the course of pregnancy are quite small compared to the large changes in insulin sensitivity. This plasticity of β-cell function in the face of progressive insulin resistance is the hallmark of normal glucose regulation during pregnancy.

GDM results from an endogenous insulin supply that is inadequate to meet tissue insulin demands. It has long been thought and taught that GDM occurs in women who are not able to increase their insulin supply as demands rise during pregnancy. Serial studies of insulin sensitivity and secretion during and after pregnancy in normal women, and in women with GDM (Fig. 8.1) now reveal this assumption to be false. The curved lines in Fig. 8.1 represent reciprocal relationships between insulin sensitivity and insulin secretion, reflecting β-cell compensation for insulin resistance as described by Bergman.[7] In normal women, insulin secretion moves along one curve as insulin sensitivity changes. Women with GDM move as well, but along a curve that reflects lower secretion for any degree of insulin sensitivity.

As the data described below indicate, the routine glucose screening that is used to detect GDM also detects women with chronic β-cell dysfunction, rather than development of relative insulin deficiency as insulin resistance increases during pregnancy. β-cell compensation for insulin resistance can be quantified as the product of insulin sensitivity and insulin response.[7] Compensation is reduced to a similar degree during and after pregnancy (Fig. 8.1, left, reductions of 39 and 47%, during and after pregnancy[8]; Fig. 8.1, right; reductions of 69 and 62%, respectively[9]). These findings are consistent with earlier studies.[10,11] Together, the available data indicate that GDM represents detection of chronic β-cell dysfunction, rather than development of relative insulin deficiency as insulin

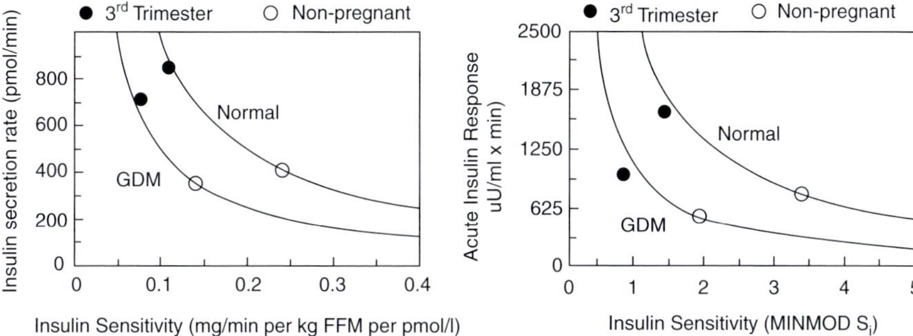

Fig. 8.1 *Left panel*: Relationships between pre-hepatic insulin secretion rates and insulin sensitivity measured during steady-state hyperglycemia (3-h, 180 mg/dL) in women with GDM ($n=7$) or normal glucose tolerance during pregnancy ($n=8$). Data are from Homko et al.[8] *Right panel*: Relationships between acute insulin response to intravenous glucose (AIRg) and insulin sensitivity (minimal model SI) Hispanic women with GDM ($n=99$) or normal glucose tolerance during and after pregnancy ($n=7$). Curved lines represent insulin sensitivity-secretion relationships defined by the product of sensitivity and secretion in each study group. Reproduced from Buchanan et al[9]

resistance increases during pregnancy. Thus, the routine glucose screening that is used to detect GDM also detects women with chronic β-cell dysfunction.

While the full array of causes of β-cell dysfunction in humans remains to be determined, clinical classification of diabetes mellitus outside of pregnancy is based on three general categories of dysfunction: (a) autoimmune, (b) monogenic, and (c) associated with insulin resistance. Each of these categories appears to contribute to β-cell dysfunction in GDM, as discussed in the next section.

8.4 GDM and Autoimmunity to β-cells

A small minority (≤10% in most studies) of women with GDM have circulating antibodies to pancreatic islets or to β-cell antigens such as glutamic acid decarboxylase.[12–18] Although detailed physiological studies are lacking in these women, they most likely have inadequate insulin secretion resulting from autoimmune damage to β cells. They have evolving type 1 diabetes that comes to clinical attention through routine glucose screening during pregnancy. Whether pregnancy initiates or accelerates islet-directed autoimmunity is unknown. The frequency of islet autoimmunity in GDM tends to parallel ethnic trends in the prevalence of type 1 diabetes outside of pregnancy. Patients are often, but not invariably, lean and of European ancestry. They can have a rapidly progressive course to overt diabetes after pregnancy.[14]

8.5 GDM and Monogenic Diabetes

Monogenic forms of diabetes follow two general inheritance patterns – autosomal dominant (Maturity Onset Diabetes of the Young or "MODY" with genetic subtypes MODY1, MODY2, etc.) and maternal (maternally inherited diabetes due to mutations in mitochondrial DNA). The age at onset/detection tends to be young relative to other forms of nonimmune diabetes and patients tend not to be obese or insulin resistant. Both features point to abnormalities in β-cell mass and/or function that are severe enough to cause hyperglycemia in the diabetic range. Mutations that cause several subtypes of MODY have been found in women with GDM: glucokinase (MODY 2),[13,19–21] hepatocyte nuclear factor 1α (MODY 3),[13] and insulin promoter factor 1 (MODY 4).[13] Mitochondrial gene mutations have also been found in small numbers of patients with GDM.[22] These monogenic forms of GDM appear to account for only a small fraction of cases of GDM.[13,19–22] They likely represent examples of preexisting diabetes that are first detected by routine glucose screening during pregnancy.

8.6 GDM in the Context of Chronic Insulin Resistance

Insulin Resistance: GDM is diagnosed during pregnancy, when insulin sensitivity is quite low in everyone. However, insulin resistance is slightly greater in women with GDM than in normal pregnant women.[15,23] The additional resistance occurs in glucose uptake (predominantly skeletal muscle),[10,15] glucose production (primarily liver),[10,15] and fatty acid levels (adipose tissue).[15] After pregnancy, insulin sensitivity rises to a greater extent in normal women than in women who had GDM. In addition, serial measurements of insulin sensitivity starting before pregnancy demonstrate insulin resistance before conception and at the beginning of the second trimester in women with GDM.[10,11]Thus, most women with GDM have a separate, chronic form of insulin resistance compared with normal women.[24–30]

Given that GDM represents a cross section of glucose intolerance in young women, mechanisms that lead to chronic insulin resistance in GDM are likely as varied as they are in the general population. Obesity is a common antecedent of GDM and many of the biochemical mediators of insulin resistance that occur in obesity have been identified in small studies of women with GDM or a history thereof. These mediators include increased circulating levels of leptin[31] and the inflammatory markers TNF-α[32] and C-reactive protein[33]; decreased levels of adiponectin[34,35]; and increased fat in liver[36] and muscle.[37] In vitro studies of adipose tissue and skeletal muscle from women with GDM or a history thereof have revealed abnormalities in the insulin signaling pathway,[6,38–41] abnormal subcellular localization of GLUT4 transporters,[42] and decreased expression of PPAR-γ,[38] over-expression of membrane glycoprotein 1,[40] all of which could contribute to the observed reductions in insulin-mediated glucose transport. The abnormalities in insulin signaling are the same ones reported in association with obesity, a common feature of women who develop GDM.

Due to the very small sample sizes in these in vitro studies, it is not clear whether any of these abnormalities represent universal or even common abnormalities underlying the chronic insulin resistance that is very frequent in GDM.

β-cell Compensation: There are two time frames in which β-cell compensation for insulin resistance must be considered in GDM. In the short term (months), women with GDM appear to be able to increase insulin secretion reciprocally to changes in insulin sensitivity (Fig. 8.1, references[8–11]). They do so along an insulin sensitivity-secretion relationship that are ~40–70% lower (i.e., 40–70% less insulin for any degree of insulin resistance) than the relationship in normal women. In the long-term (years), a large majority of women with GDM manifest progressive loss of β-cell compensation for insulin resistance (Fig. 8.2, left) that is associated with and most likely causes the progressive hyperglycemia that becomes diabetes (Fig. 8.2, right). Taken together, the short- and long-term characteristics of β-cell compensation in women with GDM are most consistent with chronically falling β-cell function that is identified "mid stream" along the progression to type 2 diabetes because routine glucose screening is applied during pregnancy.

The etiology of falling β-cell function that occurs against a background of chronic insulin resistance is not known. Two observations that we have made in Hispanic women with prior GDM indicate that insulin resistance may be an important cause of falling β-cell function. First, an additional pregnancy, which represents an additional period of severe insulin resistance, tripled the risk of diabetes after GDM even after adjusting for the impact of pregnancy on weight gain.[43] Second, treatment with insulin-sensitizing thiazolidinedione drugs slowed or stopped the loss of β-cell function, thereby delaying or preventing diabetes.[44–46] β-cell protection and diabetes prevention were closely related to reduced insulin secretory demands that occurred when insulin resistance was ameliorated. These findings suggest that Hispanic women who develop GDM do not tolerate high levels of

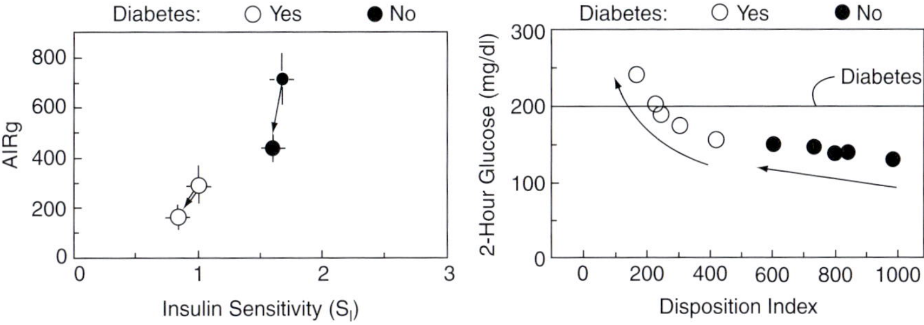

Fig. 8.2 *Left Panel*: Coordinate changes in S_I and AIRg, as defined in Fig. 8.1, in 71 nonpregnant Hispanic women with prior GDM. IVGTTs were performed at 15-month intervals for up to 5 years after index pregnancies. Symbols are mean (±se) values at initial and final visits. Median follow-up was 44 months in 24 women who developed diabetes and 47 months in 47 women who did not. Adapted from Buchanan et al.[9] *Right Panel*: Coordinate changes in β-cell compensation for insulin resistance (disposition index) and 2-h glucose levels from 75-g oral glucose tolerance tests in the same 71 women. Symbols represent mean data at 15-month intervals, ordered relative to final visits. Arrows denote direction of change over time. Adapted from Xiang et al.[61] Reproduced from Buchanan et al[9]

insulin secretion for prolonged periods of time. Chronic insulin resistance (e.g., from obesity) and short-term resistance (e.g., from pregnancy) increase demands, an effect which may cause loss of β-cell function. The biology underlying poor tolerance of high rates of insulin secretion remains to be defined. Likely candidates include susceptibility to β-cell apoptosis due to endoplasmic reticulum stress and abnormal protein folding,[47–49] islet-associated amyloid polypeptide, which is co-secreted with insulin and can be β-cell toxic,[50,51] and/or oxidative stress.[52] Of note, we have observed that changes in β-cell compensation have also been linked to weight gain, an effect that is explained by insulin resistance, reductions in the adipose tissue hormone adiponectin, and changes in C-reactive protein, a marker of low-grade inflammation associated with obesity. Thus, there may be many signals that, in combination with individual susceptibilities, promote the loss of β-cell mass and function that lead to type 2 diabetes.

8.7 Implications for Diabetes Prevention

In a minority of women diagnosed with GDM, hyperglycemia is already severe enough to meet criteria for diabetes outside of pregnancy. The rest (i.e., the majority) have a form of glucose intolerance that could be (a) limited to pregnancy, (b) chronic and stable, or (c) a stage in progression to diabetes. As reviewed by Kim et al,[53] long-term follow-up studies reveal that most, but probably not all women with GDM go on to develop diabetes outside of pregnancy (Fig. 8.3). Thus, in most women GDM is a stage in the evolution of diabetes mellitus, leading to recommendations that women with GDM be tested for diabetes soon

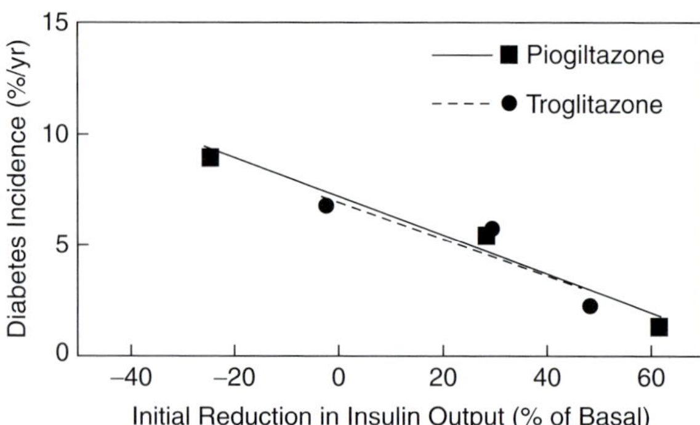

Fig. 8.3 Relationship between initial fractional reduction in insulin secretory demand and corresponding diabetes incidence rates during drug treatment in the troglitazone arm of the TRIPOD study (*round symbols*; median treatment 31 months) and in the PIPOD study (*square symbols*; median treatment 35 months). Insulin output was assessed as the total area under the insulin curve during intravenous glucose tolerance tests performed at enrollment and then at initial on-treatment IVGTT, which occurred after 3 months in TRIPOD and after 1 year in PIPOD. Symbols represent the low, middle and high tertiles of change in each study. Lines represent best linear fits of data for each study. Reproduced from Xiang et al[44]

after pregnancy and periodically thereafter. Optimal timing of such testing has not been established. Diabetes prevalence rates of ~10% in the first few months postpartum[54] support testing at that time. Diabetes incidence rates in the range of 5–10% per year (Fig. 8.3) support annual retesting. Oral glucose tolerance tests are more sensitive for detecting diabetes, as it is currently defined, than is measurement of fasting glucose levels.[55]

The type of diabetes that develops after GDM has generally not been rigorously investigated. It is reasonable to assume that the factors that contribute to poor β-cell compensation in GDM (discussed above) are likely to be involved in the pathogenesis of diabetes after GDM as well. Type 2 diabetes almost certainly predominates, given the overall prevalence of the disease in relation to other forms of diabetes and the fact that risk factors such as obesity, weight gain, and relatively older age are shared between GDM and type 2 diabetes. However, immune and monogenic forms of diabetes occur as well. These latter subtypes of diabetes should be considered in women who do not appear to be insulin resistant (e.g., lean patients). Antibodies to glutamic acid decarboxylase 65 (GAD-65) can be measured clinically and can identify women who likely have evolving type 1 diabetes. While there is as yet no specific intervention to delay or prevent that disease, patients should be followed closely for development of hyperglycemia, which may occur relatively rapidly after pregnancy.[14] If unrecognized and untreated, the condition can deteriorate to life-threatening ketoacidosis.

Clinical testing for variants that cause monogenic forms of diabetes is becoming available, but interpretation of the results can be complicated; consultation with an expert in monogenic diabetes is advised. Early-onset diabetes with an appropriate family history — autosomal dominant inheritance for MODY, maternal inheritance for mitochondrial mutations — may provide a clue to the presence of a monogenic etiology. Like autoimmune diabetes, there is no specific disease-modifying treatment for these forms of diabetes, although patients with MODY due to mutations in hepatic nuclear factor 1-alpha appear to respond well to treatment with insulin secretagogues.[56] Patients with mutations in glucokinase (MODY 2) tend to have a relatively mild and nonprogressive form of hyperglycemia. Also, their genetic information may be useful in future pregnancies. Fetuses who inherit the MODY 2 mutation are relatively resistant to the growth-promoting effects of maternal diabetes; they do not require the same aggressive glycemic management usually recommended for diabetic pregnancies.[57] Thus, genetic counseling may be appropriate for patients with monogenic diabetes and their families.

Results from the Diabetes Prevention Program (DPP), and the Troglitazone in Prevention of Diabetes (TRIPOD) and Pioglitazone in Prevention of Diabetes (PIPOD) studies suggest approaches that can be used to delay or prevent diabetes in women whose clinical characteristics suggest a risk of type 2 diabetes. In the DPP,[58] intensive lifestyle modification to promote weight loss and increased physical activity resulted in a 58% reduction in the risk of type 2 diabetes in adults with impaired glucose tolerance. GDM was one of the risk factors that led to inclusion in the study. Protection against diabetes was observed in all ethnic groups. Treatment with metformin in the same study also reduced the risk of diabetes, but to a lesser degree, and primarily in the youngest and most overweight participants. Analysis of data from parous women who entered the DPP with or without a history of GDM[59] revealed that (a) the women with prior GDM were younger than women with no history of GDM, (b) the women with prior GDM had a 60% greater cumulative incidence of diabetes after three years of follow-up, (c) intensive lifestyle modification reduced the risk of diabetes by a similar degree in women with and without prior GDM, and (d) metformin was more effective in reducing the risk of diabetes in women with a history of GDM than in women who had no such history (50 vs. 14% risk reductions, respectively).

In the TRIPOD study, assignment of Hispanic women with prior GDM to treatment with the insulin-sensitizing thiazolidinedione drug, troglitazone, was associated with a 55% reduction in the incidence of diabetes. As discussed above, protection from diabetes was closely linked to initial reductions in endogenous insulin requirements (Fig. 8.3) and ultimately associated with stabilization of pancreatic β cell function.[46] Stabilization of β cell function was also observed when troglitazone treatment was started at the time of initial detection of diabetes by annual glucose tolerance testing.[60]

In the PIPOD study, administration of another thiazolidinedione drug, pioglitazone, revealed a low diabetes rate and stabilization of β-cell function that had been falling during placebo treatment in the TRIPOD Study.[61] Again, there was a close association between reduced insulin requirements and a low risk of diabetes (Fig. 8.3). The DPP, TRIPOD, and PIPOD studies support clinical management that focuses on aggressive treatment of insulin resistance to reduce the risk of type 2 diabetes after GDM. Treatment options include weight loss and exercise, which compose the initial therapy of choice, and metformin and/or thiazolidinedione drugs if weight loss fails to prevent diabetes. Monitoring of glycemia (e.g., A1C levels) may be useful in assessing response to these interventions. However, the focus in this context is not a particular target A1C, as is the case for prevention of diabetic complications, but stabilization of A1C at a low risk level, reflecting stabilization of β-cell compensation for insulin resistance.

8.8 Summary and Future Directions

Available data suggest that GDM results from a spectrum of metabolic abnormalities that is representative of causes of hyperglycemia in relatively young individuals. In most women with GDM, the abnormalities are chronic in nature and detected by routine glucose screening in pregnancy. The abnormalities are frequently progressive, leading to rising glucose levels and, eventually, to diabetes mellitus. Thus, GDM can be viewed largely as diabetes in evolution that is detected during pregnancy. As such, GDM offers an important opportunity for the development, testing, and implementation of clinical strategies for diabetes prevention.

Acknowledgments Work cited in this chapter was supported by research grants from the National Institutes of Health (R01DK46374, R01DK61628, and M01-RR00043), the American Diabetes Association (Distinguished Clinical Scientist Award to TAB), Parke-Davis Pharmaceutical Research (the TRIPOD study) and Takeda Pharmaceuticals North America (the PIPOD Study).

References

1. Metzger BE, Lowe LP, Dyer AR, et al. HAPO, Study Cooperative Research Group: Hyperglycemia and adverse pregnancy outcomes. *N Engl J Med*. 2008;358:1991-2002.

2. Beck P, Daughaday WH. Human placental lactogen: Studies of its acute metabolic effects and disposition in normal man. *J Clin Invest.* 1967;46:103-109.
3. Handwerger S, Freemark M. The roles of placental growth hormone and placental lactogen in the regulation of human fetal growth and development. *J Pediatr Endocrinol Metab.* 2000;13:343-356.
4. Barbour LA, Shao J, Qiao L, et al. Human placental growth hormone causes severe insulin resistance in transgenic mice. *Am J Obstet Gynecol.* 2002;186:512-517.
5. Kirwan JP, Haugel-De Mouzon S, Lepercq J, et al. TNF-alpha is a predictor of insulin resistance in human pregnancy. *Diabetes.* 2002;51:2207-2213.
6. Barbour LA, McCurdy CE, Hernandez TL, Kirwan JP, Catalano PM, Friedman JE. Cellular mechanisms for insulin resistance in normal pregnancy and gestational diabetes. *Diab Care.* 2007;30(Suppl 2):S112-S119.
7. Bergman RN. Toward a physiological understanding of glucose tolerance: minimal model approach. *Diabetes.* 1989;38:1512-1528.
8. Homko C, Sivan E, Chen X, Reece EA, Boden G. Insulin secretion during and after pregnancy in patients with gestational diabetes mellitus. *J Clin Endocrinol Metab.* 2001;86:568-573.
9. Buchanan TA, Xiang AH, Kjos SL, Watanabe RM. What is gestational diabetes? *Diab Care.* 2007;30(suppl 2):S105-S111.
10. Catalano PM, Huston L, Amini SB, Kalhan SC. Longitudinal changes in glucose metabolism during pregnancy in obese women with normal glucose tolerance and gestational diabetes. *Am J Obstet Gynecol.* 1999;180:903-916.
11. Catalano PM, Tzybir ED, Wolfe RR, et al. Carbohydrate metabolism during pregnancy in control subjects and women with gestational diabetes. *Am J Physiol.* 1993;264:E60-E67.
12. Petersen JS, Dyrberg T, Damm P, Kuhl C, Molsted-Pedersen L, Buschard K. GAD65 autoantibodies in women with gestational or insulin dependent diabetes mellitus diagnosed during pregnancy. *Diabetologia.* 1996;39:1329-1333.
13. Weng J, Ekelund M, Lehto M, et al. Screening for MODY mutations, GAD antibodies, and type 1 diabetes–associated HLA genotypes in women with gestational diabetes mellitus. *Diab Care.* 2002;25:68-71.
14. Mauricio D, Corcoy RM, Codina M, et al. Islet cell antibodies identify a subset of gestational diabetic women with higher risk of developing diabetes shortly after pregnancy. *Diab Nutr Metab.* 1992;5:237-241.
15. Xiang AH, Peters RK, Trigo E, Kjos SL, Lee WP, Buchanan TA. Multiple metabolic defects during late pregnancy in women at high risk for type 2 diabetes mellitus. *Diabetes.* 1999;48:848-854.
16. Catalano PM, Tyzbir ED, Sims EAH. Incidence and significance of islet cell antibodies in women with previous gestational diabetes. *Diab Care.* 1990;13:478-482.
17. Jarvela IY, Juutinen J, Koskela P, et al. Gestational diabetes identifies women at risk for permanent type 1 and type 2 diabetes in fertile age. *Diab Care.* 2006;29:612.
18. Lobner K, Knopff A, Baumgarten A, et al. Predictors of postpartum diabetes in women with gestational diabetes mellitus. *Diabetes.* 2006;55:792-797.
19. Kousta E, Ellard S, Allen LI, et al. Glucokinase mutations in a phenotypically selected multiethnic group of women with a history of gestational diabetes. *Diabet Med.* 2001;18:683-684.
20. Ellard S, Beards F, Allen LI, et al. A high prevalence of glucokinase mutations in gestational diabetic subjects selected by clinical criteria. *Diabetologia.* 2000;43:250-253.
21. Saker PJ, Hattersley AT, Barrow B, et al. High prevalence of a missense mutation of the glucokinase gene in gestational diabetic patients due to a founder-effect in a local population. *Diabetologia.* 1996;39:1325-1328.
22. Chen Y, Liao WX, Roy AC, Loganath A, Ng SC. Mitochondrial gene mutations in gestational diabetes mellitus. *Diab Res Clin Pract.* 2000;48:29-35.
23. Catalano PM, Tyzbir ED, Roman NM, Amini SB, Sims EA. Longitudinal changes in insulin release and insulin resistance in nonobese pregnant women. *Am J Obstet Gynecol.* 1991; 165:1667-1672.

24. Ward WK, Johnston CLW, Beard JC, Benedetti TJ, Halter JB, Porte D. Insulin resistance and impaired insulin secretion in subjects with a history of gestational diabetes mellitus. *Diabetes*. 1985;34:861-869.
25. Ward WK, Johnston CLW, Beard JC, Benedetti TJ, Porte D Jr. Abnormalities of islet *B*cell function, insulin action and fat distribution in women with a history of gestational diabetes: relation to obesity. *J Clin Endocrinol Metab*. 1985;61:1039-1045.
26. Catalano PM, Bernstein IM, Wolfe RR, Srikanta S, Tyzbir E, Sims EAH. Subclinical abnormalities of glucose metabolism in subjects with previous gestational diabetes. *Am J Obstet Gynecol*. 1986;155:1255-1263.
27. Ryan EA, Imes S, Liu D, et al. Defects in insulin secretion and action in women with a history of gestational diabetes. *Diabetes*. 1995;44:506-512.
28. Kautzky-Willer A, Prager R, Waldhausl W, et al. Pronounced insulin resistance and inadequate betacell secretion characterize lean gestational diabetes during and after pregnancy. *Diab Care*. 1997;20:1717-1723.
29. Damm P, Vestergaard H, Kuhl C, Pedersen O. Impaired insulin-stimulated nonoxidative glucose metabolism in glucose-tolerant women with previous gestational diabetes. *Am J Obstet Gynecol*. 1996;174:722-729.
30. Osei K, Gaillard TR, Schuster DP. History of gestational diabetes leads to distinct metabolic alterations in nondiabetic African-American women with a parental history of type 2 diabetes. *Diab Care*. 1998;21:1250-1257.
31. Kautzky-Willer A, Pacini G, Tura A, et al. Increased plasma leptin in gestational diabetes. *Diabetologia*. 2001;44:164-172.
32. Winkler G, Cseh K, Baranyi E, et al. Tumor necrosis factor system and insulin resistance in gestational diabetes. *Diab Res Clin Pract*. 2002;56:93-99.
33. Retnakaran R, Hanley AJ, Raif N, Connelly PW, Sermer M, Zinman B. C-reactive protein and gestational diabetes: the central role of maternal obesity. *J Clin Endocrinol Metab*. 2003; 88:3507-3512.
34. Retnakaran R, Hanley AJ, Raif N, Connelly PW, Sermer M, Zinman B. Reduced adiponectin concentration in women with gestational diabetes: a potential factor in progression to type 2 diabetes. *Diab Care*. 2004;27:799-800.
35. Williams MA, Qiu C, Muy-Rivera M, Vadachkoria S, Song T, Luthy DA. Plasma adiponectin concentrations in early pregnancy and subsequent risk of gestational diabetes mellitus. *J Clin Endocrinol Metab*. 2004;89:2306-2311.
36. Tiikkainen M, Tamminen M, Hakkinen AM, et al. Liver-fat accumulation and insulin resistance in obese women with previous gestational diabetes. *Obes Res*. 2002;10:859-867.
37. Kautzky-Willer A, Krssak M, Winzer C, et al. Increased intramyocellular lipid concentration identifies impaired glucose metabolism in women with previous gestational diabetes. *Diabetes*. 2003;52(2):244-251.
38. Catalano PM, Nizielski SE, Shao J, Preston L, Qiao L, Friedman JE. Downregulated IRS-1 and PPARgamma in obese women with gestational diabetes: relationship to FFA during pregnancy. *Am J Physiol*. 2002;282:E522-E533.
39. Shao J, Yamashita H, Qiao L, Draznin B, Friedman JE. Phosphatidylinositol 3-kinase redistribution is associated with skeletal muscle insulin resistance in gestational diabetes mellitus. *Diabetes*. 2002;51:19-29.
40. Shao J, Catalano PM, Yamashita H, et al. Decreased insulin receptor tyrosine kinase activity and plasma cell membrane glycoprotein-1 over expression in skeletal muscle from obese women with gestational diabetes (GDM): evidence for increased serine/threonine phosphorylation in pregnancy and GDM. *Diabetes*. 2000;49:603-610.
41. Friedman JE, Ishizuka T, Shao J, et al. Impaired glucose transport and insulin receptor tyrosine phosphorylation in skeletal muscle from obese women with gestational diabetes. *Diabetes*. 1999;48:1807-1814.

42. Garvey WT, Maianu L, Zhu JH, et al. Multiple defects in the adipocyte glucose transport system cause cellular insulin resistance in gestational diabetes. *Diabetes*. 1993;42:1773-1785.
43. Peters RK, Kjos SL, Xiang A, Buchanan TA. Long-term diabetogenic effect of a single pregnancy in women with prior gestational diabetes mellitus. *Lancet*. 1996;347:227-230.
44. Xiang AH, Peters RK, Kjos SL, et al. Effect of pioglitazone on pancreatic β-cell function and diabetes risk in Hispanic women with prior gestational diabetes. *Diabetes*. 2006;55:517-522.
45. Xiang AH, Peters RK, Kjos SL, et al. Pharmacological treatment of insulin resistance at two different stages in the evolution of type 2 diabetes: impact on glucose tolerance and β-cell function. *J Clin Endocrinol Metab*. 2004;89:2846-2851.
46. Buchanan TA, Xiang AH, Peters RK, et al. Preservation of pancreatic β-cell function and prevention of type 2 diabetes by pharmacological treatment of insulin resistance in high-risk hispanic women. *Diabetes*. 2002;51:2796-2803.
47. Cnop M, Welsh N, Jonas NC, Jorns A, Lenzen S, Eizirik DL. Mechanisms of pancreatic beta-cell death in type 1 and type 2 diabetes: Many differences, few similarities. *Diabetes*. 2005;54(Suppl 2):S97-S107.
48. Scheuner D, Kaufman RJ. The unfolded protein response: a pathway that links insulin demand with beta cell failure and diabetes. *Endo Rev*. 2008;29:317-333.
49. Eizirik DL, Cardoza AK, Cnop M. The role for endoplasmic reticulum stress in diabetes mellitus. *Endo Rev*. 2008;29:42-61.
50. Janson J, Soeller WC, Roche PC, et al. Spontaneous diabetes mellitus in transgenic mice expressing human islet amyloid polypeptide. *Proc Nat Acad Sci*. 1996;93:7283-7288.
51. Verchere CB, D'Alessio DA, Palmiter RD, et al. Islet amyloid formation associated with hyperglycemia in transgenic mice with pancreatic beta cell expression of human islet amyloid polypeptide. *Proc Nat Acad Sci*. 1996;93:3492-3496.
52. Fridlyand LE, Philipson LH. Reactive species, cellular repair, and risk factors in the onset of type 2 diabetes mellitus: review and hypothesis. *Curr. Diabetes Rev*. 2006;2:241-259.
53. Kim C, Newton KM, Knopp RH. Gestational diabetes and the incidence of type 2 diabetes. *Diab Care*. 2002;25:1862-1868.
54. Kjos SL, Buchanan TA, Greenspoon JS, Montoro M, Bernstein GS, Mestman JH. Gestational diabetes mellitus: the prevalence of glucose intolerance and diabetes mellitus in the first two months postpartum. *Am J Obstet Gynecol*. 1990;163:93-98.
55. Kousta E, Lawrence NJ, Penny A, et al. Implications of new diagnostic criteria for abnormal glucose homeostasis in women with previous gestational diabetes. *Diab Care*. 1998;22:933-937.
56. Pearson ER, Starkey BJ, Powell RJ, Gribble FM, Clark PM, Hattersley AT. Genetic causes of hyperglycaemia and response to treatment in diabetes. *Lancet*. 2003;362:1275-1281.
57. Spyer G, Hattersley AT, Sykes JE, Sturley RH, MacLeod KM. Influence of maternal and fetal glucokinase mutations in gestational diabetes. *Am J Obstet Gynecol*. 2001;185:240-241.
58. Diabetes Prevention Program Research Group. Reduction in the incidence of type 2 diabetes with lifestyle intervention or metformin. *N Engl J Med*. 2002;346:393-403.
59. Ratner RE, Christophi CA, Metzger BE, et al. Diabetes Prevention Program Research Group: Prevention of diabetes in women with a history of gestational diabetes: effects of metformin and lifestyle intervention. *J Clin Endocrinol Metab*. 2008;93:4774-4779.
60. Xiang AH, Peters RK, Kjos SL, et al. Pharmacological treatment of insulin resistance at two different stages in the evolution of type 2 diabetes: impact on glucose tolerance and beta-cell function. *J Clin Endocrinol Metab*. 2004;89:2846-2851.
61. Xiang AH, Wang C, Peters RK, Trigo E, Kjos SL, Buchanan TA. Coordinate changes in plasma glucose and pancreatic beta cell function in Latino women at high risk for type 2 diabetes. *Diabetes*. 2006;55:1074-1079.
62. Buchanan TA. Pancreatic B-cell defects in gestational diabetes: implications for the pathogenesis and prevention of type 2 diabetes. *J Clin Endocrinol Metab*. 2001;86:989-993.

Mechanisms Underlying Insulin Resistance in Human Pregnancy and Gestational Diabetes Mellitus

9

Carrie E. McCurdy and Jacob E. Friedman

Abbreviations

GDM	Gestational diabetes mellitus
IR	Insulin receptor
IRS1	Insulin receptor substrate
PI 3-Kinase	Phosphatidylinositol 3-kinase
T2DM	Type 2 diabetes mellitus
hPL	human Placental Lactogen
hPGH	human Placental Growth Hormone
GH	Growth hormone
HSL	Hormone sensitive lipase
PD3B	cAMP-Phosphodiesterase 3B
FFA	Free fatty acid
TG	Triglyceride
TNFα	Tumor necrosis factor alpha
IGT	Impaired Glucose tolerance
MAPK	Mitogen-activated protein kinase
PDK1	3-Phosphoinositide-dependent kinase
AMPK	Adenosine monophosphate kinase
PPARα	Peroxisome proliferator-activated receptor alpha
JNK1	cJun N-terminal kinase 1
NFkB	Nuclear factor kappa B
PKCθ	Protein kinase C theta
mTor	Mammalian target of rapamyacin

C.E. McCurdy (✉)
Department of Pediatrics, University of Colorado Denver,
School of Medicine, Aurora, CO, USA
e-mail: carrie.mccurdy@ucdenver.edu

C. Kim and A. Ferrara (eds.), *Gestational Diabetes During and After Pregnancy*,
DOI: 10.1007/978-1-84882-120-0_9,

9.1 Development of Insulin Resistance During Pregnancy

Pregnancy is characterized as an insulin resistant state. While 90–95% of all women retain normal glucose tolerance, approximately 5–10% develop GDM.[1,2] The development of insulin resistance during pregnancy is usually compensated by a considerable increase in insulin secretion. However, in women diagnosed with GDM, insulin resistance is more profound, and this challenge, combined with decreased pancreatic β-cell reserve, triggers impaired glucose tolerance.[3] Catalano et al reported the first prospective longitudinal studies in women with normal glucose tolerance using the euglycemic-hyperinsulinemic clamp.[4] There was a significant 47% decrease in insulin sensitivity in obese women during late pregnancy and 56% decrease in lean women during pregnancy compared to preconception.[4,5] Other investigators have reported that insulin sensitivity significantly decreased (40–80%) with advancing gestation.[6–8] Skeletal muscle is the principal site of whole-body glucose disposal, and along with adipose tissue becomes severely insulin resistant as gestation progresses. Using isolated skeletal muscle fibers from the rectus abdominis obtained during elective caesarian-section or other elective surgery, Friedman et al demonstrated that pregnancy results in a marked 40% reduction in insulin-stimulated glucose transport in skeletal muscle compared to obese nonpregnant women. This impairment is significantly worse in GDM subjects (65% reduced) compared with obese nonpregnant subjects.[9] These results are analogous to Garvey et al,[10] who measured glucose transport in isolated adipocytes and found a more severe decrease in glucose transport in obese GDM subjects, although these were compared with lean (nonobese) pregnant controls. Regarding basal endogenous (hepatic) glucose production, hepatic glucose output is less suppressed during euglycemic-hyperinsulinemic clamp in lean and obese with GDM compared with each control group.[4,5] Overall, these results indicate that all three major insulin target tissues including liver, skeletal muscle, and adipose tissue develop marked insulin resistance in women during normal pregnancy, and to an even greater extent in obese women with GDM.

9.1.1 Hormone and Metabolic Factors Contributing to Insulin Resistance in Pregnancy and GDM

Beginning in mid-pregnancy, placental-derived hormones reprogram maternal physiology to achieve an insulin resistant state, reducing insulin sensitivity ~50% in the last trimester (Fig. 9.1). These hormones also contribute to altered β-cell function. Human placental lactogen (hPL) increases up to 30-fold throughout pregnancy and induces insulin release from the pancreas; studies outside of pregnancy find that they can cause peripheral insulin resistance.[11,12] Another major hormone implicated in insulin resistance during pregnancy is human placental growth hormone (hPGH). hPGH increases 6–8-fold during gestation and replaces normal pituitary growth hormone (GH) in the maternal circulation by ~20 weeks gestation.[13] Because hPGH is difficult to assay in human serum, and the gene is absent in other species, the potential role of hPGH in pregnancy-induced insulin resistance is not well studied. Much like the well documented effects of excess normal GH on insulin sensitivity however, over-expression

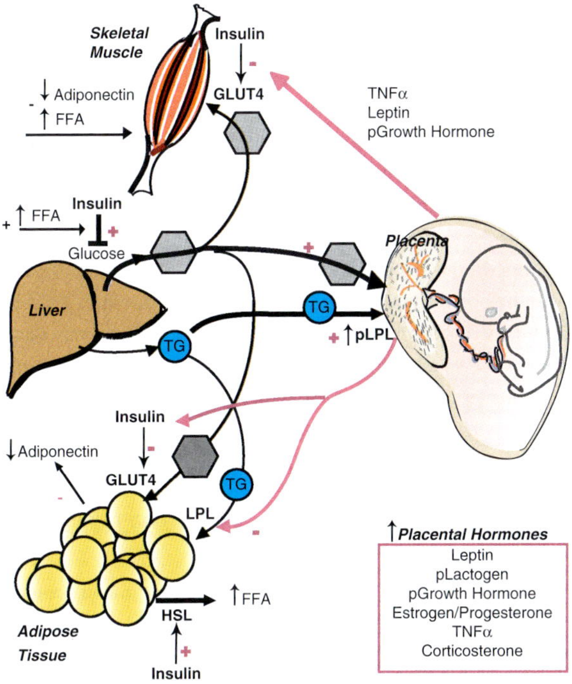

Fig. 9.1 A rise in placental hormones suppresses maternal insulin sensitivity to shuttle necessary fuels to the fetus. Increased production of placental hormones, including pGrowth Hormone, pLactogen, leptin, and potentially TNFα, act on maternal insulin-responsive tissues, the liver, skeletal muscle, and adipose tissue, to decrease insulin responsiveness. In adipose tissue, insulin's ability to suppress hormone-sensitive lipase (HSL) and stimulate adipose tissue LPL activity results in increased maternal free fatty acids (FFA) and a production of maternal triglycerides (TG) to the placenta for fetal use. In addition to placental hormones, the increased flux of FFA from maternal adipose tissue negatively impacts insulin signaling in both liver and skeletal muscle. In skeletal muscle, there is a reduction in insulin-stimulated glucose uptake and, in the liver, insulin fails to suppress glucose production. In combination, the insulin resistance in maternal liver and skeletal muscle in late pregnancy accelerates fuel availability to the fetus. In GDM, prior insulin resistance is compounded by the normal insulin resistance of pregnancy, resulting in a greater shunting of excess fuels to the fetus, which can lead to fetal overgrowth

of hPGH in transgenic mice comparable to levels seen in the third trimester of pregnancy causes severe peripheral insulin resistance.[14] The impact of hPGH on the insulin signaling cascade in skeletal muscle has been studied in vivo and in vitro in both skeletal muscle and adipose tissue, and appears to interfere with insulin signaling by a unique mechanism involving PI 3-kinase,[15–17] as discussed below. One other potentially important hormone, which increases about 2.5-fold in pregnancy, is maternal cortisol.[18] Glucocorticoids are well known to interfere with insulin signaling in skeletal muscle by postreceptor mechanisms and could, in addition to hPGH, be involved in suppressing insulin sensitivity in pregnancy.[19]

Similar to its effect on skeletal muscle, placental hormones interfere with insulin-stimulated glucose uptake into adipose tissue for esterification, as well as interfere with insulin's ability to suppress lipolysis through the enzyme hormone-sensitive lipase (HSL).[20] The normal suppression of lipolysis involves insulin-mediated phosphorylation of cAMP-phosphodiesterase 3B (PDE3B), which causes a reduction in cAMP levels to suppress lipolysis. The decrease in cAMP levels inhibits the activity of HSL, thereby reducing triglyceride (TG) breakdown in adipocytes, principally during early pregnancy. In late pregnancy, failure to fully inhibit lipolysis results in increased release of free fatty acids (FFA), which in obese individuals with GDM results in elevated fasting FFA.[20] Thus, insulin resistance in adipose tissues plays an important role in increasing circulating FFA that can accumulate in nonadipose depots, like skeletal muscle and the liver, enhancing insulin resistance in the mother, as well as providing fuel for the growth of the fetus. In women with pre-existing obesity, insulin resistance prior to gestation worsens further during pregnancy and this can lead to an elevation in maternal/fetal TG, which may play an important role in excessive adiposity in babies born to overweight/obese mothers.[21]

9.1.2 New Factors Involved in Insulin Resistance in Pregnancy

During pregnancy, the placenta and adipose tissue become significant sources of many cytokines and adipocytokines, whose expression is dysregulated by maternal diabetes and obesity.[22,23] Tumor necrosis factor alpha (TNF-α) is a cytokine produced not only from monocytes and macrophages within the adipocyte, but from T cells, neutrophils, and fibroblasts within the placenta. Obese animals and humans show a positive correlation between TNF-α levels and body mass index (BMI) and hyperinsulinemia.[24,25] Infusion of TNFα, results in increased insulin resistance in rat and in human skeletal muscle cells incubated in culture.[26,27] Although the concentration of circulating TNFα in plasma of obese patients is extremely low compared with that found in burn patients and patients with cachexia, recent evidence indicates that skeletal muscle expresses TNFα mRNA and that it may act in a paracrine fashion.[26,27] Studies report that changes in insulin sensitivity from early (22–24w) to late gestation (34–36w) are correlated with changes in plasma TNFα (r=0.45) and that circulating TNFα may be produced by the placenta to exacerbate insulin resistance, through mechanisms discussed below. Lastly, there appears to be a local fivefold increase in TNFα mRNA in skeletal muscle from obese women with GDM that persists postpartum which could be involved in producing chronic local subclinical inflammation and insulin resistance in this population.[28]

Adiponectin is a secreted globular protein synthesized exclusively in adipocytes and has been shown to correlate highly with whole-body insulin sensitivity through its receptors in skeletal muscle and liver.[29] Adiponectin can increase glucose uptake in skeletal muscle and suppress hepatic glucose production through its effect on stimulation of AMP Kinase.[30] Studies have also demonstrated that adiponectin stimulates fatty acid oxidation through activation of peroxisome proliferator-activated receptor alpha (PPARα) in liver and skeletal muscle.[31] Adiponectin levels are reduced in GDM patients, which could contribute to the reduced insulin sensitivity in women with GDM.[32]

Plasma leptin levels are elevated significantly in pregnant women compared with nonpregnant women.[33,34] Masuzaki et al found that plasma leptin levels were elevated significantly during second trimester and remained high during the third trimester.[35] Plasma leptin levels

24-h after placental delivery were reduced below those measured during the first trimester. Highman et al[34] showed that maternal plasma leptin increased significantly during early pregnancy, before any major changes in body fat and resting metabolic rate, suggesting that pregnancy is a leptin-resistant state. In humans, the higher leptin levels in umbilical veins than in umbilical arteries, and the marked decreased during the neonatal period, suggests that the placenta is one of the major sources of leptin in the fetal circulation.[36] This is in contrast to mouse and rat pregnancies, which show an increase in plasma leptin levels during pregnancy but no increase in leptin mRNA in the placentas,[37] suggesting that leptin production may be differentially regulated across species during pregnancy. Cord blood leptin levels are positively correlated with birth weight and ponderal index (kg/m^3), but also with length and head circumference.[38, 39] Cord leptin levels, but not insulin, were negatively related to weight gain from birth to 4 months.[38] Leptin may thus have an important role for fetal growth and maternal glucose metabolism. Whether leptin directly regulates fetal growth, or regulates insulin signaling and energy balance during pregnancy, remains an unanswered question.

9.1.3
Cellular Pathways Underlying Insulin Resistance in Pregnancy and GDM

In nonpregnant individuals, obesity is described as a low-grade inflammatory condition associated with an increased production of proinflammatory factors that originate from macrophage infiltration of adipose tissue.[40] Women with GDM, particularly those who are diagnosed early in pregnancy, have more severe insulin resistance that is not specifically related to pregnancy.[4, 5] Further, in women with a history of GDM, there is a significantly increased risk of the subsequent development of Type 2 diabetes (T2DM), estimated to be about 2–3% per year of follow-up.[41] Thus, it seems likely that in most women, GDM represents an unmasking of the genetic predisposition of T2DM, induced by the hormonal milieu of pregnancy, often together with the inflammatory state of obesity. This section will focus on the cellular impairments in insulin signaling underlying the insulin resistance of normal pregnancy and the mechanisms that define the excessive insulin resistance found in GDM.

9.1.3.1
The IR/IRS is a Critical Node in the Insulin Signaling Network and is Inhibited in Human Pregnancy and GDM

Insulin stimulates growth and affects metabolism through two major pathways: the mitogen-activated protein kinase (MAPK) and the phosphatidylinositol 3-kinase (PI 3-kinase) pathway. The MAPK pathway is mainly involved in insulin-mediated growth effects, while the activation of PI 3-kinase is critical for insulin-mediated metabolic effects like glucose uptake, glycogen synthesis, and regulation of protein translation initiation.[42] It should be noted that in states of insulin resistance, the mitogenic aspects of insulin signaling through the MAPK pathway is often not dampened, while insulin signaling through the PI 3-kinase pathway for glucose metabolism is severely impaired.[43] There are three major molecules/nodes involved in the insulin signaling pathway for glucose uptake in skeletal muscle and adipose tissue, and for insulin suppression of lipolysis in adipose tissue and suppression of hepatic glucose production. A critical node is defined as a point in a signaling network that is essential for the biological function of receptor signaling pathway but also allows for crosstalk between pathways that can fine-tune the response to insulin.[44]

The insulin receptor (IR)/insulin receptor substrate (IRS) tandem is the first critical node in the insulin signaling cascade (Fig. 9.2a). The IR is composed of two extracellular alpha subunits, each linked by disulfide bonds to an intracellular beta subunit that can act as a tyrosine kinase. Insulin binding causes a conformational change in the IR and leads activation and auto (self) phosphorylation of the beta subunit of the IR. The autophosphorylation of the IR on tyrosine leads to recruitment and binding of intracellular substrates. Six of the known substrates belong to the IRS protein family, which bind to IR via pleckstrin-homology and phosphotyrosine-binding domains. IRS proteins (IRS1–6) have unique tissue distribution and signaling functions.[45] IRS1 and IRS2 are the mostly widely distributed, with IRS1 playing a major role in skeletal muscle and adipose signaling for glucose transport. Once insulin binds, the IRS is recruited to bind to the IR, and IRS proteins are tyrosine phosphorylated on up to 20 known sites, thereby serving as large docking proteins for subsequent downstream targets of the IR.

Initial studies of mechanisms for pregnancy induced insulin resistance investigated the IR/IRS critical node. Most studies have found no significant decrease in insulin ability to bind its receptor and no decrease in IR abundance in pregnancy or GDM.[46, 47] However, in both pregnant rats and in obese pregnant humans, there is a significant decrease in insulin-stimulated tyrosine phosphorylation (activation) of the IR and in IRS1.[9, 47] In GDM, compared with normal pregnancy, tyrosine phosphorylation of IR and IRS1 was even further reduced.[9, 48] The decrease in tyrosine phosphorylation of IR and IRS1 in response to insulin during pregnancy is likely due to impaired IR tyrosine kinase activity as opposed to upregulation of a protein tyrosine phosphatase that dephosphorylate these proteins.[48-50] The reduction in IR activity is reversible postpartum in women with normal glucose tolerance, but not obese GDM subjects who continue to gain weight postpartum.[28, 51]

9.1.3.2 Negative Regulation of Insulin Signaling by Serine Phosphorylation at IR and IRS in Pregnancy and GDM

In contrast to phosphorylation on tyrosine, phosphorylation at serine residues on both IR and IRS proteins dampen the insulin signaling cascade by three mechanisms (Fig. 9.2b): (1) chronic serine phosphorylation can induce a conformational change in the IR or IRS that prevents ATP from phosphorylating tyrosine residues on the IR/IRS necessary for full activity, (2) the reduced level of tyrosine phosphorylation prevents association between IR/IRS and docking of PI 3-kinase to IRS, and (3) increased serine phosphorylation on IRS can trigger IRS protein degradation by the proteosomal degradation pathway.[52,53]

Using an in vitro assay on isolated IR from skeletal muscle that were pretreated with an alkaline phosphatase to dephosphorylate serine/threonine residues, there was a significant improvement in insulin's ability to stimulate tyrosine kinase activity in IR from skeletal muscle of obese pregnant and GDM women.[48] This implicates excessive serine phosphorylation as

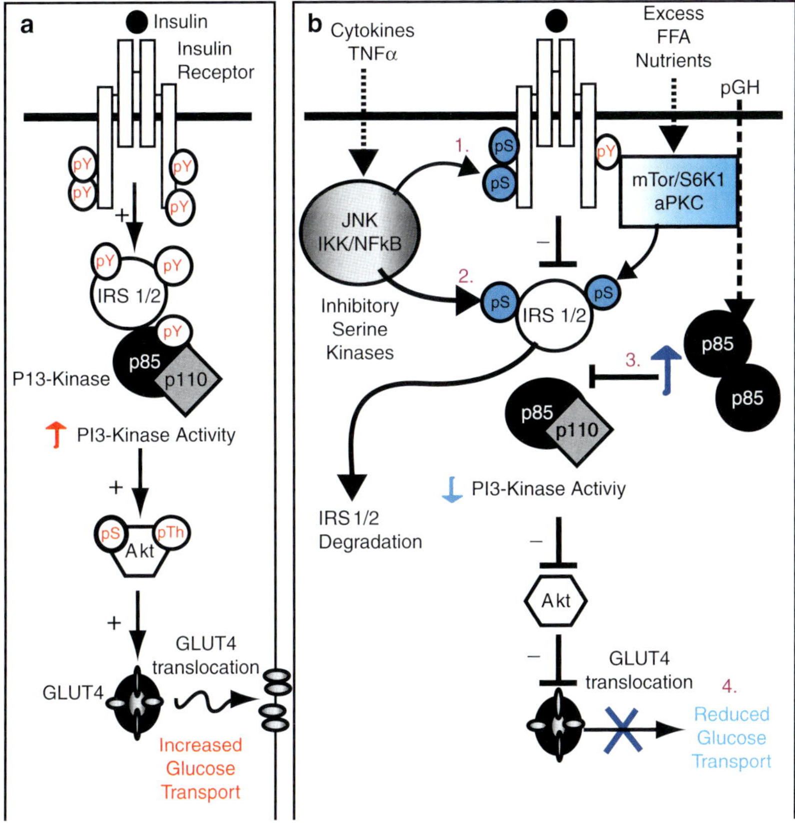

Fig. 9.2 Insulin signaling for glucose uptake. (**a**) Insulin binds to its receptor causing a conformational change in the receptor that activates its intrinsic tyrosine kinase activity. Activation of the tyrosine kinase leads to auto-phosphorylates on tyrosine residues of the beta-chain of the insulin receptor (IR). Tyrosine phosphorylation of IR recruits IR substrate 1/2 (IRS1/2) proteins to bind at these tyrosine residues on IR. IRS proteins are then phosphorylated on tyrosine residues by IR and act as large docking proteins for downstream signaling. The key regulatory (p85) subunit of PI 3-kinase (p85–p110) binds to tyrosine phosphorylated IRS allowing IR to tyrosine phosphorylate p85 and activate the catalytic (p110) subunit. Increased PI 3-kinase activity leads to activation of several downstream signaling proteins which phosphorylate and activate Akt. Akt activation is required for translocation of GLUT4 to the plasma membrane. Translocation of GLUT4 to the membrane allows glucose to enter the cells. (**b**) With GDM several of the key steps in insulin signaling for glucose transport are suppressed by a predominance of negative regulatory mechanisms. (Points 1/2) Serine phosphorylation of both the IR and IRS block tyrosine phosphorylation on IR and IRS1/2 leading to a decrease in IR-IRS1/2 association and recruitment of PI 3-kinase. Activation of serine kinases can be caused by an upregulation in inflammatory cytokines, like TNFα, or due to increased nutrient flux into the cell that can cause negative feedback on IRS-1. (Point 2) Increased serine phosphorylation on IRS1/2 promotes protein degradation and decreases the abundance of IRS1/2. (Point 3) In both pregnancy and GDM, pGH is upregulated, which increases the expression of the regulatory (p85) subunit of PI 3-kinase. Increased p85 competes with the enzymatically functional p85–p110 for binding sites on IRS1/2, thereby acting in a dominant negative fashion to dampen the effect of insulin to promote PI 3-kianse activity and, ultimately leading to (Point 4) a decrease in insulin-stimulated glucose uptake into skeletal muscle and adipose tissue

an underlying cause of the reduction in IR activity during pregnancy. Increased serine phosphorylation can be due to activation of a number of stress kinase signaling pathways induced by inflammatory cytokines or increased flux of fatty acids into cells. TNFα a potent activator of serine kinases in skeletal muscle, is increased in plasma during pregnancy, and is highly correlated with the severity of insulin resistance in pregnancy.[28, 54] Another possible mediator of serine kinase activation may be FFAs, which are elevated in pregnancy due to a failure to adequately suppress lipolysis late in pregnancy.[20, 55]

Increased basal serine phosphorylation of IRS1, specifically at IRS1 (S307 mice/S312 humans) has recently been observed in skeletal muscle from mouse and humans with GDM.[28,50,51] Although the specific serine kinase responsible for increased IR/IRS1 serine phosphorylation during pregnancy is not known, several possible candidates have been identified, including increased activation of JNK1 NFkB, PKCθ and p70 S6 Kinase.[53,56] In a genetic mouse model of spontaneous GDM (Lepr$^{db/+}$ heterozygous mouse), the increase in IRS1(S307/312) serine phosphorylation during pregnancy corresponded to an upregulation in basal and insulin-stimulated phosphorylation of p70 S6Kinase (Thr421/Ser424), but not PKCλ/ζ.[50] Similar results showing increased phosphorylation on IRS1(Ser307/312) and increased phosphorylation of p70 S6 kinase were reported recently in skeletal muscle biopsies obtained from pregnant GDM subjects compared with pregnant control subjects matched for obesity.[57] The increase in p70 S6 kinase 1 (S6K) is normally a major downstream effector of the mammalian target of rapamycin (mTOR) and PI 3-kinase pathway, primarily implicated in the control of protein synthesis, cell growth, and proliferation in response to insulin. However, S6K phosphorylation also operates, at least partly, by counteracting positive signals induced by hormones and nutrients and thus might be involved in suppressing IRS-1 function due to nutrient excess through serine phosphorylation of IRS1.[58,59]

The changes in IR and IRS1 observed in pregnancy are generally reversible in women who return to normal glucose tolerance postpartum, suggesting a pregnancy-specific mechanism.[51] However, the increase in IRS1 serine phosphorylation remained elevated in former GDM subjects with impaired glucose tolerance (IGT) postpartum.[28,57] Increased serine phosphorylation on IRS1 is associated with degradation of the protein in skeletal muscle[9,47,50] and in adipose tissue,[20] particularly in GDM subjects, and contributes to the severe insulin resistance to glucose uptake. Taken together, these data suggest that a persistence in IRS1 serine phosphorylation in skeletal muscle may underlie chronic insulin resistance in GDM women and, in some cases, is likely to underlie their increased risk for progression to type 2 diabetes.

9.1.3.3
PI 3-Kinase is Suppressed in States of Insulin Resistance by a Dominant Negative Mechanism

PI 3-kinase is a class IA heterodimer composed of a regulatory subunit that binds to IRS proteins and a catalytic subunit. There are at least five known protein isoforms of the regulatory subunit encoded on three separate genes that were identified by molecular weight (p85α and its splice variants p55α and p50α, p85β and p55γ) and three isoforms of the catalytic subunit (p110α, p110β and p110γ), all of which have unique tissue distribution and signaling functions.[60–62] The regulatory subunits p85α and p85β are ubiquitously expressed in tissues with the p85α subunit making up 65–75% of the regulatory subunit pool.[63] Interestingly, the pool of regulatory subunits exists in excess of the pool of catalytic subunits and because unbound p85α monomers compete for the same IRS1 binding sites as the holoenzyme (p85–p110), the monomers can inhibit PI 3-kinase activity by preventing binding of catalytically functional heterodimers (p85–p110). Therefore, the activity of the PI 3-kinase holoenzyme (and therefore insulin sensitivity) can be controlled by the ratio of the abundance of the regulatory to catalytic subunits. Thus, it was discovered that decreasing any of the regulatory subunits by genetic deletion in mouse models or by siRNA in cell models leads to enhanced PI 3-kinase activity and downstream signaling,[64,65] whereas an increase in the expression of p85α paradoxically reduces insulin-stimulated PI 3-kinase activity.[17,66] In human studies, p85α abundance is increased 1.5–2-fold in obese pregnant as compared with obese nonpregnant control in skeletal muscle and adipose tissue biopsies[9, 20,28] and returned to normal levels postpartum.[28,51] No difference was noted between control pregnant and GDM in the level of increase in p85α, suggesting the increased p85α is a mechanism for the normal insulin resistance of pregnancy. Interestingly, in transgenic mice engineered to over-express hPGH variant there is a lean phenotype with extreme insulin resistance.[14] This is associated with a significant increase in p85α subunit of PI 3-kinase and striking decrease in IRS-1-associated PI 3-kinase activity in skeletal muscle.[15] Conversely, mice with a heterozygous deletion of p85α are protected from GH-induced insulin resistance in skeletal muscle,[17] demonstrating that the level of p85α is inversely related to PI 3-kinase activity and insulin sensitivity. Thus, p85α may be acting as a dominant negative during pregnancy, and can be viewed as a potential nutrient or hormonal sensor in skeletal muscle.

9.1.3.4
Akt is the Third Critical Node in the Insulin Signaling Pathway

Perhaps the most critical mediator for insulin action immediately downstream of PI 3-Kinase is 3-phosphoinositide-dependent kinase 1 (PDK1), which is responsible for activation of Akt and aPKCζ. Akt (or PKB) is a serine/threonine kinase that signals most of insulin's metabolic actions downstream of PI3K, including activation of glucose transport, increasing protein synthesis and increasing glycogen synthesis in skeletal muscle, and suppression of gluconeogenesis in liver. In skeletal muscle and adipose tissue, insulin stimulates PI 3-Kinase to phosphorylate kinase 1 (PDK1), which is responsible for activation of Akt and aPKCζ. Activation of Akt requires phosphorylation of a threonine residue by PDK1 and a serine residue by the mTor/Rictor complex (mTORC1). There are three Akt isoforms (Akt1–3) with distinct but partially redundant signaling functions.[67] In contrast to the other isoforms, only loss of Akt2 function results in dysregulation of glucose metabolism and insulin resistance.[68-70] In signaling for glucose transport, Akt phosphorylates and inhibits AS160, a Rab-GTPase, permitting GLUT4 translocation to the plasma membrane. In skeletal muscle and adipose tissue from pregnant subjects, Akt levels are normal (unpublished observations), as are the levels of insulin-responsive glucose transporter GLUT4.[9]

9.2 Summary: Postpartum and Beyond

The impact of GDM on both the health of the mother and the offspring has been shown to last well beyond delivery. Women with a history of GDM are at much higher risk of developing T2DM,[41] while children born to these GDM mothers have an increased risk of childhood obesity and early onset of T2DM.[71,72] With GDM increasing rapidly due to the maternal obesity epidemic, identification of the major defects in the insulin signaling pathway during pregnancy is essential for understanding what factors (genetic and environmental) trigger excessive insulin resistance. These triggers may underlie excess fuel transfer to the fetus and the vicious cycle of maternal diabetes transmission to the offspring. Whether our efforts should be focused on reducing maternal adipose tissue inflammation or simply improving skeletal muscle insulin signaling as a therapeutic target is still an open question. Human studies have shown that a major defect in GDM involves the inability of insulin to stimulate glucose transport into skeletal muscle. The mechanisms for this severe insulin resistance are not completely understood, but involve a defect in the IR, IRS1, and an unknown post-receptor defect(s), perhaps caused by interaction between inflammation and serine kinases in skeletal muscle and adipose tissue. In obese women, there is an upregulation in inflammatory cytokines and adipokines that are thought to increase serine phosphorylation of the IRS proteins, while in women with GDM this defect is more severe and more likely to persist postpartum. Although potential candidates for both the inflammatory cytokine mediator(s) and the activated serine kinase have been identified, there is still very little understanding of what initiates these defects during pregnancy and beyond. A persistent dampening in skeletal muscle insulin signaling in cultured myocytes or adipocytes from GDM women, for example, would be an excellent candidate for a primary genetic or perhaps epigenetic mechanism that contributes to insulin resistance of GDM women. Future questions to be addressed include: What is the contribution of skeletal muscle TNFα production as a mechanism for greater insulin resistance in women with GDM? What is the role of the p70 S6 kinase-1 signaling pathway as a potential mediator of maternal insulin resistance independent of PI 3-kinase? Is the infiltration of macrophage into skeletal muscle or adipose tissue accelerated by pregnancy, and if so by what mechanism? Ultimately, answers to these questions should provide us with a better understanding of the cellular factors that trigger human GDM.

References

1. King H. Epidemiology of glucose intolerance and gestational diabetes in women of childbearing age. *Diabetes Care.* 1998;21(suppl 2):B9-B13.
2. Engelgau MM, Herman WH, Smith PJ, German RR, Aubert RE. The epidemiology of diabetes and pregnancy in the U.S., 1988. *Diabetes Care.* 1995;18:1029-1033.
3. Kuhl C. Insulin secretion and insulin resistance in pregnancy and GDM. Implications for diagnosis and management. *Diabetes.* 1991;40(suppl 2):18-24.

4. Catalano PM, Tyzbir ED, Roman NM, Amini SB, Sims EA. Longitudinal changes in insulin release and insulin resistance in nonobese pregnant women. *Am J Obstet Gynecol.* 1991; 165:1667-1672.
5. Catalano PM, Huston L, Amini SB, Kalhan SC. Longitudinal changes in glucose metabolism during pregnancy in obese women with normal glucose tolerance and gestational diabetes mellitus. *Am J Obstet Gynecol.* 1999;180:903-916.
6. Ryan EA, O'Sullivan MJ, Skyler JS. Insulin action during pregnancy. Studies with the euglycemic clamp technique. *Diabetes.* 1985;34:380-389.
7. Sivan E, Chen X, Homko CJ, Reece EA, Boden G. Longitudinal study of carbohydrate metabolism in healthy obese pregnant women. *Diabetes Care.* 1997;20:1470-1475.
8. Buchanan TA, Metzger BE, Freinkel N, Bergman RN. Insulin sensitivity and B-cell responsiveness to glucose during late pregnancy in lean and moderately obese women with normal glucose tolerance or mild gestational diabetes. *Am J Obstet Gynecol.* 1990;162:1008-1014.
9. Friedman JE, Ishizuka T, Shao J, Huston L, Highman T, Catalano P. Impaired glucose transport and insulin receptor tyrosine phosphorylation in skeletal muscle from obese women with gestational diabetes. *Diabetes.* 1999;48:1807-1814.
10. Garvey WT, Maianu L, Zhu JH, Hancock JA, Golichowski AM. Multiple defects in the adipocyte glucose transport system cause cellular insulin resistance in gestational diabetes. Heterogeneity in the number and a novel abnormality in subcellular localization of GLUT4 glucose transporters. *Diabetes.* 1993;42:1773-1785.
11. Beck P, Daughaday WH. Human placental lactogen: studies of its acute metabolic effects and disposition in normal man. *J Clin Invest.* 1967;46:103-110.
12. Brelje TC, Scharp DW, Lacy PE, et al. Effect of homologous placental lactogens, prolactins, and growth hormones on islet B-cell division and insulin secretion in rat, mouse, and human islets: implication for placental lactogen regulation of islet function during pregnancy. *Endocrinology.* 1993;132:879-887.
13. Handwerger S, Freemark M. The roles of placental growth hormone and placental lactogen in the regulation of human fetal growth and development. *J Pediatr Endocrinol Metab.* 2000; 13:343-356.
14. Barbour LA, Shao J, Qiao L, et al. Human placental growth hormone causes severe insulin resistance in transgenic mice. *Am J Obstet Gynecol.* 2002;186:512.
15. Barbour LA, Shao J, Qiao L, et al. Human placental growth hormone increases expression of the p85 regulatory unit of phosphatidylinositol 3-kinase and triggers severe insulin resistance in skeletal muscle. *Endocrinology.* 2004;145:1144-1150.
16. del Rincon J-P, Iida K, Gaylinn BD, et al. Growth hormone regulation of p85{alpha} expression and phosphoinositide 3-kinase activity in adipose tissue: mechanism for growth hormone-mediated insulin resistance. *Diabetes.* 2007;56:1638-1646.
17. Barbour LA, Rahman SM, Gurevich I, et al. Increased P85alpha is a potent negative regulator of skeletal muscle insulin signaling and induces in vivo insulin resistance associated with growth hormone excess. *J Biol Chem.* 2005;280:37489-37494.
18. Hornnes PJ, Kuhl C. Gastrointestinal hormones and cortisol in normal pregnant women and women with gestational diabetes. *Acta Endocrinol Suppl (Copenh).* 1986;277:24-26.
19. Giorgino F, Almahfouz A, Goodyear LJ, Smith RJ. Glucocorticoid regulation of insulin receptor and substrate IRS-1 tyrosine phosphorylation in rat skeletal muscle in vivo. *J Clin Invest.* 1993;91:2020-2030.
20. Catalano PM, Nizielski SE, Shao J, Preston L, Qiao L, Friedman JE. Downregulated IRS-1 and PPARgamma in obese women with gestational diabetes: relationship to FFA during pregnancy. *Am J Physiol Endocrinol Metab.* 2002;282:E522-E533.
21. Schaefer-Graf UM, Graf K, Kulbacka I, et al. Maternal lipids as strong determinants of fetal environment and growth in pregnancies with gestational diabetes mellitus. *Diabetes Care.* 2008;31:1858-1863.

22. Hauguel-de Mouzon S, Guerre-Millo M. The placenta cytokine network and inflammatory signals. *Placenta* 2006;27:794-798
23. Stewart FM, Freeman DJ, Ramsay JE, Greer IA, Caslake M, Ferrell WR. Longitudinal assessment of maternal endothelial function and markers of inflammation and placental function throughout pregnancy in lean and obese mothers. *J Clin Endocrinol Metab.* 2007;92: 969-975.
24. Hotamisligil GS, Shargill NS, Spiegelman BM. Adipose expression of tumor necrosis factor-alpha: direct role in obesity-linked insulin resistance. *Science.* 1993;259:87-91.
25. Hotamisligil GS, Peraldi P, Budavari A, Ellis R, White MF, Spiegelman BM. IRS-1-mediated inhibition of insulin receptor tyrosine kinase activity in TNF-alpha- and obesity-induced insulin resistance. *Science.* 1996;271:665-668.
26. Ofei F, Hurel S, Newkirk J, Sopwith M, Taylor R. Effects of an engineered human anti-TNF-alpha antibody (CDP571) on insulin sensitivity and glycemic control in patients with NIDDM. *Diabetes.* 1996;45:881-885.
27. Frost RA, Lang CH. Skeletal muscle cytokines: regulation by pathogen-associated molecules and catabolic hormones. *Curr Opin Clin Nutr Metab Care.* 2005;8:255-263.
28. Friedman JE, Kirwan JP, Jing M, Presley L, Catalano PM. Increased skeletal muscle tumor necrosis factor-{alpha} and impaired insulin signaling persist in obese women with gestational diabetes mellitus 1 year postpartum. *Diabetes.* 2008;57:606-613.
29. Weyer C, Funahashi T, Tanaka S, et al. Hypoadiponectinemia in obesity and type 2 diabetes: close association with insulin resistance and hyperinsulinemia. *J Clin Endocrinol Metab.* 2001;86:1930-1935.
30. Long YC, Zierath JR. AMP-activated protein kinase signaling in metabolic regulation. *J Clin Invest.* 2006;116:1776-1783.
31. Yamauchi T, Nio Y, Maki T, et al. Targeted disruption of AdipoR1 and AdipoR2 causes abrogation of adiponectin binding and metabolic actions. *Nat Med.* 2007;13:332-339.
32. Worda C, Leipold H, Gruber C, Kautzky-Willer A, Knofler M, Bancher-Todesca D. Decreased plasma adiponectin concentrations in women with gestational diabetes mellitus. *Am J Obstet Gynecol.* 2004;191:2120-2124.
33. Henson MC, Swan KF, O'Neil JS. Expression of placental leptin and leptin receptor transcripts in early pregnancy and at term. *Obstet Gynecol.* 1998;92:1020-1028.
34. Highman TJ, Friedman JE, Huston LP, Wong WW, Catalano PM. Longitudinal changes in maternal serum leptin concentrations, body composition, and resting metabolic rate in pregnancy. *Am J Obstet Gynecol.* 1998;178:1010-1015.
35. Masuzaki H, Ogawa Y, Sagawa N, et al. Nonadipose tissue production of leptin: leptin as a novel placenta-derived hormone in humans. *Nat Med.* 1997;3:1029-1033.
36. Yura S, Sagawa N, Mise H, et al. A positive umbilical venous-arterial difference of leptin level and its rapid decline after birth. *Am J Obstet Gynecol.* 1998;178:926-930.
37. Kawai M, Yamaguchi M, Murakami T, Shima K, Murata Y, Kishi K. The placenta is not the main source of leptin production in pregnant rat: gestational profile of leptin in plasma and adipose tissues. *Biochem Biophys Res Commun.* 1997;240:798-802.
38. Ong KK, Ahmed ML, Sherriff A, et al. Cord blood leptin is associated with size at birth and predicts infancy weight gain in humans. ALSPAC Study Team. Avon Longitudinal Study of Pregnancy and Childhood. *J Clin Endocrinol Metab.* 1999;84:1145-1148.
39. Tamura T, Goldenberg RL, Johnston KE, Cliver SP. Serum leptin concentrations during pregnancy and their relationship to fetal growth. *Obstet Gynecol.* 1998;91:389-395.
40. Schenk S, Saberi M, Olefsky JM. Insulin sensitivity: modulation by nutrients and inflammation. *J Clin Invest.* 2008;118:2992-3002.
41. Diabetes Prevention Program Research G. Reduction in the incidence of type 2 diabetes with lifestyle intervention or metformin. *N Engl J Med.* 2002;346:393-403
42. Shepherd PR, Withers DJ, Siddle K. Phosphoinositide 3-kinase: the key switch mechanism in insulin signalling. *Biochem J.* 1998;333(pt 3):471-490.

43. Cusi K, Maezono K, Osman A, et al. Insulin resistance differentially affects the PI 3-kinase- and MAP kinase-mediated signaling in human muscle. *J Clin Invest.* 2000;105:311-320.
44. Taniguchi CM, Emanuelli B, Kahn CR. Critical nodes in signalling pathways: insights into insulin action. *Nat Rev Mol Cell Biol.* 2006;7:85-96.
45. Kerouz NJ, Horsch D, Pons S, Kahn CR. Differential regulation of insulin receptor substrates-1 and -2 (IRS-1 and IRS-2) and phosphatidylinositol 3-kinase isoforms in liver and muscle of the obese diabetic (ob/ob) mouse. *J Clin Invest.* 1997;100:3164-3172.
46. Andersen O. Insulin receptor binding and glucose metabolism in normal human pregnancy and gestational diabetes mellitus. A review. *Dan Med Bull.* 1990;37:492-501.
47. Saad MJ, Maeda L, Brenelli SL, Carvalho CR, Paiva RS, Velloso LA. Defects in insulin signal transduction in liver and muscle of pregnant rats. *Diabetologia.* 1997;40:179-186.
48. Shao J, Catalano PM, Yamashita H, Ishizuka T, Friedman JE. Vanadate enhances but does not normalize glucose transport and insulin receptor phosphorylation in skeletal muscle from obese women with gestational diabetes mellitus. *Am J Obstet Gynecol.* 2000;183:1263-1270.
49. Shao J, Catalano PM, Yamashita H, et al. Decreased insulin receptor tyrosine kinase activity and plasma cell membrane glycoprotein-1 overexpression in skeletal muscle from obese women with gestational diabetes mellitus (GDM): evidence for increased serine/threonine phosphorylation in pregnancy and GDM. *Diabetes.* 2000;49:603-610.
50. Shao J, Yamashita H, Qiao L, Draznin B, Friedman JE. Phosphatidylinositol 3-kinase redistribution is associated with skeletal muscle insulin resistance in gestational diabetes mellitus. *Diabetes.* 2002;51:19-29.
51. Kirwan JP, Varastehpour A, Jing M, et al. Reversal of insulin resistance postpartum is linked to enhanced skeletal muscle insulin signaling. *J Clin Endocrinol Metab.* 2004;89:4678-4684.
52. Craparo A, Freund R, Gustafson TA. 14-3-3 (epsilon) Interacts with the insulin-like growth factor i receptor and insulin receptor substrate I in a phosphoserine-dependent manner. *J Biol Chem.* 1997;272:11663-11669.
53. Zick Y. Ser/Thr phosphorylation of IRS proteins: a molecular basis for insulin resistance. *Science's STKE.* 2005;2005:pe4
54. Kirwan JP, Hauguel-De Mouzon S, Lepercq J, et al. TNF-{alpha} is a predictor of insulin resistance in human pregnancy. *Diabetes.* 2002;51:2207-2213.
55. Sivan E, Homko CJ, Chen X, Reece EA, Boden G. Effect of insulin on fat metabolism during and after normal pregnancy. *Diabetes.* 1999;48:834-838.
56. Barbour LA, McCurdy CE, Hernandez TL, Kirwan JP, Catalano PM, Friedman JE. Cellular mechanisms for insulin resistance in normal pregnancy and gestational diabetes. *Diabetes Care.* 2007;30:S112-S119.
57. Barbour L, McCurdy CM, Hernadez, TL, et al. Reduced IRS1 and increased serine IRS1 phosphorylation in skeletal muscle of women with GDM. *Diabetes.* 2006;55(suppl 1):A39
58. Um SH, Frigerio F, Watanabe M, et al. Absence of S6K1 protects against age- and diet-induced obesity while enhancing insulin sensitivity. *Nature.* 2004;431:200-205
59. Um SH, D'Alessio D, Thomas G. Nutrient overload, insulin resistance, and ribosomal protein S6 kinase 1, S6K1. *Cell Metab.* 2006;3:393-402.
60. Shepherd PR, Nave BT, Rincon J, et al. Differential regulation of phosphoinositide 3-kinase adapter subunit variants by insulin in human skeletal muscle. *J Biol Chem.* 1997;272:19000-19007.
61. Inukai K, Funaki M, Anai M, et al. Five isoforms of the phosphatidylinositol 3-kinase regulatory subunit exhibit different associations with receptor tyrosine kinases and their tyrosine phosphorylations. *FEBS Lett.* 2001;490:32-38.
62. Brachmann SM, Ueki K, Engelman JA, Kahn RC, Cantley LC. Phosphoinositide 3-kinase catalytic subunit deletion and regulatory subunit deletion have opposite effects on insulin sensitivity in mice. *Mol Cell Biol.* 2005;25:1596-1607.
63. Lefai E, Roques M, Vega N, Laville M, Vidal H. Expression of the splice variants of the p85alpha regulatory subunit of phosphoinositide 3-kinase in muscle and adipose tissue of healthy subjects and type 2 diabetic patients. *Biochem J.* 2001;360:117-126.

64. Ueki K, Algenstaedt P, Mauvais-Jarvis F, Kahn CR. Positive and negative regulation of phosphoinositide 3-kinase-dependent signaling pathways by three different gene products of the p85alpha regulatory subunit. *Mol Cell Biol.* 2000;20:8035-8046.
65. Mauvais-Jarvis F, Ueki K, Fruman DA, et al. Reduced expression of the murine p85alpha subunit of phosphoinositide 3-kinase improves insulin signaling and ameliorates diabetes. *J Clin Invest.* 2002;109:141-149.
66. Bandyopadhyay GK, Yu JG, Ofrecio J, Olefsky JM. Increased p85/55/50 expression and decreased phosphotidylinositol 3-kinase activity in insulin-resistant human skeletal muscle. *Diabetes.* 2005;54:2351-2359.
67. Kim Y, Peroni O, Franke T, Kahn B. Divergent regulation of Akt1 and Akt2 isoforms in insulin target tissues of obese Zucker rats. *Diabetes.* 2000;49:847-856.
68. Cho H, Thorvaldsen JL, Chu Q, Feng F, Birnbaum MJ. Akt1/PKBalpha is required for normal growth but dispensable for maintenance of glucose homeostasis in mice. *J Biol Chem.* 2001; 276:38349-38352.
69. Bae SS, Cho H, Mu J, Birnbaum MJ. Isoform-specific regulation of insulin-dependent glucose uptake by Akt/protein kinase B. *J Biol Chem.* 2003;278:49530-49536.
70. Brozinick JT Jr, Roberts BR, Dohm GL. Defective signaling through Akt-2 and -3 but not Akt-1 in insulin-resistant human skeletal muscle: potential role in insulin resistance. *Diabetes.* 2003;52:935-941.
71. Dabelea D, Knowler WC, Pettitt DJ. Effect of diabetes in pregnancy on offspring: follow-up research in the Pima Indians. *J Matern Fetal Med.* 2000;9:83-88.
72. Dabelea D, Hanson RL, Lindsay RS, et al. Intrauterine exposure to diabetes conveys risks for type 2 diabetes and obesity: a study of discordant sibships. *Diabetes.* 2000;49:2208-2211.

Inflammation, Adipokines, and Gestational Diabetes Mellitus

10

Ravi Retnakaran

10.1 Introduction

In the past decade, advances in our understanding of the pathophysiology of type 2 diabetes (T2DM) have identified chronic subclinical inflammation and dysregulation of adipocyte-derived proteins (adipokines) as pathologic processes that may contribute to the development of metabolic and vascular disease. Characterized by abnormal circulating concentrations of inflammatory proteins and adipokines, these processes have been linked to both the underlying pathophysiology and development of incident T2DM. As such, they may be relevant to populations at high-risk of developing T2DM, such as women with GDM. In this chapter, we address the relationships between these factors and GDM, both during and after pregnancy. We begin by reviewing current concepts regarding inflammation and adipokines in relation to T2DM and the central role of obesity in this context. We then examine the growing body of evidence linking these factors to GDM and the associated implications for insulin resistance and pancreatic beta-cell function in pregnancy. Finally, we consider the limited data currently available from the postpartum period, which suggest that previous GDM may be associated with chronic subclinical inflammation and adipokine dysregulation. It emerges that inflammatory proteins and adipokines clearly warrant further study both during, and particularly after pregnancy complicated by GDM, as these factors may provide (1) insight into the pathophysiology of GDM and T2DM, (2) risk stratification of a patient population at high risk of developing future diabetes, and (3) potential therapeutic targets for the amelioration of this risk.

10.2 Pathophysiologic Similarity Between GDM and Type 2 Diabetes

As discussed in the preceding chapters, GDM and T2DM share considerable pathophysiologic similarity. In particular, both conditions are characterized by two main metabolic

R. Retnakaran
Leadership Sinai Centre for Diabetes,
Toronto, ON, Canada
e-mail: rretnakaran@mtsinai.on.ca

C. Kim and A. Ferrara (eds.), *Gestational Diabetes During and After Pregnancy*,
DOI: 10.1007/978-1-84882-120-0_10, © Springer-Verlag London Limited 2010

defects: (1) target cell resistance to the activity of insulin (*insulin resistance*) and (2) insufficient secretion of insulin by the pancreatic beta cells to compensate for this peripheral tissue resistance (*beta-cell dysfunction*).[1–3] Insight regarding the pathophysiology of T2DM may be relevant to GDM and vice versa.[4]

Consistent with its being a high-risk state for later T2DM, GDM is characterized by chronic insulin resistance and beta-cell dysfunction.[4] Normal pregnancy is characterized by progressive insulin resistance from mid-gestation onwards, with overall reductions in insulin sensitivity of 50–60%.[5] Women with GDM, however, have greater reductions in insulin sensitivity than do pregnant women with NGT.[6] This finding reflects these patients' chronic insulin resistance that likely exists prior to pregnancy and is known to persist postpartum.[4,7–10]

Against this background of insulin resistance, women with GDM have a chronic defect in beta-cell function.[4,11] In normal physiology, insulin secretion is linked to insulin sensitivity through a postulated negative feedback loop that allows the beta cells to compensate for any change in whole-body insulin sensitivity through a proportionate and reciprocal change in insulin secretion.[12–14] Accordingly, in pregnancy, the beta cells must increase their secretion of insulin in order to overcome declining insulin sensitivity and maintain normoglycemia. Women with GDM, however, have a chronic underlying beta-cell defect such that their compensatory increase in insulin secretion is not sufficient to fully offset the insulin resistance of pregnancy, resulting in the hyperglycemia that defines GDM.[4,11] Importantly, for women with a history of GDM, even in the postpartum when their glucose tolerance may appear to be normal, beta-cell function remains abnormal. This becomes apparent when insulin secretion is appropriately adjusted for ambient insulin resistance.[11]

10.2.1 Role of Obesity

Recognizing (1) that GDM is associated with subsequent T2DM and (2) that these two conditions share pathophysiologic similarity, research interest has focussed on risk factors linking GDM and T2DM, as these factors may provide insight relating to the development of both conditions.[4] Clinical factors that have been reported to predict the development of T2DM in women with a history of GDM include high prepregnancy body mass index (BMI), elevated fasting glucose and degree of hyperglycemia in pregnancy, earlier gestational age at diagnosis, recurrent GDM, nonwhite ethnicity, dysglycemia at 1–4 months postpartum, and additional pregnancies.[15–25] Of note, prepregnancy BMI is a particularly important risk factor, having emerged as the factor accounting for the highest attributable risk fraction in multivariate analysis.[25] As such, considerable attention has been focused on the pathologic effects of obesity and how they may relate to insulin resistance, beta-cell dysfunction, and the clinical development of GDM and T2DM. In this context, two pathologic sequelae of obesity have emerged as processes that may potentially link adiposity with the development of GDM and T2DM: (1) chronic subclinical inflammation and (2) dysregulation of adipokines.[26,27] These processes are characterized by abnormal serum concentrations of (1) inflammatory biomarkers, such as C-reactive protein (CRP) and (2) adipokines, such as adiponectin and leptin, respectively. These proteins have thus emerged as novel, nontraditional risk factors for T2DM (discussed in the next section) and GDM (discussed in Sects. 10.4 and 10.5).

10.3 Inflammatory Proteins and Adipokines as Nontraditional Risk Factors for T2DM

The emergence of inflammatory proteins and adipokines as novel risk factors for metabolic disease originated with recognition of their associations with T2DM. As such, before considering their relevance to GDM, it is informative to first review these associations with T2DM.

10.3.1 Inflammatory Proteins and T2DM

In the past decade, evidence has emerged indicating that obesity is a state of subclinical inflammation, as reflected by chronic, low-grade activation of the acute-phase response.[26, 28] The acute-phase response, as manifested by the dramatic change in serum concentration of certain proteins (acute-phase proteins) in the setting of stressors, such as inflammation and infection, is part of the innate immune system. In the short term, the acute-phase response has survival value in restoring homeostasis after environmental stress. Long-term activation of this system, however, has been proposed as an etiologic factor in disease, including T2DM and cardiovascular disease (CVD).[26]

It is now recognized that the expansion of visceral fat mass is associated with the infiltration of adipose tissue by macrophages, which may be recruited by adipocyte necrosis, hypoxia, or specific chemokines, such as monocyte chemo-attractant protein-1.[29] These macrophages release proinflammatory cytokines that act upon adipose tissue, ultimately resulting in the increased secretion of several inflammatory proteins, including interleukin-6 (the main upstream regulator of the hepatic acute-phase response) and CRP (the prototypical acute-phase protein). This adiposity-related inflammation may then be a factor that links obesity with increased risk of T2DM.

The suggestion that inflammation may play a role in the pathogenesis of T2DM is based on experimental, cross-sectional, and prospective evidence linking increased serum concentrations of acute-phase proteins, such as CRP, IL-6, and plasminogen activator inhibitor-1 (PAI-1), with the metabolic defects of hyperglycemia, insulin resistance, and overt T2DM.[26, 30–32] Indeed, several prospective studies have shown that elevated serum levels of CRP, IL-6, and PAI-1 can independently predict the development of incident T2DM in a variety of populations, including healthy middle-aged women (Women's Health Study), middle-aged men (West of Scotland Coronary Prevention Study), elderly subjects (Cardiovascular Health Study) and a large, multiethnic cohort (Insulin Resistance Atherosclerosis Study (IRAS)).[33–36] These associations linking CRP and incident T2DM have been robust to adjustment for typical diabetes risk factors, although it should be noted that in all but IRAS, the adjustment for obesity was made by accounting for BMI (which reflects total body adiposity), rather than waist circumference (i.e., which may better reflect visceral adiposity). In this context, it is noteworthy that, in IRAS, after adjustment for waist circumference and insulin sensitivity, the significant association between CRP and risk of diabetes was markedly attenuated, while PAI-1 remained an independent predictor of incident T2DM.[36] In general, these data are consistent with a model in which increased visceral fat is associated with subclinical inflammation that may then contribute to insulin resistance and the development of T2DM.

10.3.2 Adipokines and T2DM

Once considered a passive storage depot for triglycerides, adipose tissue is now recognized as an active endocrine organ, responsible for the secretion of several metabolically important proteins called adipokines. The growing list of adipokines includes adiponectin, leptin, tumor necrosis factor alpha (TNFα), retinol-binding protein-4 (RBP-4), resistin, and visfatin. In general, obesity is associated with dysregulation of the secretion of these proteins by adipose tissue, leading to their over-abundance in the circulation (with the notable exception of adiponectin, as discussed below) and potential pathologic effects.

One of the best-studied adipokines related to T2DM is adiponectin, a collagen-like plasma protein with putative insulin-sensitizing, antiatherogenic and anti-inflammatory properties.[37] Secreted exclusively by adipocytes, adiponectin circulates at relatively high concentration in oligomeric complexes, consisting of trimers, hexamers, and high-molecular-weight (HMW) multimers of 12–18 subunits.[38, 39] Unlike other adipokines, total serum adiponectin concentration (i.e., consisting of all multimeric forms) decreases as visceral fat mass expands.[40] Accordingly, central obesity, insulin resistance, and T2DM are all characterized by hypoadiponectinemia.[40–42] In a longitudinal investigation of adiponectin and the deterioration of glucose tolerance in rhesus monkeys, Hotta et al found that adiponectin levels begin to decline at an early stage in the pathogenesis of diabetes, in parallel with increases in adiposity and reductions in insulin sensitivity, and prior to the appearance of frank hyperglycemia.[43] Indeed, in human studies, low serum concentration of adiponectin has predicted the future development of insulin resistance in the Pima Indian population[44] and has been associated with beta-cell dysfunction in limited studies.[45, 46] Furthermore, hypoadiponectinemia has been shown to predict the future development of incident T2DM in various populations, including Pima Indians, Caucasians, Japanese, and South Asians.[47–50] Taken together, these data are consistent with a role for adiponectin deficiency early in the pathogenesis of diabetes.

Experimental evidence suggests that hypoadiponectinemia is a pathologic factor in diabetogenesis rather than a marker of risk alone. In animal models of obesity and diabetes, the administration of adiponectin has been shown to ameliorate insulin resistance, enhance hepatic insulin action, and lower glucose levels.[38, 51, 52] Furthermore, transgenic over-expression of globular adiponectin afforded diabetes-prone *ob/ob* mice protection from diabetes that was accompanied by enhancement of both insulin sensitivity and secretion, suggestive of improved beta-cell function.[53]

In contrast to adiponectin, circulating concentrations of other adipokines are increased in the setting of obesity. Leptin is an adipocyte-derived hormone that controls food intake and energy expenditure, with circulating levels that generally parallel fat stores.[29] While leptin also affects the reproductive and central nervous systems, the complex physiology of this hormone in relation to insulin sensitivity and beta-cell function remains to be fully elucidated. Similarly, TNFα is a multifunctional circulating cytokine that is upregulated in obesity and may have varying effects on insulin sensitivity in different tissues (e.g., muscle, liver, pancreatic beta-cells).[27] Circulating levels of the newer adipokines RBP-4 and resistin have also both been reported to be increased with obesity and linked to insulin resistance, although conflicting evidence exists regarding these associations.[29] Finally, the relationships between visfatin and both obesity and T2DM are similarly unclear, although recent evidence implicates a potential proinflammatory role for this adipokine.[54]

In general, in the setting of obesity, it is apparent that adipokine dysregulation and inflammation are not isolated processes, but rather are closely interrelated. For example, obesity is characterized by low circulating concentrations of adiponectin (which has putative anti-inflammatory activity) and increased levels of adipokines that have been linked to inflammatory effects (e.g. TNFα, resistin and visfatin). While our understanding of the relationships between these processes and T2DM continues to evolve, it should be noted that inflammation and adipokine dysregulation are both relevant to GDM as well, as will be reviewed in the following sections.

10.4 Inflammation During Pregnancy in Women with GDM

10.4.1 C-Reactive Protein and Other Inflammatory Proteins

As with T2DM, the strongest evidence linking inflammation to GDM is derived from studies of CRP. Indeed, prospective nested case-control studies in pregnancy cohorts have shown that increased CRP concentration in the first trimester is associated with a significantly increased risk of subsequent GDM.[55,56] Of note, in the Massachusetts General Hospital Obstetric Maternal Study, this association was attenuated by adjustment for BMI.[55] Increased serum CRP in women with GDM has also been reported in some,[57,58] although not all cross-sectional studies later in pregnancy.[59] These differing results may be due to changes in CRP levels late in gestation.[58] It is more likely, however, that these differences reflect the dominant effect of maternal obesity on circulating CRP levels, a consistent finding in previous reports.[55,59,60] Specifically, as may be anticipated based on the pathologic effects of adiposity discussed earlier, maternal obesity has emerged as a principal determinant of CRP concentration in pregnancy.[59]

Besides CRP, other markers of inflammation have also been linked to GDM. In first trimester, increased leukocyte count, an inflammatory marker previously associated with T2DM, has been shown to independently predict subsequent GDM.[61] In cross-sectional studies, upregulation of the proinflammatory cytokine IL-6 has been reported in women with GDM.[62,63] Increased ferritin early in pregnancy has been shown to predict subsequent GDM, although this relationship was again attenuated by adjustment for pregravid BMI.[64] In women from Hong Kong, the association between ferritin and GDM has been partly explained by maternal carriage of hepatitis B surface antigen.[65] Finally, heterozygosity for the 5G allele of the PAI-1 gene has been related to GDM, potentially consistent with a pathophysiologic role for PAI-1 in this setting.[66]

10.4.2
Pathophysiologic Implications of Inflammation in GDM

In the nonpregnant state, obesity-mediated subclinical inflammation is believed to contribute to insulin resistance.[28] Similarly, in pregnancy, CRP (principally driven by obesity, as noted above) has been linked to insulin resistance.[59] Indeed, after adjustment for covariates (including BMI), CRP concentration in pregnancy has been shown to be independently and significantly associated with fasting insulin, a surrogate measure of insulin resistance.[59] Overall, these data support a model in which maternal obesity mediates a chronic systemic inflammatory response, with possible downstream metabolic sequelae, including insulin resistance and gestational dysglycemia.[59]

10.5
Adipokines During Pregnancy in Women with GDM

10.5.1
Adiponectin and Other Adipokines

As with T2DM, low circulating adiponectin has been strongly linked to GDM. First, several clinical studies have demonstrated that serum levels of total adiponectin are decreased in women with GDM compared with pregnant women with normal glucose tolerance.[67–73] Furthermore, hypoadiponectinemia in the first trimester independently predicts the subsequent development of GDM later in the pregnancy, after adjustment for known GDM risk factors.[74] In addition, the high molecular weight (HMW) form of adiponectin has been specifically implicated in GDM.[75] In the nonpregnant state, it is believed that the insulin-sensitizing and antidiabetic activity of adiponectin is mediated by its HMW form. Consistent with this concept, the hypoadiponectinemia of GDM has been characterized by decreased levels of HMW adiponectin.[75] Overall, as with T2DM in the nonpregnant state, the relationship between decreased adiponectin and GDM has been consistent across numerous studies.

Interestingly, women of South Asian descent (who have a well-established increased risk of both GDM and T2DM) exhibit markedly decreased circulating levels of both total and HMW adiponectin in pregnancy, compared with Caucasian women.[76, 77] It has thus been hypothesized that hypoadiponectinemia may be a factor contributing to the increased metabolic and vascular risk faced by this patient population.[78]

There have been fewer studies addressing other adipokines in GDM, although their findings have been generally concordant with expectations. Indeed, women with GDM have been shown to exhibit increased circulating levels of TNFα.[62, 72] Similarly, recent reports have documented increased concentrations of RBP-4 in women with GDM compared with their peers.[79, 80] GDM has also been associated with higher levels of visfatin,[81] although the implications of this observation are not clear.

In contrast to the generally consistent findings that have been reported for the preceding adipokines, studies of leptin and resistin in GDM have offered some conflicting results. Specifically, whereas two studies noted increased leptin in women with GDM compared to women with normal glucose tolerance in pregnancy,[82, 83] Festa et al reported relative hypoleptinemia in subjects with GDM compared with peers, after adjustment for BMI and insulin resistance.[84] Similarly, there have been conflicting reports of both increased and decreased resistin levels in women with GDM.[85, 86]

10.5.2 Pathophysiologic Implications of Adipokine Dysregulation in GDM

Adipokine dysregulation may hold several pathophysiologic implications in GDM. As in the nonpregnant state, both total and HMW adiponectin are independently and inversely related to insulin resistance in pregnancy.[67, 75] Indeed, the longitudinal changes in maternal circulating adiponectin during normal pregnancy (levels of which reach a nadir in the third trimester) are strongly associated with the physiologic changes in insulin sensitivity that occur during gestation (i.e., lowest in third trimester).[87] Importantly, as shown in Fig. 10.1, hypoadiponectinemia in pregnancy has also been associated with beta-cell dysfunction.[46] Furthermore, the relationship between decreased total adiponectin and beta-cell dysfunction in pregnant women has been shown to be independent of covariate adjustment, raising the possibility that it may reflect a pathophysiologic association.[46] More recently, a similar independent relationship was demonstrated between decreased circulating levels of HMW adiponectin (as in GDM) and beta-cell dysfunction in pregnancy.[75] Overall, these data suggest that, as with T2DM, hypoadiponectinemia (and specifically deficiency of HMW adiponectin) may be a pathophysiologic factor contributing to the development of insulin resistance, beta-cell dysfunction, and ultimately GDM in affected women.

Besides adiponectin, other adipokines have also been linked to insulin resistance in GDM. The correlation between TNFα and insulin resistance in pregnancy is particularly noteworthy.[57, 72, 88, 89] Interestingly, in contrast to the classical teaching implicating placental hormones, Kirwan et al[90] demonstrated that, amongst candidate hormones (including estrogen,

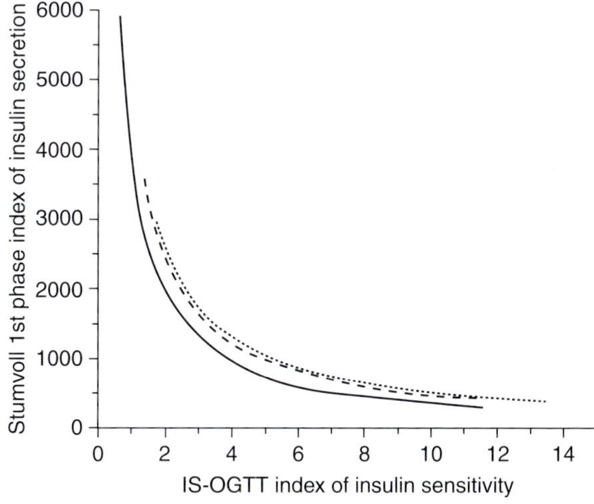

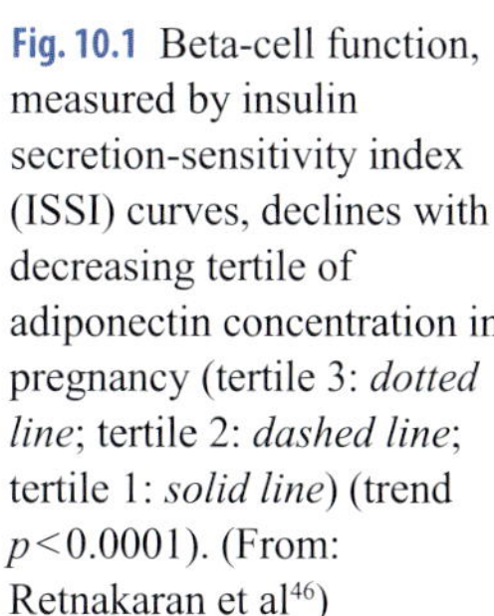
Fig. 10.1 Beta-cell function, measured by insulin secretion-sensitivity index (ISSI) curves, declines with decreasing tertile of adiponectin concentration in pregnancy (tertile 3: *dotted line*; tertile 2: *dashed line*; tertile 1: *solid line*) (trend $p<0.0001$). (From: Retnakaran et al[46])

progesterone, human placental lactogen, and cortisol), the change in TNFα from pre-gravid to late pregnancy was the most significant independent predictor of the longitudinal change in insulin sensitivity over this period of time (even after adjustment for fat mass) in a study of 15 women (5 with GDM) assessed before pregnancy, at 12–14 weeks gestation, and at 34–36 weeks gestation. It should be noted that adiponectin was not measured in this study. In other studies, leptin has been consistently associated with insulin resistance in pregnancy.[82–84] Finally, the effects of RBP-4 and visfatin in GDM remain to be fully elucidated.

10.6 Inflammatory Proteins and Adipokines in the Postpartum Following GDM

By testing the capacity for beta-cell compensation in the context of the significant acquired insulin resistance of pregnancy, a woman's glucose tolerance in pregnancy can provide unique insight into her future risk of T2DM. It has long been recognized that women who develop GDM have a substantial risk of developing T2DM in the future. In fact, it has recently emerged that any degree of abnormal glucose homeostasis in pregnancy (i.e., not just GDM) predicts an increased risk of prediabetes or diabetes in the postpartum (Fig. 10.2) and that this risk is proportional to the degree of antepartum dysglycemia.[91–93] Women with GDM thus represent the highest level on this continuum of future diabetic risk. As such, they constitute an important patient population in whom evaluation in the years following the index pregnancy may

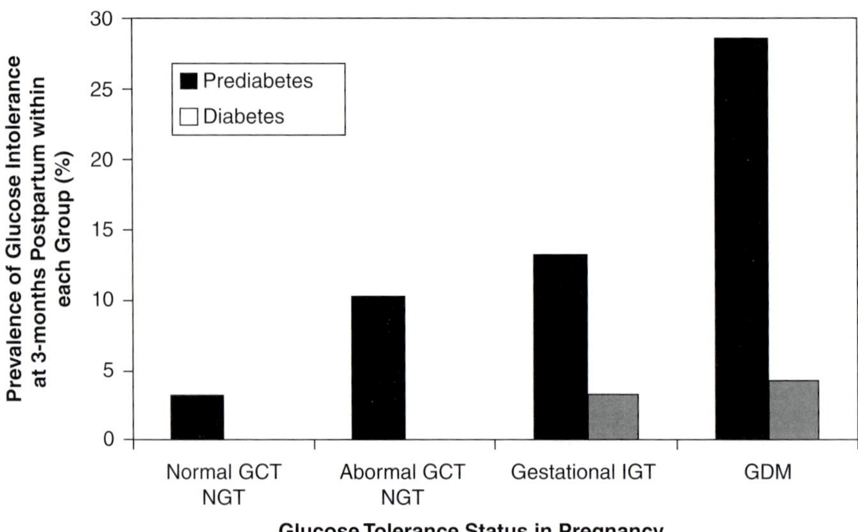

Fig. 10.2 Prevalence of glucose intolerance (prediabetes or diabetes) in four groups of women with varying degrees of glucose tolerance in pregnancy: (1) normal glucose challenge test (GCT) with normal glucose tolerance (NGT) on OGTT; (2) abnormal GCT with NGT; (3) gestational impaired glucose tolerance (GIGT); and (4) GDM (trend $p<0.0001$). (From: Retnakaran et al[91])

provide insight into key factors that mediate a woman's risk of developing T2DM. Given their emerging associations with both GDM and T2DM, inflammatory proteins and adipokines have recently begun to garner interest as factors of particular interest.

Consistent with the evidence of inflammation in women with GDM in pregnancy, several studies have reported increased levels of inflammatory proteins in this patient population following pregnancy. In a study of 96 women (46 with previous GDM and 50 without) evaluated at 7-years postpartum, Sriharan et al demonstrated increased levels of total sialic acid (a measure of the acute-phase response) in women with previous GDM that correlated with the metabolic syndrome and its components.[94] Similarly, circulating PAI-1 is also elevated in women with a history of GDM compared with their peers.[95] Further, increased CRP levels have been consistently reported in women with previous GDM[96–99] and, as with sialic acid, correlated with the metabolic syndrome.[99] A recurrent finding in these studies has been the significant association between CRP and central obesity.[97,99] Indeed, in the population-based Third National Health and Nutrition Survey Examination (NHANES III), adjustment for waist circumference attenuated differences in CRP levels between women with previous GDM and women without such a history.[100] At present, from limited studies to date, it appears that women with a history of GDM exhibit evidence of chronic subclinical inflammation following the index pregnancy, but further study is needed to determine if this relationship is entirely driven by a tendency towards visceral fat accumulation and central obesity in this population.

There has been very little study thus far of adipokines in women with previous GDM. In a study of 89 women with previous GDM, compared with 19 controls, the former exhibited significantly lower levels of adiponectin and higher leptin concentration at 3-months postpartum.[96] The observed hypoadiponectinemia in women with previous GDM persisted even after adjustment for body fat mass. Moreover, low adiponectin was independently associated with decreased insulin sensitivity and low HDL. While further study is needed, these data suggest that hypoadiponectinemia may be a factor contributing to the risk of T2DM in women with a history of GDM.

It is readily apparent that the literature on inflammation and adipokines following GDM is limited, with the few reports thus far generally modest in size and cross-sectional in design. Nevertheless, their characterization of the post-GDM postpartum as a state of subclinical inflammation and hypoadiponectinemia is intriguing when considering that (1) these features are associated with incident T2DM,[33–36,47–50] (2) treatment with a thiazolidinedione significantly reduced the risk of T2DM following GDM in the TRoglitazone In the Prevention Of Diabetes (TRIPOD) study,[101] and (3) TZD therapy decreases concentrations of inflammatory proteins and increases adiponectin levels.[102,103] These findings, in conjunction with the pathophysiologic effects of inflammation and adipokine dysregulation discussed earlier, suggest that inflammatory proteins and adipokines may play an important role in the development of T2DM in women with previous GDM by contributing to the progressive worsening of insulin resistance, beta-cell dysfunction, and dysglycemia, in the years following the index pregnancy. Given the substantial risk of T2DM in women with a history of GDM, the results of large-scale prospective longitudinal studies evaluating the potential contributions of inflammatory proteins and adipokines will be welcomed. These ongoing studies[91] may also provide insight into the relevance of these factors to cardiovascular risk, as GDM is also associated with an increased risk of CVD.[104]

10.7 Conclusions and Future Research

As reviewed in this chapter, chronic subclinical inflammation and adipokine dysregulation are pathologic effects of central obesity that may relate to insulin resistance and beta-cell dysfunction and thereby contribute to the development of GDM and T2DM in at-risk individuals. At present, these processes have been linked to both GDM and T2DM. However, their potential contribution to the risk of progression to T2DM in women with a history of GDM has not yet been studied.

The importance of further clarifying their role in this patient population is underscored by the potential implications that such insight may hold for basic science, public health, and clinical practice. First, such study could help to elucidate key mechanisms underlying the pathophysiology of both GDM and T2DM. Second, if inflammatory proteins or adipokines are indeed important to the development of T2DM in women with a history of GDM, then these factors may provide a simple means of stratifying patients who are at the highest risk of progression to T2DM. Further, this insight may inform the identification of relevant therapeutic targets and effective interventions prior to the onset of clinical disease. Notably, both lifestyle modification targeting weight loss and certain medications can decrease levels of inflammatory proteins and increase adiponectin levels.[102, 103, 105]

In conclusion, evidence to date suggests that, in women at risk of GDM, subclinical inflammation and adipokine dysregulation may be relevant in both pregnancy and in the postpartum. As women with a history of GDM face a high risk of both T2DM and vascular disease, further study is needed to clarify the effects of inflammatory proteins and adipokines in this context. Ultimately, such study may help to elucidate the shared pathophysiology of GDM and T2DM and may inform the clinical care of this high-risk patient population.

References

1. Kahn SE. The relative contributions of insulin resistance and beta-cell dysfunction to the pathophysiology of type 2 diabetes. *Diabetologia*. 2003;46:3-19.
2. Bergman RN, Finegood DT, Kahn SE. The evolution of beta-cell dysfunction and insulin resistance in type 2 diabetes. *Eur J Clin Invest*. 2002;32(suppl 3):35-45.
3. Lyssenko V, Almgren P, Agnevski D, et al. Predictors of and longitudinal changes in insulin sensitivity and secretion preceding onset of type 2 diabetes. *Diabetes*. 2005;54:166-174.
4. Buchanan TA, Xiang AH. Gestational diabetes mellitus. *J Clin Invest*. 2005;115:485-491.
5. Kuhl C. Etiology and pathogenesis of gestational diabetes. *Diabetes Care*. 1998;21:B19-B26.
6. Catalano PM, Tyzbir ED, Wolfe RR, et al. Carbohydrate metabolism during pregnancy in control subjects and women with gestational diabetes. *Am J Physiol*. 1993;264:E60-E67.
7. Ward WK, Johnston CL, Beard JC, Benedetti TJ, Halter JB, Porte D Jr. Insulin resistance and impaired insulin secretion in subjects with histories of gestational diabetes mellitus. *Diabetes*. 1985;34:861-869.
8. Byrne MM, Stuns J, OMeara NM, Polonsky KS. Insulin secretion in insulin-resistant women with a history of gestational diabetes. *Metabolism*. 1995;44:1067-1073.

9. Ryan EA, Imes S, Liu D, et al. Defects in insulin secretion and action in women with a history of gestational diabetes. *Diabetes*. 1995;44:506-512.
10. Homko C, Sivan E, Chen X, Reece EA, Boden G. Insulin secretion during and after pregnancy in patients with gestational diabetes mellitus. *J Clin Endocrinol Metab*. 2001;86: 568-573.
11. Buchanan TA. Pancreatic β-cell defects in gestational diabetes: implications for the pathogenesis and prevention of type 2 diabetes. *J Clin Endocrinol Metab*. 2001;86:989-993.
12. Bergman RN, Phillips LS, Cobelli C. Physiologic evaluation of factors controlling glucose tolerance in man: measurement of insulin sensitivity and β-cell glucose sensitivity from the response to intravenous glucose. *J Clin Invest*. 1981;68:1456-1467.
13. Kahn SE, Prigeon RL, McCulloch DK, et al. Quantification of the relationship between insulin sensitivity and β-cell function in human subjects: evidence for a hyperbolic function. *Diabetes*. 1993;42:1663-1672.
14. Retnakaran R, Shen S, Hanley AJ, Vuksan V, Hamilton JK, Zinman B. Hyperbolic relationship between insulin secretion and sensitivity on oral glucose tolerance test. *Obesity*. 2008;16:1901-1907.
15. Damm P, Kuhl C, Bertelsen A, Molsted-Pedersen L. Predictive factors for the development of diabetes in women with previous gestational diabetes mellitus. *Am J Obstet Gynecol*. 1992; 167:607-616.
16. Metzger BE, Cho NH, Roston SM, Radvany R. Prepregnancy weight and antepartum insulin secretion predict glucose tolerance five years after gestational diabetes mellitus. *Diabetes Care*. 1993;16:1598-1605.
17. Kjos SL, Peters RK, Xiang A, Henry OA, Montoro M, Buchanan TA. Predicting future diabetes in Latino women with gestational diabetes. Utility of early postpartum glucose tolerance testing. *Diabetes*. 1995;44:586-591.
18. Peters RK, Kjos SL, Xiang A, Buchanan TA. Long-term diabetogenic effect of single pregnancy in women with previous gestational diabetes mellitus. *Lancet*. 1996;347:227-230.
19. Kjos SL, Peters RK, Xiang A, Thomas D, Schaefer U, Buchanan TA. Contraception and the risk of type 2 diabetes mellitus in Latina women with prior gestational diabetes mellitus. *JAMA*. 1998;280:533-538.
20. Buchanan TA, Xiang A, Kjos SL, et al. Gestational diabetes: antepartum characteristics that predict postpartum glucose intolerance and type 2 diabetes in Latino women. *Diabetes*. 1998;47:1302-1310.
21. Pallardo F, Herranz L, Garcia-Ingelmo T, et al. Early postpartum metabolic assessment in women with prior gestational diabetes. *Diabetes Care*. 1999;22:1053-1058.
22. Buchanan TA, Xiang AH, Kjos SL, Trigo E, Lee WP, Peters RK. Antepartum predictors of the development of type 2 diabetes in Latino women 11-26 months after pregnancies complicated by gestational diabetes. *Diabetes*. 1999;48:2430-2436.
23. Schaefer-Graf UM, Buchanan TA, Xiang AH, et al. Clinical predictors for a high risk for the development of diabetes mellitus in the early pueperium in women with recent gestational diabetes mellitus. *Am J Obstet Gynecol*. 2002;186:751-756.
24. Sinha B, Brydon P, Taylor RS, et al. Maternal ante-natal parameters as predictors of persistent postnatal glucose intolerance: a comparative study between Afro-Caribbeans, Asians and Caucasians. *Diabet Med*. 2003;20:382-386.
25. Albareda M, Caballero A, Badell G, et al. Diabetes and abnormal glucose tolerance in women with previous gestational diabetes. *Diabetes Care*. 2003;26:1199-1205.
26. Pickup JC, Crook MA. Is Type 2 DM a disease of the innate immune system? *Diabetologia*. 1998;41:1241-1248.
27. Greenberg AS, McDaniel ML. Identifying the links between obesity, insulin resistance and beta-cell function: potential role of adipocyte-derived cytokines in the pathogenesis of type 2 diabetes. *Eur J Clin Invest*. 2002;32(suppl 3):24-34.

28. Yudkin JS, Stehouwer CDA, Emeis JJ, Coppack SW. C-reactive protein in healthy subjects: associations with obesity, insulin resistance and endothelial dysfunction. *Arterioscler Thromb Vasc Biol*. 1999;19:972-978.
29. Rasouli N, Kern PA. Adipocytokines and the metabolic complications of obesity. *J Clin Endocrinol Metab*. 2008;93(11 Suppl 1):S64-S73.
30. Mattock PJC, MB CGD, Burt D. NIDDM as a disease of the innate immune system: association of acute-phase reactants and interleukin-6 with metabolic syndrome X. *Diabetologia*. 1997;40:1286-1292.
31. Festa A, D'Agostino R Jr, Howard G, Mykkänen L, Tracy RP, Haffner SM. Chronic subclinical inflammation as part of the insulin resistance syndrome: the Insulin Resistance Atherosclerosis Study (IRAS). *Circulation*. 2000;102:42-47.
32. Pickup JC. Inflammation and activated innate immunity in the pathogenesis of type 2 diabetes. *Diabetes Care*. 2004;27:813-823.
33. Pradham AD, Manson JE, Rifai N, Buring J, Ridker PM. C-reactive protein, interleukin 6 and risk of developing type 2 diabetes mellitus. *JAMA*. 2001;286:327-334.
34. Freeman DJ, Norrie J, Caslake MJ, et al. West of Scotland Coronary Prevention Study. C-reactive protein is an independent predictor of risk for the development of diabetes in the West of Scotland Coronary Prevention Study. *Diabetes*. 2002;51:1596-1600.
35. Barzilay JI, Abraham L, Heckbert SR, et al. The relation of markers of inflammation to the development of glucose disorders in the elderly: the Cardiovascular Health Study. *Diabetes*. 2001;50:2384-2389.
36. Festa A, D'Agostino R Jr, Tracy RP, Haffner SM. Elevated levels of acute-phase proteins and plasminogen activator inhibitor-1 predict the development of type 2 diabetes. The Insulin Resistance Atherosclerosis Study. *Diabetes*. 2002;51:1131-1137.
37. Goldstein BJ, Scalia R. Adiponectin: a novel adipokine linking adipocytes and vascular function. *J Clin Endocrinol Metab*. 2004;89:2563-2568.
38. Pajvani UB, Hawkins M, Combs T, et al. Complex distribution, not absolute amount of adiponectin, correlates with thiazolidinedione-mediated improvement in insulin sensitivity. *J Biol Chem*. 2004;279:12152-12162.
39. Liu Y, Retnakaran R, Hanley A, Tungtrongchitr R, Shaw C, Sweeney G. Total and high molecular weight but not trimeric or hexameric forms of adiponectin correlate with markers of the metabolic syndrome and liver injury in Thai subjects. *J Clin Endocrinol Metab*. 2007;92: 4313-4318.
40. Cnop C, Havel PJ, Utzschneider K, et al. Relationship of adiponectin to body fat distribution, insulin sensitivity and plasma lipoproteins: evidence for independent roles of age and sex. *Diabetologia*. 2003;46:459-469.
41. Weyer C, Funahashi T, Tanaka S, et al. Hypoadiponectinemia in obesity and type 2 diabetes: close association with insulin resistance and hyperinsulinemia. *J Clin Endocrinol Metab*. 2001;86:1930-1935.
42. Hotta K, Funahashi T, Arita Y, et al. Plasma concentrations of a novel, adipose-specific protein, adiponectin, in type 2 diabetic patients. *Arterioscler Thromb Vasc Biol*. 2000;20: 1595-1599.
43. Hotta K, Funahashi T, Bodkin NL, et al. Circulating concentrations of the adipocyte protein adiponectin are decreased in parallel with reduced insulin sensitivity during the progression to type 2 diabetes in rhesus monkeys. *Diabetes*. 2001;50:1126-1133.
44. Stefan N, Vozarova B, Funahashi T, et al. Plasma adiponectin concentration is associated with skeletal muscle insulin receptor tyrosine phosphorylation, and low plasma concentration precedes a decrease in whole-body insulin sensitivity in humans. *Diabetes*. 2002;51:1884-1888.
45. Musso G, Gambino R, Biroli G, et al. Hypoadiponectinemia predicts the severity of hepatic fibrosis and pancreatic Beta-cell dysfunction in nondiabetic nonobese patients with nonalcoholic steatohepatitis. *Am J Gastroenterol*. 2005;100:2438-2446.

46. Retnakaran R, Hanley AJ, Raif N, et al. Adiponectin and beta-cell dysfunction in gestational diabetes: pathophysiological implications. *Diabetologia*. 2005;48:993-1001.
47. Lindsay RS, Funahashi T, Hanson RL, et al. Adiponectin and development of type 2 diabetes in the Pima Indian population. *Lancet*. 2002;360:57-58.
48. Spranger J, Kroke A, Mohlig M. Adiponectin and protection against type 2 diabetes mellitus. *Lancet*. 2003;361:226-228.
49. Daimon M, Oizumi T, Saitoh T, et al. Decreased serum levels of adiponectin are a risk factor for the progression to type 2 diabetes in the Japanese Population: the Funagata study. *Diabetes Care*. 2003;26:2015-2020.
50. Snehalatha C, Mukesh B, Simon M, et al. Plasma adiponectin is an independent predictor of type 2 diabetes in Asian Indians. *Diabetes Care*. 2003;26:3226-3229.
51. Yamauchi T, Kamon J, Waki H, et al. The fat-derived hormone adiponectin reverses insulin resistance associated with both lipoatrophy and obesity. *Nat Med*. 2001;7:941-946.
52. Berg AH, Combs TP, Du X, Brownlee M, Schere PE. The adipocyte-secreted protein Acrp30 enhances hepatic insulin action. *Nat Med*. 2001;7:947-953.
53. Yamauchi T, Kamon J, Waki H, et al. Globular adiponectin protected ob/ob mice from diabetes and ApoE-deficient mice from atherosclerosis. *J Biol Chem*. 2003;278:2461-2468.
54. Retnakaran R, Youn BS, Liu Y, et al. Correlation of circulating full-length visfatin (PBEF/NAMPT) with metabolic parameters in subjects with and without diabetes: a cross-sectional study. *Clin Endocrinol*. 2008;69:885-893.
55. Wolf M, Sandler L, Hsu K, et al. First-trimester C-reactive protein and subsequent gestational diabetes. *Diabetes Care*. 2003;26:819-824.
56. Qiu C, Sorensen TK, Luthy DA, et al. A prospective study of maternal serum C-reactive protein (CRP) concentrations and risk of gestational diabetes mellitus. *Paediatr Perinat Epidemiol*. 2004;18:377-384.
57. Bo S, Signorile A, Menato G, et al. C-reactive protein and tumor necrosis factor-alpha in gestational hyperglycemia. *J Endocrinol Invest*. 2005;28:779-786.
58. Leipold H, Worda C, Gruber CJ, et al. Gestational diabetes mellitus is associated with increased C-reactive protein concentrations in the third but not second trimester. *Eur J Clin Invest*. 2005;35:752-757.
59. Retnakaran R, Hanley AJG, Raif N, Connelly PW, Sermer M, Zinman B. C-reactive protein and gestational diabetes: the central role of maternal obesity. *J Clin Endocrinol Metab*. 2003;88:3507-3512.
60. Ramsay JE, Ferrell WR, Crawford L, Wallace AM, Greer IA, Sattar N. Maternal obesity is associated with dysregulation of metabolic, vascular, and inflammatory pathways. *J Clin Endocrinol Metab*. 2002;87:4231-4237.
61. Wolf M, Sauk J, Shah A, et al. Inflammation and glucose intolerance: a prospective study of gestational diabetes mellitus. *Diabetes Care*. 2004;27:21-27.
62. Ategbo JM, Grissa O, Yessoufou A, et al. Modulation of adipokines and cytokines in gestational diabetes and macrosomia. *J Clin Endocrinol Metab*. 2006;91:4137-4143.
63. Kuzmicki M, Telejko B, Zonenberg A, et al. Circulating pro- and anti-inflammatory cytokines in Polish women with gestational diabetes. *Horm Metab Res*. 2008;40:556-560.
64. Chen X, Scholl TO, Stein TP. Association of elevated serum ferritin levels and the risk of gestational diabetes mellitus in pregnant women: The Camden study. *Diabetes Care*. 2006;29:1077-1082.
65. Lao TT, Tse KY, Chan LY, Tam KF, Ho LF. HBsAg carrier status and the association between gestational diabetes with increased serum ferritin concentration in Chinese women. *Diabetes Care*. 2003;26:3011-3016.
66. Leipold H, Knoefler M, Gruber C, Klein K, Haslinger P, Worda C. Plasminogen activator inhibitor 1 gene polymorphism and gestational diabetes mellitus. *Obstet Gynecol*. 2006;107:651-656.

67. Retnakaran R, Hanley AJ, Raif N, Connelly PW, Sermer M, Zinman. Reduced adiponectin concentration in women with gestational diabetes: a potential factor in progression to type 2 diabetes. *Diabetes Care*. 2004;27:799-800.
68. Cseh K, Baranyi E, Melczer Z, et al. Plasma adiponectin and pregnancy-induced insulin resistance. *Diabetes Care*. 2004;27:274-275.
69. Rainheim T, Haugen F, Staff AC, et al. Adiponectin is reduced in gestational diabetes mellitus in normal weight women. *Acta Obstet Gynecol Scand*. 2004;83:341-347.
70. Worda C, Leipold H, Gruber C, et al. Decreased plasma adiponectin concentrations in women with gestational diabetes mellitus. *Am J Obstet Gynecol*. 2004;191:2120-2124.
71. Thyfault JP, Hedberg EM, Anchan RM, et al. Gestational diabetes is associated with depressed adiponectin levels. *J Soc Gynecol Investig*. 2005;12:41-45.
72. Kinalski M, Telejko B, Kuzmicki M, et al. Tumor necrosis factor alpha system and plasma adiponectin concentration in women with gestational diabetes. *Horm Metab Res*. 2005;37: 450-454.
73. Tsai PJ, Yu CH, Hsu SP, et al. Maternal plasma adiponectin concentrations at 24 to 31 weeks of gestation: negative association with gestational diabetes mellitus. *Nutrition*. 2005;21: 1095-1099.
74. Williams MA, Qiu C, Muy-Rivera M, et al. Plasma adiponectin concentrations in early pregnancy and subsequent risk of gestational diabetes mellitus. *J Clin Endocrinol Metab*. 2004;89:2306-2311.
75. Retnakaran R, Connelly PW, Maguire G, Sermer M, Zinman B, Hanley AJ. Decreased high molecular weight adiponectin in gestational diabetes: implications for the pathophysiology of type 2 diabetes. *Diabetic Med*. 2007;24:245-252.
76. Retnakaran R, Hanley AJ, Raif N, Connelly PW, Sermer M, Zinman B. Hypoadiponectinemia in South Asian women during pregnancy: evidence of ethnic variation in adiponectin concentration. *Diabetic Med*. 2004;21:388-392.
77. Retnakaran R, Hanley AJ, Connelly PW, Maguire G, Sermer M, Zinman B. Low serum levels of high molecular weight adiponectin in Indo-Asian women during pregnancy: evidence of ethnic variation in adiponectin isoform distribution. *Diabetes Care*. 2006;29:1377-1379.
78. Retnakaran R, Hanley AJ, Zinman B. Does hypoadiponectinemia explain the increased risk of diabetes and cardiovascular disease in South Asians? *Diabetes Care*. 2006;29:1950-1954.
79. Chan TF, Chen HS, Chen YC, et al. Increased serum retinol-binding protein 4 concentrations in women with gestational diabetes mellitus. *Reprod Sci*. 2007;14:169-174.
80. Lewandowski KC, Stojanovic N, Bienkiewicz M, et al. Elevated concentrations of retinol-binding protein-4 (RBP-4) in gestational diabetes mellitus: negative correlation with soluble vascular cell adhesion molecule-1 (sVCAM-1). *Gynecol Endocrinol*. 2008;24:300-305.
81. Lewandowski KC, Stojanovic N, Press M, et al. Elevated serum levels of visfatin in gestational diabetes: a comparative study across various degrees of glucose tolerance. *Diabetologia*. 2007;50:1033-1037.
82. Kautzky-Willer A, Pacini G, Tura A, et al. Increased plasma leptin in gestational diabetes. *Diabetologia*. 2001;44:164-172.
83. Vitoratos N, Salamalekis E, Kassanos D, et al. Maternal plasma leptin levels and their relationship to insulin and glucose in gestational-onset diabetes. *Gynecol Obstet Invest*. 2001;51:17-21.
84. Festa A, Shnawa N, Krugluger W, Hopmeier P, Schernthaner G, Haffner SM. Relative hypoleptinaemia in women with mild gestational diabetes mellitus. *Diabet Med*. 1999;16:656-662.
85. Chen D, Fang Q, Chai Y, Wang H, Huang H, Dong M. Serum resistin in gestational diabetes mellitus and early postpartum. *Clin Endocrinol*. 2007;67:208-211.
86. Megia A, Vendrell J, Gutierrez C, et al. Insulin sensitivity and resistin levels in gestational diabetes mellitus and after parturition. *Eur J Endocrinol*. 2008;158:173-178.

87. Catalano PM, Hoegh M, Minium J, et al. Adiponectin in human pregnancy: implications for regulation of glucose and lipid metabolism. *Diabetologia*. 2006;49:1677-1685.
88. Winkler G, Cseh K, Baranyi E, et al. Tumor necrosis factor system in insulin resistance in gestational diabetes. *Diabetes Res Clin Pract*. 2002;56:93-99.
89. Cseh K, Baranyi E, Melczer Z, et al. The pathophysiological influence of leptin and the tumor necrosis factor system on maternal insulin resistance: negative correlation with anthropometric parameters of neonates in gestational diabetes. *Gynecol Endocrinol*. 2002;16:453-460.
90. Kirwan JP, Hauguel-De Mouzon S, Lepercq J, et al. TNF-alpha is a predictor of insulin resistance in human pregnancy. *Diabetes*. 2002;51:2207-2213.
91. Retnakaran R, Qi Y, Sermer M, Connelly PW, Hanley AJ, Zinman B. Glucose intolerance in pregnancy and future risk of pre-diabetes or diabetes. *Diabetes Care*. 2008;31:2026-2031.
92. Retnakaran R, Qi Y, Sermer M, Connelly PW, Zinman B, Hanley AJ. Isolated hyperglycemia at 1-hour on oral glucose tolerance test in pregnancy resembles gestational diabetes in predicting postpartum metabolic dysfunction. *Diabetes Care*. 2008;31:1275-1281.
93. Retnakaran R, Qi Y, Sermer M, Connelly PW, Zinman B, Hanley AJ. An abnormal screening glucose challenge test in pregnancy predicts postpartum metabolic dysfunction, even when the antepartum oral glucose tolerance test is normal. *Clin Endocrinol*. 2009;71:208-214, doi: 10.1111/j.1365-2265.2008.03460.x.
94. Sriharan M, Reichelt AJ, Opperman ML, et al. Total sialic acid and associated elements of the metabolic syndrome in women with and without previous gestational diabetes. *Diabetes Care*. 2002;25:1331-1335.
95. Farhan S, Winzer C, Tura A, et al. Fibrinolytic dysfunction in insulin-resistant women with previous gestational diabetes. *Eur J Clin Invest*. 2006;36:345-352.
96. Winzer C, Wagner O, Festa A, et al. Plasma adiponectin, insulin sensitivity, and subclinical inflammation in women with prior gestational diabetes mellitus. *Diabetes Care*. 2004;27:1721-1727.
97. Di Benedetto A, Russo GT, Corrado F, et al. Inflammatory markers in women with a recent history of gestational diabetes mellitus. *J Endocrinol Invest*. 2005;28:34-38.
98. Di Cianni G, Lencioni C, Volpe L, et al. C-reactive protein and metabolic syndrome in women with previous gestational diabetes. *Diabetes Metab Res Rev*. 2007;23:135-140.
99. Ferraz TB, Motta RS, Ferraz CL, Capibaribe DM, Forti AC, Chacra AR. C-reactive protein and features of metabolic syndrome in Brazilian women with previous gestational diabetes. *Diabetes Res Clin Pract*. 2007;78:23-29.
100. Kim C, Cheng YJ, Beckles GL. Inflammation among women with a history of gestational diabetes mellitus and diagnosed diabetes in the Third National Health and Nutrition Examination Survey. *Diabetes Care*. 2008;31:1386-1388.
101. Buchanan TA, Xiang AH, Peters RK, et al. Preservation of pancreatic beta-cell function and prevention of type 2 diabetes by pharmacological treatment of insulin resistance in high-risk Hispanic women. *Diabetes*. 2002;51:2796-2803.
102. Yu JG, Javorschi S, Hevener AL, et al. The effect of thiazolidinediones on plasma adiponectin levels in normal, obese and type 2 diabetic subjects. *Diabetes*. 2002;51:2968-2974.
103. Haffner S, Greenberg AS, Weston WM, et al. Effect of rosiglitazone treatment on nontraditional markers of cardiovascular disease in patients with type 2 diabetes mellitus. *Circulation*. 2002;106:679-684.
104. Shah BR, Retnakaran R, Booth GL. Increased risk of cardiovascular disease in young women following gestational diabetes mellitus. *Diabetes Care*. 2008;31:1668-1669.
105. Bobbert T, Rochlitz H, Wegewitz U, et al. Changes of adiponectin oligomer composition by moderate weight reduction. *Diabetes*. 2005;54:2712-2719.

Lipids in Gestational Diabetes: Abnormalities and Significance

11

Robert H. Knopp, Elizabeth Chan, Xiaodong Zhu, Pathmaja Paramsothy, and Bartolome Bonet

11.1 Introduction and Overview

Cholesterol and essential fatty acids are required for fetal development. In mammals, this requirement is met in the mother by an increase in all lipoprotein fractions under the influence of estrogen. Plasma triglycerides and low density lipoprotein (LDL) increase in proportion to gestational age, while high density lipoprotein (HDL) peaks in midgestation and then declines. As a generalization, gestational diabetes (GDM) exaggerates the triglyceride increase and decreases HDL, but without an increase in LDL cholesterol. The dyslipidemia of GDM affects fetal and maternal health in at least four ways: (1) triglyceride increases are associated with increased birth weight, (2) hyperlipidemia in pregnancy predicts elevated maternal lipids in later life, just as GDM predicts diabetes, (3) GDM is associated with increased susceptibility of LDL to oxidative stress, and (4) elevated triglycerides are associated with occurrence of preeclampsia. Clinical management focuses on excellent diabetes management, with consideration of a moderate allowable fat diet and omega-3 fatty acid supplements. Triglyceride elevations exceeding 1,000 mg/dL justify high dose fish oil or fibric acid treatment to prevent pancreatitis, the major therapeutic priority of lipid management in pregnancy. Further research is needed to determine the extent to which the dyslipidemia of GDM drives lipoprotein oxidation, inflammation, preeclampsia, divergent effects on birth weight, malformations, and transmission of acquired traits to the next generation, and to what extent altering lipid levels can modify these predispositions. Devising dietary and pharmacologic therapies for disorders linked to dyslipidemia in GDM are challenges for the future.

E. Chan (✉)
Northwest Lipid Research Clinic, Division of Metabolism, Endocrinology and Nutrition, Division of Cardiology, University of Washington, Seattle, WA, USA
e-mail: gkuroishi@pcamailbox.com

C. Kim and A. Ferrara (eds.), *Gestational Diabetes During and After Pregnancy*, DOI: 10.1007/978-1-84882-120-0_11, © Springer-Verlag London Limited 2010

11.2 Lipid Metabolism in Normal Pregnancy

Hyperlipidemia in pregnancy is a physiological adaptation to the altered hormonal milieu of pregnancy. The progression of maternal lipid elevations is predominately regulated by estrogen, which stimulates the production of very low density lipoprotein (VLDL), inducing hypertriglyceridemia in proportion to the growth of the placenta (Fig. 11.1).[1] Triglyceride levels rise gradually to a maximum 2–4-fold (Fig. 11.2). Likewise, the levels of LDL cholesterol at term increase 25–50% above baseline.[2, 3] Concomitantly, the activity of lipoprotein lipase (LPL) to remove triglyceride by maternal tissues is reduced, especially in the third trimester[4] while placental LPL activity increases.[5] The net effect is to favor lipid delivery, and especially chylomicron triglyceride fatty acid delivery, to the placenta. The importance of essential fatty acid supply to the fetus is underscored by the positive association of placental fatty acid transport protein (FATP) mRNA expression with maternal, placental, and umbilical cord blood phospholipid docosahexanoic acid (DHA).[6] In addition, reduced fetal growth has been observed in mothers with an adverse fatty acid profile including increased trans-, arachidonic, and most n-6 fatty acids, and decreased n-3 fatty acids.[7] In addition, the incidence of small for gustational age (SGA) was increased twofold among the 7% of mothers with the most adverse fatty acid profile.[7]

HDL protects against oxidative[8] and inflammatory stress[9, 10] as well as accomplishing reverse cholesterol transport.[11] Very little study has gone into the effects on the placenta in normal pregnancy. What is known is that the buoyant subfraction of HDL, HDL_2, can both deliver cholesterol for progesterone synthesis[12] and facilitate the removal of cholesterol from tissues, primarily by the ABC-A1 and ABC-G1 transporter proteins.[13–15] Descriptively, HDL cholesterol reaches a peak at midgestation that is about 25 mg/dL higher than nonpregnant baseline (about 80 mg/dL) and then declines in the second half of gestation to about half of the midterm increase (about 65 mg/dL). It is speculated that the midterm HDL peak is estrogen driven while the partial decline in the second half of gestation is related to the contra-insulin hormones of gestation which peak in late gestation. Notably, apoproteins (apo) A-I and A-II levels do not fall like HDL cholesterol in the last half of

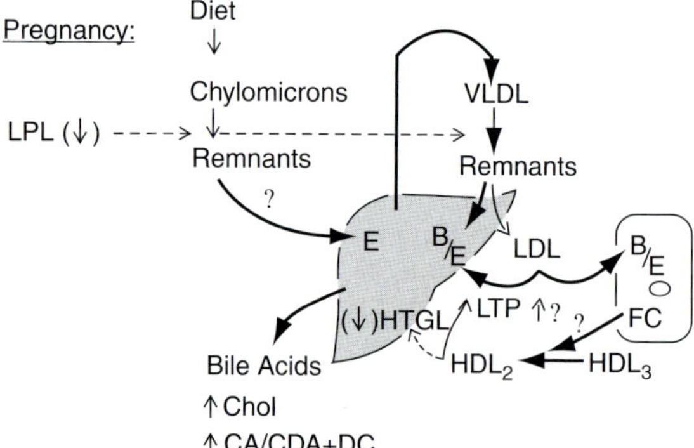

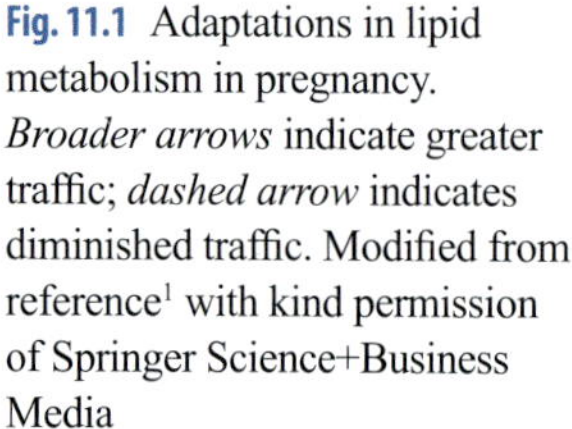
Fig. 11.1 Adaptations in lipid metabolism in pregnancy. *Broader arrows* indicate greater traffic; *dashed arrow* indicates diminished traffic. Modified from reference[1] with kind permission of Springer Science+Business Media

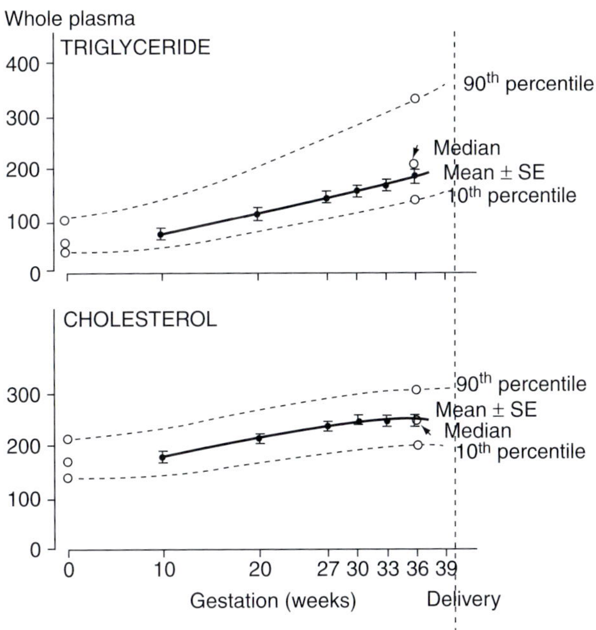

Fig. 11.2 Plasma triglyceride and cholesterol in normal pregnancy: 10th median and 90th percentile values. Reproduced from *Heart* 92, *1529-1534,* 2006 with permission from BMJ Publishing Group Ltd

gestation. Apo A-I may help to maintain the anti-oxidant, progesterone secretory, and reverse cholesterol transport functions of HDL, despite the fall in HDL cholesterol.[9, 10]

11.3 Placental Lipid Transport in Normal Pregnancy

The metabolism of lipids by the placenta is illustrated in Fig. 11.3. Triglyceride is metabolized to free fatty acids (FFAs) and transported across the placenta with chylomicron triglyceride metabolized more rapidly than VLDL triglyceride. Cholesterol can enter the placenta from VLDL remnants, the classical LDL receptor, or select fractions of HDL, probably by the scavenger receptor, SR-B1.[12] Cholesterol is most likely transferred to fetal HDL by ABC-A1 and G1 cholesterol transporters residing on the placental endothelium on the fetal surface of the placenta.[15] Apo B is made by the placenta[16] but its role in cholesterol transfer to the fetus has not been demonstrated.[13] It appears that the supply of cholesterol to the placenta and fetus is conserved and redundant.

Essential fatty acid transport to the fetus is among the most important lipid metabolic functions of the placenta. It was shown long ago that polyunsaturated fatty acids cross the subhuman primate placenta more rapidly and in proportion to chain length[17] than do saturated fatty acids. This property is likely due to the greater fluidity of the polyunsaturates and would specifically favor transplacental transport of the omega-3 series and particularly docosahexanoic acid (DHA) (22:6), important for central nervous system development and in particular, vision.

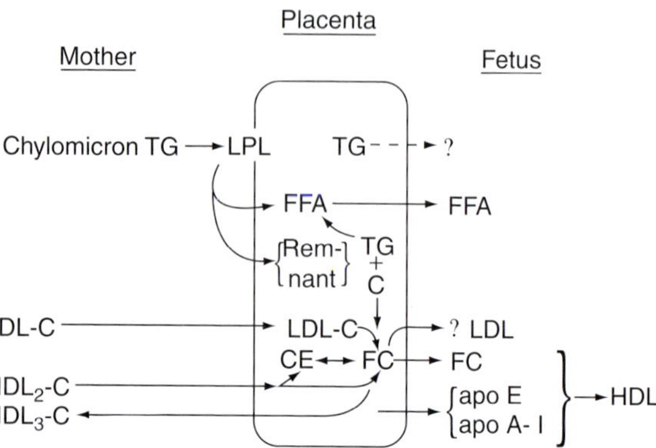

Fig. 11.3 Transplacental lipid transport. Modified from reference[1] with kind permission of Springer Science+Business Media

Other proteins control placental fatty acid transport as in other tissues, including fatty acid binding protein[18] and the fatty acid transport proteins FATP-1 and FATP-4. FATP-4 is especially correlated with DHA concentrations in cord blood phospholipids.[6,19] Finally, placental LPL activity is threefold elevated at term compared to the first trimester, thereby augmenting placental provision of fatty acids from lipoproteins including essential fatty acids from chylomicrons during rapid fetal growth.[5]

11.4 Effects of Maternal Lipids and Lipoproteins on Birth Weight in Normal, Unselected Pregnancies

We examined the relationship of birth weight in healthy pregnancy to fuels and hormones, including fasting glucose, insulin, FFAs, progesterone, estradiol, estriol, and human placental lactogen (HPL). Only HPL was significantly associated ($p<0.01$) with birth weight ratio and birth length,[20] possibly due to its contrainsulin effect or as a barometer of placental size. Birth weight variation explained by other categories of predictors (R^2) was 14% for lipoprotein lipids, 8% for apoproteins, and 33% for maternal characteristics.[20]

VLDL triglyceride was a positive but not significant weight predictor ($p=0.14$) in this healthy cohort of subjects[20] (mean 36-week triglyceride was 209 mg/dL, 10th to 90th percentile confidence interval 146–341 mg/dL).[2] More surprising was the *negative* association of apo A-II with birth weight and length.[20] Apo A-II is primarily associated with HDL_3; it associates with enhanced and pro-inflammatory HDL in transgenic models[21] and accelerates apo A-I catabolism.[22] Conversely, the positive association of apo A-I with birth weight and length underscores the positive effects of HDL in pregnancy, including cholesterol transport to the fetus, support of placental progesterone synthesis,[12] anti-inflammatory and anti-oxidative effects in the maternal circulation and possibly in the placenta,[8,9] and support of innate immunity.[10]

In a later study, the association of triglyceride to birth weight ratio was maximal at a triglyceride level of 200 mg/dL (~80th percentile at 36 weeks) and a birth weight ratio of

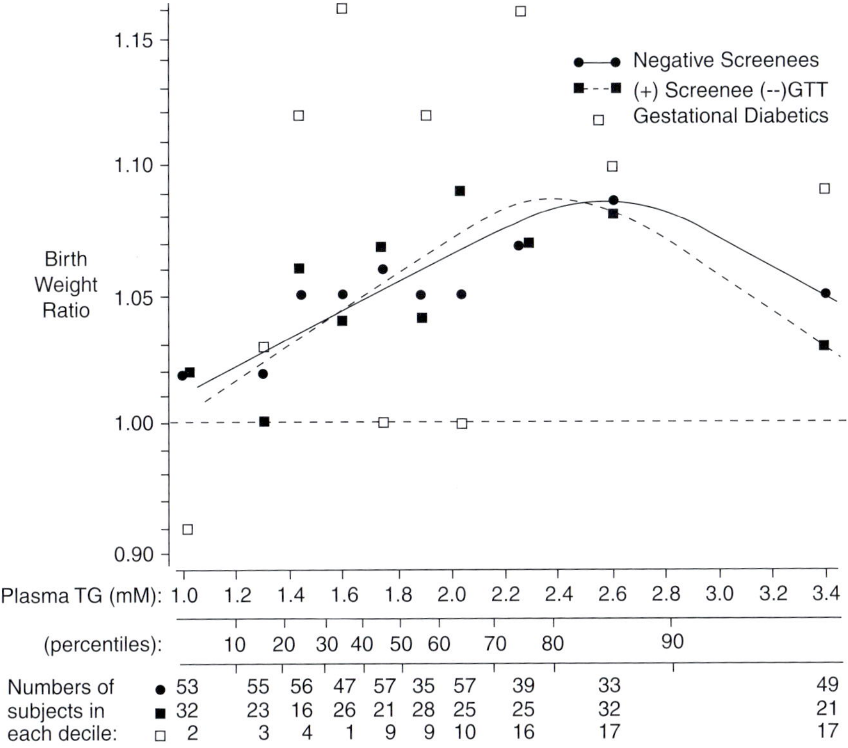

Fig. 11.4 Relationship of birthweight ratio to plasma triglycerides. Copyright 1992 American Diabetes Association from Diabetes Care®, Volume 15, 1992; 1605–1613. Modified with permission from *The American Diabetes Association*

1.08 (Fig. 11.4).[23] Unexpectedly, higher triglyceride concentrations were associated with progressively lower birth weight ratios (Fig. 11.4). This hyperbolic trend was superimposable in normal and positive glucose screen, negative GTT pregnancies.[23] This relationship suggests a toxic effect of major hypertriglyceridemia on fetal growth and development in late gestation, even in otherwise healthy pregnancies. Possible mechanisms include the toxicity of diabetic VLDL to vascular endothelium,[24] the association of elevated triglyceride levels with preeclampsia[25] and oxidative stress from obesity and the metabolic syndrome,[26] for which triglyceride is a marker.

11.5 Dyslipidemia in Pregnancy

Because the hyperlipidemia of pregnancy is a normal adaptation, normal reference values are useful to judge degrees of abnormality as a function of gestational age. The 90th percentile values are provided in Table 11.1.[2, 3] A greater than 90th percentile value for

Table 11.1 Upper limits of normal for plasma total triglyceride, total cholesterol and LDL-C in normal pregnancy

	90th Percentile			10th Percentile
Gestational week	Triglyceride	Cholesterol	LDL-C	HDL-C
0	115	225	140	40
10	140	230	143	50
20	210	275	165	62
27	265	290	180	61
30	300	295	186	58
33	315	300	192	52
36	340	300	200	46
39	370	300	204	45

triglyceride approaches 400 mg/dL in late gestation and the triglyceride elevations of gestational diabetic pregnancy can be interpreted in this light.

A clinical indication for triglyceride-lowering is a triglyceride level above 1,000 mg/dL, as it is in nonpregnant individuals, on the rationale of preventing pancreatitis, usually due to LPL deficiency or uncontrolled diabetes.[27] Severe pancreatitis and at the extreme, hemorrhagic pancreatitis in pregnancy can be lethal for the fetus and a potential cause of long-term disability in the mother if it becomes chronic and recurrent. Fortunately, cases usually do not reach this level of severity, but present with gradual onset of abdominal pain rather than sudden, acute pancreatitis. A slower onset allows time for triglycerides to be checked and treatment to be initiated. An immediate clue to severe hypertriglyceridemia is lipemic plasma at the time of blood draw or in the lab report. Typically, the lipemia interferes with measurements in aqueous plasma, causing reductions in electrolytes and lower than expected or even normal amylase levels.

A first choice for treatment of hypertriglyceridemia is high dose omega-3 fatty acids on the order of 8–10 g/day and avoidance of dietary fat. An example of this treatment for recurrent pancreatitis is given in Table 11.2. This 28-year-old nondiabetic woman was having low-grade mid-abdominal pain radiating to the back, similar to but less severe than that experienced in her first pregnancy. Ascending doses of fish oil extract containing EPA and DHA to 10 g/day resulted in a 57% decrease in triglyceride levels between weeks 30 and 38 and resolution of the abdominal pain between 30 and 34 weeks. Fibrates and low fat diet are two other choices for triglyceride management.[27] This complication is more often due to LPL deficiency than GDM or overt diabetes.[27]

Heterozygous familial hypercholesterolemia and LDL elevations 2–4 times normal are not associated with decreased reproductive efficiency as far as we are aware. However, maternal hypercholesterolemia is associated with cholesterol and fatty streak deposition and monocyte and oxidation markers in fetal, newborn, and childhood aortae, even in the absence of offspring hypercholesterolemia.[28,29] Whether the dyslipidemia of GDM

Table 11.2 Effects of ω-3 fatty acids in severe hypertriglyceridemia*

Weeks gestation	20–26	30	34	35	36	37	38
Triglyceride (mg/dL)	2,152–4,040	6,480	4,860	4,904	3,480	3,147	2,791
ω-3 fatty acids (g/d)[a]	0	0	2	4	6	8	10

[a]Semipurified fish oil extracts; courtesy Virginia Stout, PhD, NOAA, Seattle, WA

*28-year-old, pancreatitis in first pregnancy with triglycerides ~10,000 mg/dL, delivered at 38 weeks; patient had gnawing abdominal pain at week 30

(see below) has similar association with perinatal and childhood vasculopathy has not been studied to our knowledge.

A final reason to obtain plasma lipid levels in pregnancy is that they provide a clue to the existence of disordered lipid metabolism post-partum, just as GDM predicts the evolution to overt diabetes in about 50% of subjects postpartum.[3, 30]

11.6 Lipoprotein Lipids in GDM

Effects of GDM on lipid and lipoprotein levels compared to normal pregnancy are reviewed in Table 11.3. In the first trimester, triglycerides were 14 gm/dL higher at 15 weeks gestation in one study.[31] Second trimester elevations were 101, 38, 43, 35 mg/dL (mean of 54 mg/dL in four studies).[31–33] Third trimester elevations were 42, 18, 42, 47, 77, 59, and 35 mg/dL (mean of 48 mg/dL in seven studies).[23,31–37] The unweighted grand mean triglyceride level in GDM in the third trimester is 232 mg/dL (Table 11.3). This elevation is ~50 mg/dL compared to both second and third trimester non-GDM comparators (Table 11.3) and 23 mg/dL above the 36 week median,[2,37] but this reference group did not exclude GDM and diabetes.[2] The triglyceride distribution in GDM is shifted generally upward compared to all deciles of the triglyceride distribution in normal pregnancy (see horizontal axis, Fig. 11.4).

Regarding cholesterol levels, first trimester values are higher in GDM compared with non-GDM (33 mg/dL in one study), slightly higher in the second trimester (10 mg/dL in three studies), but slightly lower in the third trimester (13.4 mg/dL in seven studies). In contrast, LDL-C levels are lower in GDM in the second trimester by 20 and 4 mg/dL and more so in third trimester GDM by 19–54 mg/dL (mean of 27.5 mg/dL in four studies (Table 11.3).

Because cholesterol carried in LDL is shifted to VLDL in hypertriglyceridemic states, LDL can be an inexact measure of atherogenic lipoprotein levels. To quantify this shift, the sum of VLDL and LDL cholesterol (calculated as non-HDL-C) is a more accurate measure of atherogenicity in hypertriglyceridemia. Non-HDL-C is higher in GDM by 6 and 13 mg/dL (two studies) in the second trimester (Table 11.3), but lower in the third trimester, 11–38 mg/dL in four studies (mean 23 mg/dL). The higher non-HDL-C value in second trimester GDM is potentially important, as vascular lesions in the

Table 11.3 Mean lipoprotein lipids in normal (Nl) and GDM pregnancy and postpartum

		Weeks							
		15		24–27		32–39		12–14 post	
Year [Reference]		Nl	GDM	Nl	GDM	Nl	GDM	Nl	GDM
1972[37]	(*n*)					(14)	(11)		
	Triglyceride					186	228		
	Cholesterol					278	193		
1977[34]	(*n*)					(38)	(22)		
	Triglyceride					189	207		
	Cholesterol					211	209		
1980[35]	Fasting glucose					≤85	≥85		
	(*n*)					(327)	(23)		
	Triglyceride					232	274		
	Cholesterol					266	255		
	LDL-C					155	136		
	Non-HDL-C					202	191		
	HDL-C					64.1	63.8		
1982[32]	(*n*)			(21)	(5)	(21)	(5)	(21)	(5)
	Triglyceride			185	286	224	271	82	148
	Cholesterol			251	241	259	224	204	208
	LDL-C[a]			165	145	162	130	145	147
	Non-HDL-C			183	189	204	172	153	163
	HDL-C[a]			68	52	55	52	51	45
1992[23]	(*n*)					(521)	(96)		
	Triglyceride					165[c]	203		
1992	(*n*)					(9)	(7)		
Unpub-	Triglyceride					143	220		
lished data	Cholesterol					247	197		
(Bonet B,	LDL-C					151	97		
Knopp	Non-HDL-C					180	142		
RH)	HDL-C					67	55		
1998[36]	(*n*)					(20)	(20)		
	Triglyceride					178	237		
	Cholesterol					232	221		
	VLDL-C					72	50		
	LDL-C					101	96		
	Non-HDL-C					162	150		
	HDL-C					70	71		
2005[33]	(*n*)			(121)	(36)				
	Triglyceride			176	219				
	Cholesterol			245	255				
	LDL-C			155	151				
	Non-HDL-C			180	193				
	HDL-C			65	62				

Table 11.3 (continued)

Year [Reference]		Weeks							
		15		24–27		32–39		12–14 post	
		Nl	GDM	Nl	GDM	Nl	GDM	Nl	GDM
2007[31]	(*n*)	(45)	(62)	(45)	(62)	(45)	(62)		
	Triglyceride	70	94	106	141	150	185		
	Cholesterol	163	198	190	220	224	274		
Grand	(*n*)	(45)	(62)	(1461)	(199)	(474)	(150)	(21)	(5)
Means	Triglyceride	70	94	158	212	186	232	82	148
	Cholesterol	163	198	229	239	238	225	204	205
Reference Values[b,2]									
	Triglyceride	98 (50–180)		140 (100–250)		209 (146–341)		77 (54–137)	
	Cholesterol	195 (140–250)		235 (190–280)		243 (161–254)		200 (161–254)	

( ) denotes numbers of subjects; *Nl* normal

[a]Values estimated from figure in reference[32]

[b]Mean (10–90th percentile ranges) extrapolated, GDM or diabetes not excluded, from reference[3]

[c]1-h post glucose screen triglyceride measurement; excludes GDM or screen (+), GTT (–)

second trimester fetus are linked to maternal hypercholesterolemia [28,29]. An additional atherosclerotic effect of hypertriglyceridemia is an increase in small dense LDL, conferring additional atherogenicity in GDM.[38]

HDL-C is antiatherogenic by its reverse cholesterol transport, anti-oxidant and anti-inflammatory effects. Typically, levels are reduced in hypertriglyceridemia and diabetes. In GDM, second trimester HDL-C levels were lower by 16 and 3 mg/dL in two studies. In third trimester, HDL-C levels were −0.3, −3, −12 and 1 mg/dL in GDM (mean of −3.6 mg/dL in four studies (Table 11.3).

The separate effects of obesity and GDM on the dyslipidemia of GDM have been addressed by Sanchez-Vera et al.[31] GDM is consistently associated with elevated triglyceride, even in the absence of obesity. On the other hand, triglyceride elevations associated with obesity diminish as gestation proceeds, indicating that the hypertriglyceridemia of GDM is more related to the GDM than to obesity.

11.7 Placental Lipid Metabolism in GDM

There is little research on placental lipid metabolism in GDM, though it is relevant to the relationship of maternal nutrient excess, including effects of maternal hypertriglyceridemia on fetal growth and development and macrosomia. In an abstract report of obesity, GDM or type 2 diabetes in pregnancy with maternal hypertriglyceridemia and cord blood hypertriglyceridemia, placental villi had increased levels of FFAs, but reduced triglycerides and no enhancement of villous droplets or lipid droplet associated proteins.[39] The data suggest that that the placenta adapts to the maternal hypertriglyceridemia with increased transport of fatty acids without becoming triglyceride enriched. These observations in GDM differ from type 1 diabetic pregnancy where placental triglyceride content increases.[40]

Another example of the maintenance of placental transport function relates to arachidonic and DHAs which are decreased in infants of GDM pregnancy compared with normal pregnancy.[41] However, when umbilical arterial and umbilical venous arachidonic acid (AA) and DHA levels in GDM pregnancy were compared with normal pregnancy, venous plasma levels were normal but arterial values were reduced.[41] These results indicate that fetal AA and DHA levels are reduced by fetal consumption and not deficiency of placental transport, consistent with adaptations to enhance DHA transplacental transport discussed above.[6, 19]

11.8 Dyslipidemia of GDM and Birth Weight

The importance of triglyceride elevations to increased birth weight can be judged by comparison to other predictors of birth weight. Triglyceride is positively associated with birth weight, up to a triglyceride level of 200 mg/dL in normal pregnancy, approximately 80th percentile in healthy women and then becomes negative, suggestive of a negative or toxic effect of higher triglycerides on birth weight.[23] Among second trimester, screen (+), GTT (−) women (most of whom have triglycerides OR TGs < 200 mg/dl TGs <200 mg/dL), plasma triglycerides 1-h after a 50-g glucose load are as strong a predictor of birth weight (r=0.13), as 2-h glucose concentration (r=0.15) or the sum of glucose increments (r=0.13) after a 100-g glucose tolerance test (all <0.05) in screen (+), GTT (−) women (n=264).[23] Triglyceride was not a statistically significant correlate in GDM (r=0.11) possibly due in part to GDM's association with triglyceride levels above 200 mg/dL (Fig. 11.4). The association between triglyceride and birthweight was strongest was strongest in the combined group of positive screened, negative GTT and GDM subjects (r=0.16) (p<0.01, n=360) compared with negative screenees (r=0.09) (p<0.05, n=511).

Couch et al confirmed an association of triglyceride with birth weight in normal women, along with HDL_2 (p<0.05).[36] Surprisingly, this association was not seen in GDM subjects, although the sample sizes were equal, 20 in each group. Kitajima et al also found a positive association of late second trimester fasting plasma triglyceride levels with birth-weight ratio in 146 subjects with a positive 1-h screening test but a negative 75-g oral glucose tolerance test (r=0.22, p=0.009).[42] Among measured maternal lipids, only triglyceride was associated with birth-weight in univariate analysis. Associations with maternal prepregnancy body mass index (BMI) and fasting glucose were less, r=0.18 and 0.17, respectively (p=0.04 in both instances). In logistic regression, fasting triglyceride was a predictor of large for gestational age (LGA) infants, independent of prepregnant BMI, maternal weight gain, and maternal glucose levels. Di Cianni et al performed a similar analysis in 83 women with positive screening test but with negative oral glucose tolerance tests (GTTs).[33] The R^2 association of triglyceride with birth weight was 0.09, meaning that this measure accounted for 9% of the birth weight association, while the glucose R^2 was 0.044, both $p<0.05$. In step-wise regression, only triglycerides and prepregnancy BMI remained independently associated with birth weight (F tests 4.07 and 7.26 respectively) ($p<0.01$ in both instances).

Most recently, Schaeffer-Graf et al found that maternal FFA as well as triglycerides were significantly associated with fetal abdominal circumference (AC) at 28 weeks gestation (FFA $p<0.02$ and triglyceride $p<0.001$).[43] This study also examined the cord blood lipids and found lower cord triglyceride levels in LGA babies and cord triglyceride inversely associated with birth weight and neonatal fat mass. Separately, Bomba-Opon et al found elevated FFA levels in late gestation GDM women and a positive association of FFA with birth weight.[44]

In conclusion, triglycerides are predictors of birth weight across all categories of GDM screening status and among several studies. The most consistent association is in (+) screen, (−) GTT non-GDM women. In GDM, a weaker association of TG and birth weight may be due to the larger number of GDM women with triglycerides >200 mg/dL and a negative, possibly toxic, association of higher triglycerides with birth weight.

11.9 Oxidative Stress in GDM

Because of the known association of inflammation with metabolic syndrome, GDM, and diabetes,[45–47] it is of interest to assess the role of oxidative stress in GDM, including lipoprotein susceptibility to oxidation. Sánchez-Vera et al measured LDL oxidation in 45 non-diabetic subjects and 62 women with GDM by measuring the time for LDL oxidation to begin under oxidizing conditions (lag phase).[31] A shortened lag phase reflects diminished antioxidant defense against oxidative stress due to prior antioxidant consumption in vivo. Lag phase was shortened in GDM compared to healthy pregnant women by 32, 31, and 24 % across the 3 trimesters (<0.001). These data indicate that GDM increases the susceptibility of LDL to oxidative stress by one third. LDL from non-obese GDM women were less sensitive to oxidative modification especially in the third trimester whereas obese GDM women were more-so.

Additional evidence of heightened oxidative stress and diminished antioxidant defense has been detected in GDM (see review[48]). Vitamin C levels and total antioxidant capacity levels were reduced in GDM, though oxidized lipids measured as malonyldialdehyde (MDA) and lipid hydroperoxides were unchanged. However, evidence of lipid oxidation has been found in maternal tissues and placenta in the form of lipid hydroperoxides, 8-isoprostanes and MDA with compensatory antioxidant enzyme activity including elevated activity of superoxide dismutase and glutathione peroxidase. Surprisingly, the ability of the placenta to respond to inflammatory stress was impaired with a reduced capacity to form 8-isoprostane, TNFα, and NF-kappa B.[49] Oxidative stresses can injure the placenta as seen in trophoblast cytotoxicity from oxidized LDL in primary tissue culture.[50] Also of interest is that lag phase for the oxidation of LDL is shortened in type 1 diabetic pregnancy (B Bonet and RH Knopp, unpublished observations). Enhanced oxidative stress is a well known cause of congenital malformations in animal models of diabetes.[51]

Extreme examples of oxidative stress in pregnancy are found in preeclampsia and eclampsia, where lipid hydroperoxides are in excess, the placenta is dysfunctional and newborns are SGA.[52] The lipoprotein system may play a role in propagating oxidative stress in the course of scavenging oxidized lipids from the placenta and transporting them to the liver for excretion, but, in the process, causing endothelial injury and hypertension, especially in hypertriglyceridemia.[25,53] Maternal antibodies to oxidized LDL have been found in preeclampsia.[54] Similarly, evidence of lipid peroxidation and altered anti-oxidant defense has been observed in maternal and cord plasma and placenta in severe hypercholesterolemia.[55]

11.10 Summary

The dyslipidemia of GDM is associated with ~50 mg/dL increase in triglyceride at term, ~4 mg/dL lower HDL level, lower LDL levels, and normal or reduced non-HDL-cholesterol levels. The defense of LDL against oxidation is reduced by 35% in GDM and LDL is small and dense, consistent with the hypertriglyceridemia of GDM. Increases in multiple other measures of inflammation and oxidative stress are observed in GDM pregnancy. At the extreme, the consumption of antioxidant defenses is associated with circulating lipid peroxides in preeclampsia, placental damage, endothelial injury, hypertension, and retarded fetal growth. Both hypertriglyceridemia in GDM and familial hypercholesterolemia are associated with heightened oxidative stress. Birth weight in GDM may be the result of competing effects of nutrient excess (elevated glucose and triglyceride) on the one hand, and toxic effects of enhanced oxidative stress propagated by lipid peroxidation and placental dysfunction, on the other. A challenge for the future is to understand the interplay between nutrient excess, inflammation, lipoprotein oxidation, perinatal morbidity and mortality, and to devise treatments for these pathophysiologies in GDM.

Acknowledgments This work was supported in part by NIH grant DK 035816, Clinical Nutrition Research Unit at the University of Washington.

References

1. Knopp R, Bonet B, Zhu X-D. Lipid metabolism in pregnancy. In: Cowett R, ed. *Principles of Perinatal-Neonatal Metabolism*. New York: Springer; 1998:221-258.
2. Knopp RH, Bergelin RO, Wahl PW, Walden CE, Chapman M, Irvine S. Population-based lipoprotein lipid reference values for pregnant women compared to nonpregnant women classified by sex hormone usage. *Am J Obstet Gynecol*. 1982;143:626-637.
3. Knopp R, Paramsothy P. Part 2. Management of diabetic/medical complications in pregnancy: management of hyper/dyslipidmias. In: Kitzmiller J, Jovanovic L, Brown F, Coustan D, Reader D, eds. *Managing Preexisting Diabetes and Pregnancy: Technical Reviews and Consensus Recommendations for Care*. Alexandria: American Diabetes Association; 2008:355-374.
4. Alvarez JJ, Montelongo A, Iglesias A, Lasuncion MA, Herrera E. Longitudinal study on lipoprotein profile, high density lipoprotein subclass, and postheparin lipases during gestation in women. *J Lipid Res*. 1996;37:299-308.

5. Magnusson-Olsson AL, Hamark B, Ericsson A, Wennergren M, Jansson T, Powell TL. Gestational and hormonal regulation of human placental lipoprotein lipase. *J Lipid Res*. 2006;47:2551-2561.
6. Larque E, Krauss-Etschmann S, Campoy C, et al. Docosahexaenoic acid supply in pregnancy affects placental expression of fatty acid transport proteins. *Am J Clin Nutr*. 2006;84: 853-861.
7. van Eijsden M, Hornstra G, van der Wal MF, Vrijkotte TG, Bonsel GJ. Maternal n-3, n-6, and trans fatty acid profile early in pregnancy and term birth weight: a prospective cohort study. *Am J Clin Nutr*. 2008;87:887-895.
8. Banka CL. High density lipoprotein and lipoprotein oxidation. *Curr Opin Lipidol*. 1996;7:139-142.
9. Vaisar T, Pennathur S, Green PS, et al. Shotgun proteomics implicates protease inhibition and complement activation in the antiinflammatory properties of HDL. *J Clin Invest*. 2007;117: 746-756.
10. Grunfeld C, Feingold KR. HDL and innate immunity: a tale of two apolipoproteins. *J Lipid Res*. 2008;49:1605-1606.
11. Oram JF. The ins and outs of ABCA. *J Lipid Res*. 2008;49:1150-1151.
12. Lasuncion MA, Bonet B, Knopp RH. Mechanism of the HDL2 stimulation of progesterone secretion in cultured placental trophoblast. *J Lipid Res*. 1991;32:1073-1087.
13. Woollett LA. Maternal cholesterol in fetal development: transport of cholesterol from the maternal to the fetal circulation. *Am J Clin Nutr*. 2005;82:1155-1161.
14. Schmid KE, Davidson WS, Myatt L, Woollett LA. Transport of cholesterol across a BeWo cell monolayer: implications for net transport of sterol from maternal to fetal circulation. *J Lipid Res*. 2003;44:1909-1918.
15. Stefulj J, Panzenboeck U, Becker T, et al. Human endothelial cells of the placental barrier efficiently deliver cholesterol to the fetal circulation via ABCA1 and ABCG1. *Circ Res*. 2009;104:600-608.
16. Madsen EM, Lindegaard ML, Andersen CB, Damm P, Nielsen LB. Human placenta secretes apolipoprotein B-100-containing lipoproteins. *J Biol Chem*. 2004;279:55271-55276.
17. Portman OW, Behrman RE, Soltys P. Transfer of free fatty acids across the primate placenta. *Am J Physiol*. 1969;216:143-147.
18. Campbell FM, Clohessy AM, Gordon MJ, Page KR, Dutta-Roy AK. Uptake of long chain fatty acids by human placental choriocarcinoma (BeWo) cells: role of plasma membrane fatty acid-binding protein. *J Lipid Res*. 1997;38:2558-2568.
19. Koletzko B, Larque E, Demmelmair H. Placental transfer of long-chain polyunsaturated fatty acids (LC-PUFA). *J Perinat Med*. 2007;35(suppl 1):S5-S11.
20. Knopp RH, Bergelin RO, Wahl PW, Walden CE. Relationships of infant birth size to maternal lipoproteins, apoproteins, fuels, hormones, clinical chemistries, and body weight at 36 weeks gestation. *Diabetes*. 1985;34(suppl 2):71-77.
21. Weng W, Breslow JL. Dramatically decreased high density lipoprotein cholesterol, increased remnant clearance, and insulin hypersensitivity in apolipoprotein A-II knockout mice suggest a complex role for apolipoprotein A-II in atherosclerosis susceptibility. *Proc Natl Acad Sci U S A*. 1996;93:14788-14794.
22. Kalopissis AD, Pastier D, Chambaz J. Apolipoprotein A-II: beyond genetic associations with lipid disorders and insulin resistance. *Curr Opin Lipidol*. 2003;14:165-172.
23. Knopp RH, Magee MS, Walden CE, Bonet B, Benedetti TJ. Prediction of infant birth weight by GDM screening tests. Importance of plasma triglyceride. *Diabetes Care*. 1992;15:1605-1613.
24. Arbogast BW, Lee GM, Raymond TL. In vitro injury of porcine aortic endothelial cells by very-low-density lipoproteins from diabetic rat serum. *Diabetes*. 1982;31:593-599.
25. Hubel CA, McLaughlin MK, Evans RW, Hauth BA, Sims CJ, Roberts JM. Fasting serum triglycerides, free fatty acids, and malondialdehyde are increased in preeclampsia, are positively correlated, and decrease within 48 hours post partum. *Am J Obstet Gynecol*. 1996; 174:975-982.

26. Pou KM, Massaro JM, Hoffmann U, et al. Visceral and subcutaneous adipose tissue volumes are cross-sectionally related to markers of inflammation and oxidative stress: the Framingham Heart Study. *Circulation*. 2007;116:1234-1241.
27. Knopp RH. Drug treatment of lipid disorders. *N Engl J Med*. 1999;341:498-511.
28. Napoli C, D'Armiento FP, Mancini FP, et al. Fatty streak formation occurs in human fetal aortas and is greatly enhanced by maternal hypercholesterolemia. Intimal accumulation of low density lipoprotein and its oxidation precede monocyte recruitment into early atherosclerotic lesions. *J Clin Invest*. 1997;100:2680-2690.
29. Napoli C, Glass CK, Witztum JL, Deutsch R, D'Armiento FP, Palinski W. Influence of maternal hypercholesterolaemia during pregnancy on progression of early atherosclerotic lesions in childhood: Fate of Early Lesions in Children (FELIC) study. *Lancet*. 1999;354:1234-1241.
30. Montes A, Walden CE, Knopp RH, Cheung M, Chapman MB, Albers JJ. Physiologic and supraphysiologic increases in lipoprotein lipids and apoproteins in late pregnancy and postpartum. Possible markers for the diagnosis of "prelipemia". *Arteriosclerosis*. 1984;4:407-417.
31. Sanchez-Vera I, Bonet B, Viana M, et al. Changes in plasma lipids and increased low-density lipoprotein susceptibility to oxidation in pregnancies complicated by gestational diabetes: consequences of obesity. *Metabolism*. 2007;56:1527-1533.
32. Hollingsworth DR, Grundy SM. Pregnancy-associated hypertriglyceridemia in normal and diabetic women. Differences in insulin-dependent, non-insulin-dependent, and gestational diabetes. *Diabetes*. 1982;31:1092-1097.
33. Di Cianni G, Miccoli R, Volpe L, et al. Maternal triglyceride levels and newborn weight in pregnant women with normal glucose tolerance. *Diabet Med*. 2005;22:21-25.
34. Warth MR, Knopp RH. Lipid metabolism in pregnancy. V. Interactions of diabetes, body weight, age and high carbohydrate diet. *Diabetes*. 1977;26:1056-1062.
35. Knopp RH, Chapman M, Bergelin R, Wahl PW, Warth MR, Irvine S. Relationships of lipoprotein lipids to mild fasting hyperglycemia and diabetes in pregnancy. *Diabetes Care*. 1980;3:416-420.
36. Couch SC, Philipson EH, Bendel RB, Wijendran V, Lammi-Keefe CJ. Maternal and cord plasma lipid and lipoprotein concentrations in women with and without gestational diabetes mellitus. Predictors of birth weight? *J Reprod Med*. 1998;43:816-822.
37. Knopp RH, Warth MR, Carrol CJ. Lipid metabolism in pregnancy. I. Changes in lipoprotein triglyceride and cholesterol in normal pregnancy and the effects of diabetes mellitus. *J Reprod Med*. 1973;10:95-101.
38. Qiu C, Rudra C, Austin MA, Williams MA. Association of gestational diabetes mellitus and low-density lipoprotein (LDL) particle size. *Physiol Res*. 2007;56:571-578.
39. Scifres C, Chen B, Nelson D, Sadovsky Y. The influence of maternal obesity and diabetes on placental lipi trafficking. *J Obster Gynec*. 2008;199:S22. abstract #50.
40. Lindegaard ML, Damm P, Mathiesen ER, Nielsen LB. Placental triglyceride accumulation in maternal type 1 diabetes is associated with increased lipase gene expression. *J Lipid Res*. 2006;47:2581-2588.
41. Ortega-Senovilla H, Alvino G, Taricco E, Cetin I, Herrera E. Gestational diabetes mellitus upsets the proportion of fatty acids in umbilical arterial but not venous plasma. *Diabetes Care*. 2009;32:120-122.
42. Kitajima M, Oka S, Yasuhi I, Fukuda M, Rii Y, Ishimaru T. Maternal serum triglyceride at 24–32 weeks' gestation and newborn weight in nondiabetic women with positive diabetic screens. *Obstet Gynecol*. 2001;97:776-780.
43. Schaefer-Graf UM, Graf K, Kulbacka I, et al. Maternal lipids as strong determinants of fetal environment and growth in pregnancies with gestational diabetes mellitus. *Diabetes Care*. 2008;31:1858-1863.
44. Bomba-Opon D, Wielgos M, Szymanska M, Bablok L. Effects of free fatty acids on the course of gestational diabetes mellitus. *Neuro Endocrinol Lett*. 2006;27:277-280.

45. Hansel B, Giral P, Nobecourt E, et al. Metabolic syndrome is associated with elevated oxidative stress and dysfunctional dense high-density lipoprotein particles displaying impaired antioxidative activity. *J Clin Endocrinol Metab*. 2004;89:4963-4971.
46. Tesauro M, Schinzari F, Rovella V, et al. Tumor necrosis factor-alpha antagonism improves vasodilation during hyperinsulinemia in metabolic syndrome. *Diabetes Care*. 2008;31:1439-1441.
47. Kim C, Cheng YJ, Beckles GL. Inflammation among women with a history of gestational diabetes mellitus and diagnosed diabetes in the Third National Health and Nutrition Examination Survey. *Diabetes Care*. 2008;31:1386-1388.
48. Chen X, Scholl TO. Oxidative stress: changes in pregnancy and with gestational diabetes mellitus. *Curr Diab Rep*. 2005;5:282-288.
49. Coughlan MT, Permezel M, Georgiou HM, Rice GE. Repression of oxidant-induced nuclear factor-kappaB activity mediates placental cytokine responses in gestational diabetes. *J Clin Endocrinol Metab*. 2004;89:3585-3594.
50. Bonet B, Hauge-Gillenwater H, Zhu XD, Knopp RH. LDL oxidation and human placental trophoblast and macrophage cytotoxicity. *Proc Soc Exp Biol Med*. 1998;217:203-211.
51. Wentzel P, Gareskog M, Eriksson UJ. Decreased cardiac glutathione peroxidase levels and enhanced mandibular apoptosis in malformed embryos of diabetic rats. *Diabetes*. 2008;57:3344-3352.
52. Hubel CA, Roberts JM, Taylor RN, Musci TJ, Rogers GM, McLaughlin MK. Lipid peroxidation in pregnancy: new perspectives on preeclampsia. *Am J Obstet Gynecol*. 1989;161:1025-1034.
53. Clausen T, Djurovic S, Henriksen T. Dyslipidemia in early second trimester is mainly a feature of women with early onset pre-eclampsia. *Bjog*. 2001;108:1081-1087.
54. Branch DW, Mitchell MD, Miller E, Palinski W, Witztum JL. Pre-eclampsia and serum antibodies to oxidised low-density lipoprotein. *Lancet*. 1994;343:645-646.
55. Liguori A, D'Armiento FP, Palagiano A, et al. Effect of gestational hypercholesterolaemia on omental vasoreactivity, placental enzyme activity and transplacental passage of normal and oxidised fatty acids. *Bjog*. 2007;114:1547-1556.

Blood Pressure in GDM

12

Baha Sibai and Mounira Habli

12.1 Gestational Diabetes and Hypertension During Pregnancy

There is a strong association between insulin resistance and hypertensive disorders in pregnancy,[1] both of which are associated with higher risk of cardiovascular disease later in life.[1] Because of recent trends in advanced maternal age at time of conception and the growing rate of obesity, the incidences of both chronic hypertension as well as gestational diabetes (GDM) are also increasing.[2] Therefore, the rate of pregnancies complicated by both hypertensive disorders and GDM are expected to rise. In this chapter, we discuss the classification of hypertensive disorders of pregnancy; pathophysiology of hypertension and insulin resistance; outcomes of pregnancies affected by hypertension and GDM and prevention and management strategies of hypertensive disorders with and without GDM.

12.2 Classification of Hypertensive Disorders

Hypertensive disorders are the most common medical complications of pregnancy, affecting 5–8% of all pregnancies.[2,3] Categories of hypertensive disorders in pregnancy include chronic hypertension and the group of hypertensive disorders unique to pregnancy, including gestational hypertension, with and without preeclampsia. Approximately 30% of hypertensive disorders in pregnancy are due to chronic hypertension and 70% are due to gestational hypertension.[2,3] The spectrum of disease ranges from mildly elevated blood pressures with minimal clinical significance to severe hypertension and multi-organ dysfunction. The incidence of disease is dependent upon multiple demographic parameters including maternal age, race, and associated underlying medical conditions. Understanding the disease process

B. Sibai (✉)
Department of Obstetrics and Gynecology, University of Cincinnati College of Medicine, Cincinnati, OH, USA
e-mail: sibaibm@ucmail.uc.edu

C. Kim and A. Ferrara (eds.), *Gestational Diabetes During and After Pregnancy*,
DOI: 10.1007/978-1-84882-120-0_12, © Springer-Verlag London Limited 2010

and the impact of hypertensive disorders on pregnancy is of utmost importance, because these disorders remain a major cause of maternal and perinatal morbidity and mortality worldwide.

Hypertension is defined as a systolic blood pressure (SBP) of 140 mm Hg or greater, or a diastolic blood pressure (DBP) of 90 mm Hg or greater.[2–4] These measurements must be present on at least two occasions at least 4 h apart, but no more than a week apart.[2–4] Abnormal proteinuria in pregnancy is defined as the excretion of 300 mg or more of protein in 24 h. The most accurate measurement of proteinuria is obtained with a 24-h urine collection, but in certain instances, semiquantitative dipstick measurement may be the only test available to assess urinary protein. A value of 1+ or greater correlates with 30 mg/dL. Proteinuria by dipstick is defined as 1+ or more on at least two occasions at least 4 h apart but no more than 1 week apart in the absence of urinary tract infection. The accuracy of semiquantitative dipstick measurements on spot urine samples as compared with 24-h urine collections is highly variable.[2–4] Care should be taken when obtaining urine protein measurements to use a clean sample for dipstick measurement, because blood, vaginal secretions, and bacteria can increase the amount of protein in urine. In addition, protein excretion is influenced by posture and exercise.

Edema is a common finding in the gravid patient, occurring in approximately 50–80% of normal pregnancies. Lower extremity edema is the most typical form. Pathologic edema is usually seen in nondependent regions such as the face, hands, or lungs. Excessive, rapid weight gain of five pounds or more per week is another sign of pathologic fluid retention.[2–4]

The recent classification system of hypertension in pregnancy by the American College of Obstetricians and Gynecologists Committee adopted the criteria proposed by the National High Blood Pressure Education Program Working Group in 2000. This system offers simple, concise, and clinically relevant features for each of the four major categories of hypertension[2–4] in pregnancy – gestational hypertension, preeclampsia or eclampsia, chronic hypertension, and preeclampsia superimposed on chronic hypertension.

Gestational hypertension is the most frequent cause of hypertension during pregnancy.[4] The rate ranges between 6 and 17% in healthy nulliparous women and between 2 and 4% in multiparous women based on the population studied.[4] Gestational hypertension is considered severe if there is sustained SBP to at least 160 mmHg and/or DBP to at least 110 mmHg for at least 6 h without proteinuria. Treatment generally is not warranted, because most patients have mild hypertension. However, approximately 40–50% of patients diagnosed with preterm mild gestational hypertension will develop proteinuria and progress to preeclampsia.[4] In general, the majority of cases of mild gestational hypertension are diagnosed at or beyond 37 weeks and have a pregnancy outcome similar to term normotensive pregnancies.[4]

The incidence of preeclampsia is reported to be from 5 to 8%, depending upon the population.[2–4] Preeclampsia occurs more frequently in primigravidas. The reported rate of preeclampsia ranges from 6 to 7% in primigravidas and from 3 to 4% in multiparous patients.[2–4] Advanced maternal age (≥35 years) is another risk factor especially if conception was secondary to assisted reproductive technology.[2–4] Obesity is another important factor.[2–4]

The symptoms of preeclampsia are headaches, visual changes, and epigastric or right upper quadrant pain plus nausea or vomiting.[2–4] In the absence of proteinuria, preeclampsia should be considered when gestational hypertension is associated with persistent cerebral symptoms, epigastric or right upper quadrant pain with nausea or vomiting, fetal growth restriction, thrombocytopenia or abnormal liver enzymes.[2–4]

Preeclampsia may be subdivided further into mild and severe forms. The distinction between the two is made on the basis of the degree of hypertension and proteinuria and the involvement of other organ systems.[2–4] Close surveillance of patients with either mild preeclampsia or gestational hypertension is warranted, because they may progress to fulminant disease. A particularly severe form of preeclampsia is the HELLP syndrome, an acronym for hemolysis (H), elevated liver enzymes (EL), and low platelet count (LP).[5] The acronym may be deceptive, because hypertension or proteinuria might be absent in 10–15% of women who develop HELLP and in 20–25 % of those who develop eclampsia.[5] A patient diagnosed with HELLP syndrome should be classified as having severe preeclampsia. Another severe form of preeclampsia is eclampsia, which is the occurrence of seizures not attributable to other causes.[5]

Hypertension complicating pregnancy is considered chronic if a patient was diagnosed with hypertension before pregnancy, if hypertension was present prior to 20 weeks gestation, or if it persists longer than 12 weeks after delivery.[3] Women with chronic hypertension are at risk of developing superimposed preeclampsia. The reported rate of superimposed preeclampsia ranges from 15% to 35%.[3] Superimposed preeclampsia is defined as an exacerbation of hypertension with new onset of proteinuria or symptoms of headache or epigastric pain or laboratory abnormalities as elevated liver enzymes.[3]

12.3 Pathophysiology

The etiologic agent responsible for the development of preeclampsia remains unknown.[2–4] Theories as to the causative mechanisms include placental origin, immunologic origin, abnormal angiogenesis, endothelial cell injury, alterations in nitric oxide levels, increased oxygen free radicals, abnormal cytotrophoblast invasion, dietary deficiencies, and genetic predisposition.[2–4]

Insulin resistance has long been implicated in the pathogenesis of preeclampsia. Insulin resistance and preeclampsia share several biomarkers that vary over the course of pregnancy, and both insulin resistance and cardiovascular disease share similar biomarkers with preeclampsia.[6] For example, levels of triglycerides, small dense low density lipoprotein particles, free fatty acids, plasminogen activator inhibitor-1, vascular cell adhesion molecules, and leptin normally increase in normal pregnancy with advancing gestational age and with progression of insulin resistance.[7–9] Pregnancies complicated with preeclampsia are characterized by low sex hormone binding globulin[10–12] and low serum adiponectin levels,[13,14] which are also risk factors for GDM (Table 12.1).

GDM itself may increase risk for hypertension. Suhonen et al[15] reported that women with GDM ($n=81$) as compared with controls ($n=327$) have a higher frequency of chronic hypertension (2.5 vs. 0.3%, $p<0.05$) and preeclampsia (19.8 vs. 6.1%, $p<0.001$). Hyperinsulinemia has been prospectively diagnosed before the clinical diagnosis of preeclampsia.[16] However, in the Toronto Tri-Hospital Gestational Diabetes Project, Naylor et al[17] found only a 9% incidence of preeclampsia in untreated GDM, which is comparable to the incidence reported in treated women with GDM and in women treated for type 1 or type 2 diabetes mellitus. Therefore, treatment of GDM apparently does not reduce the incidence of hypertensive

Table 12.1 Risk factors for GDM and hypertensive disorders in pregnancy

Risk factor
Multifetal gestation
Chronic vascular disease (renal disease, rheumatic disease, connective tissue disease)
Age ≥25 years
Body mass index (BMI) ≥25 kg/m^2
Ethnicity (Native American, Asian)
Type 1 or type 2 diabetes or GDM in a first degree relative
Previous history of GDM
Previous macrosomic baby
Mother's own weight <2,500 g or 10th percentile
Multiple gestation
Polycystic ovary syndrome
Family history of preeclampsia or eclampsia
Metabolic syndrome

disorders in pregnancy. No treatment studies[18–27] have corrected for age or maternal BMI, which are well established risk factors for hypertensive disorders in pregnancy. There are also no prospective observational studies or randomized trials evaluating the benefits of treating mild hypertension for prevention of GDM. Thus, whether GDM shares a common causal pathway with hypertensive disorders or is a cause of hypertensive disorders is unknown (Table 12.2).

12.4 Pregnancy Outcomes

Maternal and neonatal outcome in patients with preeclampsia with or without GDM depends on the following factors: the gestational age at delivery, severity of disease, quality of management, and presence of preexisting disease. Perinatal mortality is increased in those who develop hypertensive disease at <34 weeks. Risk to the mother can be significant and includes the possible development of disseminated intravascular coagulation, intracranial hemorrhage, renal failure, retinal detachment, pulmonary edema, liver rupture, abruptio placentae, and death.[28]

At least one study has shown an association between GDM and preexisting chronic hypertension and subsequent impact on perinatal outcomes. Schaffer found that the coexistence of chronic hypertension and GDM is associated with a higher rate of induction of labor (36.7 vs. 6.6%, $p < 0.05$) but not with increased incidence of small- or large- for gestational age deliveries or low Apgar scores as compared with nonhypertensive GDM women.[29]

Table 12.2 Percent of hypertensive disorders in pregnancies complicated with GDM

Author	N	% Gestational hypertension	% Preeclampsia
Prospective studies			
Yogev et al (2008)[18]	1,319		11.7
Metzger B et al (HAPO) (2008)[19]	25,505	5.9	4.8
Retrospective studies			
Svare JA et al (2001)[20]	323		7
Yogev et al (2004)[21]	1,813		9.6
Jacobson et al (2005)[22]	504		8.7
Shand AW et al (2008)[23]	16,727	6.9	6.7
Stella C et al (2008)[24]	14,880	21.4	
Randomized clinical trials			
Langer O et al (2000)[25]	404		6
Crowther CA et al (2005)[26]	1,030		15.1
Rowan JA et al (2008)[27]	733	5.04	6.3

12.5 Prevention of Preeclampsia

Preventive interventions for preeclampsia could impact maternal and perinatal morbidity and mortality worldwide. As a result, during the past decade several randomized trials reported methods to reduce the rate and/or severity of preeclampsia. Several trials assessed protein or low-salt diets, diuretics, bed rest, zinc, magnesium, fish oil, vitamin C and E supplementation, and heparin to prevent preeclampsia, but results showed minimal to no effects of these therapies.[28] Of note, none of these strategies were evaluated among women with coexisting GDM per se.

12.6 Management of Hypertension and GDM

There are no proven benefits of treating mild chronic hypertension or mild gestational hypertension during pregnancy, regardless of GDM.[30] On the other hand, there is general agreement regarding treatment of severe hypertension during pregnancy (chronic or gestational).[4] Informed by guidelines in persons without diabetes, the American College of Obstetricians and Gynecologists recommends that maternal blood pressure be aggressively treated to levels below 130/80 mm Hg (both systolic and diastolic) in women with type 1 and 2 diabetes mellitus.[31] While some authors recommend treating GDM women with antihypertensive medications to keep SBP <140 mm Hg and DBP <90 mm Hg, the benefits and neonatal impact of such therapy remain unclear.

Women with GDM should be evaluated for superimposed preeclampsia as soon as the diagnosis is suspected. There are no data to guide physicians regarding the proper management of chronic hypertension in patients with GDM. As such, our recommendations are empiric.

The development of superimposed preeclampsia or mild preeclampsia/gestational hypertension is an indication for hospitalization in order to maintain close observation of maternal and fetal conditions. This evaluation should include 24 h urine for protein, platelet count, liver enzymes, and attention to new onset symptoms, such as severe headaches, visual disturbances, epigastric pain, and shortness of breath. In addition, patients should receive fetal testing (ultrasound for fetal growth and amniotic fluid index, and non-stress test or biophysical profile) at the time of diagnosis. If the patient was a candidate for outpatient management, fetal testing should be performed weekly and ultrasound for fetal growth every 3 weeks. We recommend that urine and blood tests be obtained at least once every week.

If there is proteinuria (≥300 mg/24 h), thrombocytopenia (platelet count <100,000/mm^3), or elevated liver enzymes (AST or ALT >2x upper limit of normal), or signs or symptoms of severe preeclampsia, patients should be considered to have severe preeclampsia and be managed accordingly. Management strategies upon diagnosis should include intravenous magnesium sulfate, antihypertensive medications to control blood pressure in labor and delivery, and steroids for fetal lung maturity. Subsequent management will depend on response to this therapy, results of fetal and maternal evaluation, and gestational age at time of diagnosis.

Delivery is recommended for all patients with mild preeclampsia and gestational age of ≥37 weeks or in the presence of fetal or maternal indications. The presence of any of the factors listed in Table 12.3 is an indication for delivery. In addition, once the diagnosis of severe preeclampsia is established, women with gestational age greater than 24 weeks and less than 34 weeks should receive corticosteroids to accelerate fetal lung maturity and then be delivered within 48–72 h,[32] likewise, delivery at gestational age >34 weeks is the treatment of choice after maternal stabilization.

For patients with essential chronic hypertension (absent target organ damage), we recommend using a calcium channel blocker such as nifedipine or diltiazem extended release (see doses in Table 12.4) with a target goal of SBP <140 mm Hg and DBP <90 mm Hg based on the recommendations for type 2 diabetes with hypertension in nonpregnant individuals. For patients with mild gestational hypertension (absent chronic hypertension), we do not recommend antihypertensive therapy because of the concern that such therapy may mask the development of severe gestational hypertension-preeclampsia. However, if the physician elects to use antihypertensive therapy to control mild hypertension, we recommend that such patients be managed in-hospital under close medical evaluation.

It is important to note that the recommendation for achieving this target goal is empiric and is not based on validated scientific data. Indeed, our target goal for patients without GDM is to keep systolic BP below 160 mm Hg and diastolic BP below 105 mm Hg.[33] If the target goal BP is not achieved with maximum dose of nifedipine, we then add a combined β-and α- blocker such as labetalol starting with a dose of 100–200 mg twice daily for a maximum dose of 2,400 mg/day (800 mg three times daily). Failure to achieve the target blood pressure goal with maximum doses of these drugs is considered an

Table 12.3 Indications for delivery in patients with GDM and severe preeclampsia

Gestational age >34 weeks
Preterm labor or rupture of membranes
Vaginal bleeding/suspected abruption
Persistent symptoms after magnesium sulfate
Eclampsia or persistent cerebral symptoms
Thrombocytopenia (platelet count less than 100,000) or elevated liver enzymes (HELLP syndrome)
Serum creatinine of 1.5 mg/dL or more or oliguria (<0.5 mL/kg/h)
Uncontrolled severe hypertension (SBP≥160 mmHg, DBP≥110 mmHg) despite maximum doses of antihypertensive (intravenous labetalol, hydralazine, and oral nifedipine)
Non-reassuring fetal heart rate testing
Congestive heart failure or pulmonary edema
Fetal growth restriction (<5‰ for gestational age)
Oligohydramnios (fluid index of <5 cm on at last two occasions >24 h apart)
Biophysical profile <4 on two occasions at 4 h apart
Repetitive late deceleration or severe variable deceleration or loss of variability
Reverse end diastolic flow or persistent absent diastolic flow in umbilical artery Doppler studies

indication for delivery except in cases where gestational age is <30 weeks, where a third drug can be added, such as oral hydralazine.

12.7 Conclusions

While the pathophysiology and risk factors for GDM and hypertension during pregnancy overlap, the implications of this overlap for clinical management remain uncertain. Currently, management of these conditions remains separate, with hypertension and preeclampsia guidelines nearly identical in women with and without glucose intolerance during pregnancy. Future studies exploring the effects of concurrent treatment of mild hypertension and glucose intolerance are needed. Of particular importance would be studies of the impact of lifestyle interventions for both hypertension and glucose intolerance on incidence of GDM and preeclampsia. Elucidation of the common pathways of glucose intolerance and hypertension during pregnancy would address the adverse outcomes associated with these two increasingly common conditions.

Table 12.4 Antihypertensive drugs commonly used in pregnancy

Drug	Starting dose	Maximum dose		Comments
Acute treatment of severe hypertension				
Hydralazine	5–10 mg IV every 20 min	30 mg[a]		
Labetalol	20–40 mg IV every 10–15 min	220 mg[a]		Avoid in women with asthma or congestive heart failure
Nifedipine	10–20 mg oral every 30 min	50 mg[a]		
Long term treatment of hypertension			Half life	
Methyldopa	250 mg twice a day	4 g/day	2 h	Rarely indicated
Labetalol	100–200 mg twice a day	2,400 mg/day	5–8 h	First choice
Nifedipine	10 mg twice a day	120 mg/day	2 h	To be used in women with diabetes
Diltiazem	120–180 mg daily	540 mg/day	2 h	To be used in women with diabetes
Thiazide diuretic	12.5 mg twice a day	50 mg/day	3 h	Use in salt-sensitive hypertension and/or congestive heart failure May be added as second agent Not to be used if preeclampsia develops or intrauterine growth retardation present
Angiotensin converting enzyme inhibitors or angiotensin receptor blockers				Not to be used except post partum

[a]If desired blood pressure levels are not achieved, switch to another drug

References

1. Carpenter MW et al. Gestational diabetes, pregnancy hypertension, and late vascular disease. *Diabetes Care*. 2007;30:S246-S250.
2. American College of Obstetricians and Gynecologists. Diagnosis and management of preeclampsia and eclampsia. ACOG Practice Bulletin No. 33. *Obstet Gynecol*. 2002;99:159-167.
3. American College of Obstetricians and Gynecologists. Chronic hypertension in pregnancy. ACOG Practice Bulletin No. 29. *Obstet Gynecol*. 2001;98:177-185.
4. Sibai BM. Diagnosis and management of gestational hypertension and preeclampsia. *Obstet Gynecol*. 2003;102:181-192.

5. Sibai BM. Diagnosis, controversies, and management of the syndrome of hemolysis, elevated liver enzymes, and low platelet count. *Obstet Gynecol.* 2004;103:981-991.
6. Sherif K, Kushner H, Falkner BE. Sex hormone-binding globulin and insulin resistance in African-American women. *Metabolism.* 1998;47:70-74.
7. Belo L, Caslake M, Gaffney D, et al. Changes in LDL size and HDL concentration in normal and preeclamptic pregnancies. *Atherosclerosis.* 2002;162:425-432.
8. Ogura K, Miyatake T, Fukui O, Nakamura T, Kameda T, Yoshino G. Low-density lipoprotein particle diameter in normal and preeclampsia. *J Atheroscler Thromb.* 2002;9:42-47.
9. Sattar N, Greer IA, Rumley A, et al. A longitudinal study of the relationships between between haemostatic, lipid, and oestradiol changes during normal human pregnancy. *Thromb Haemost.* 1999;81:71-75.
10. Carlsen SM, Romundstad P, Jacobsen G. Early second-trimester maternal hyperandrogenemia and subsequent preeclampsia: A prospective study. *Acta Obstet Gynecol Scand.* 2005;84:117-121.
11. Spencer K, Yu CKH, Rembouskos G, et al. First trimester sex hormone-binding globulin and subsequent development of preeclampsia or other adverse pregnancy outcomes. *Hypertens Pregnancy.* 2005;24:303-311.
12. Wolf M, Sandler L, Munoz K, et al. First trimester insulin resistance and subsequent preeclampsia: A prospective study. *J Clin Endocrinol Metabol.* 2002;87:1563-1568.
13. D'Anna R, Baviera G, Corrado F, et al. Adiponectin and insulin resistance in early and late-onset pre-eclampsia. *Br J Obstet Gynaecol.* 2006;113:1264-1269.
14. Masuyama H, Nakatsukasa H, Takamoto N, Hiramatsu Y. Correlation between soluble endoglin, vascular endothelial growth factor receptor-1, and adipocytokines in preeclampsia. *J Clin Endocrinol Metab.* 2007;92:2672-2679.
15. Suhonen L, Teramo K. Hypertension and pre-eclampsia in women with gestational glucose intolerance. *Acta Obstet Gynecol Scand.* 1993;72:269-272.
16. Martinez AE, Gonzalez OM, Quinones GA, Ferrannini E. Hyperinsulinemia in glucose-tolerant women with preeclampsia. A controlled study. *Am J Hypertens.* 1996;9:610-614.
17. Naylor CD, Sermer M, Chen E, et al. Cesarean delivery in relation to birth weight and gestational glucose tolerance. Pathophysiology or practice style? *JAMA.* 1996;275:1165-1170.
18. Yogev Y, Langer O. Pregnancy outcome in obese and morbidly obese gestational diabetic women. *Eur J Obstet Gynecol Reprod Biol.* 2008;137:21-26.
19. Metzger BE, Lowe LP, Dyer AR, et al. Hyperglycemia and adverse pregnancy outcomes. *N Engl J Med.* 2008;358:1991-2002.
20. Svare JA, Hansen BB, Mølsted-Pedersen L. Perinatal complications in women with gestational diabetes mellitus. *Acta Obstet Gynecol Scand.* 2001;80:899-904.
21. Yogev Y, Xenakis EM, Langer O. The association between preeclampsia and the severity of gestational diabetes: the impact of glycemic control. *Am J Obstet Gynecol.* 2004;191: 1655-1660.
22. Jacobson GF, Ramos GA, Ching JY, Kirby RS, Ferrara A, Field DR. Comparison of glyburide and insulin for the management of gestational diabetes in a large managed care organization. *Am J Obstet Gynecol.* 2005;193:118-124.
23. Shand AW, Bell JC, McElduff A, Morris J, Roberts CL. Outcomes of pregnancies in women with pre-gestational diabetes mellitus and gestational diabetes mellitus; a population-based study in New South Wales, Australia, 1998-2002. *Diabet Med.* 2008;25:708-715.
24. Stella CL, O'Brien JM, Forrester KJ, et al. The coexistence of gestational hypertension and diabetes: influence on pregnancy outcome. *Am J Perinatol.* 2008;25:325-329.
25. Langer O, Conway DL, Berkus MD, Xenakis EM, Gonzales O. A comparison of glyburide and insulin in women with gestational diabetes mellitus. *N Engl J Med.* 2000;343:1134-1138.
26. Crowther CA, Hiller JE, Moss JR, et al. Effect of treatment of gestational diabetes mellitus on pregnancy outcomes. *N Engl J Med.* 2005;352:2477-2486.

27. Rowan JA, Hague WM, Gao W, Battin MR, Moore MP, Investigators MiG Trial. Metformin versus insulin for the treatment of gestational diabetes. *N Engl J Med*. 2008;358:2003-2015.
28. Sibai BM. Preeclampsia. *Lancet*. 2005;365:785-799.
29. Anyaegbunam AM, Scarpelli S, Mikhail MS. Chronic hypertension in gestational diabetes: influence on pregnancy outcome. *Gynecol Obstet Invest*. 1995;39:167-170.
30. Abalos E, Duley L, Steyn DW, Henderson-Smart DJ. Antihypertensive drug therapy for mild to moderate hypertension during pregnancy. *Cochrane Database Syst Rev*. 2007;(1): CD002252.
31. Whalen KL, Stewart RD. Pharmacologic management of hypertension in patients with diabetes. *Am Fam Physician*. 2008;78:1277-1282.
32. Sibai BM, Barton JR. Expectant management of severe preeclampsia remote from term: patient selection, treatment, and delivery indications. *Am J Obstet Gynecol*. 2007;196:1-9.
33. Chobian AV, Bakris GL, Black HR, et al. The Seventh Report of the Joint National Committee on Prevention, Detection, Evaluation, and Treatment of High Blood Pressure: The JNC 7 Report. *JAMA*. 2003;289:2560-2572.

Genetics of Gestational Diabetes Mellitus and Type 2 Diabetes

13

Richard M. Watanabe

13.1 Introduction

Positional cloning is the process of identifying disease susceptibility genes through various gene mapping techniques when little is known about the genes underlying the disease. The success of positional cloning in single-gene diseases led to the possibility that the same process could be used to identify genes underlying complex diseases like diabetes.[1,2]

However, years before any of the major efforts to positionally clone diabetes genes began, a book entitled "The Genetics of Diabetes Mellitus" appeared with a lead chapter prophetically entitled "Diabetes Mellitus – A Geneticist's Nightmare".[3] This chapter, written by James V. Neel, considered the father of human genetics, warned of the complexity surrounding diabetes, small gene effects, confounding due to environmental factors, and interactions among genes and environment, and the challenge that would be faced in uncovering the genetic architecture of diabetes.

Scientific and technological advances led to an explosion of discoveries regarding genes underlying type 2 diabetes mellitus (T2DM) and related traits. Unfortunately, knowledge regarding the genetic basis for gestational diabetes mellitus (GDM) lags behind that of T2DM. In this chapter, we will summarize the general state of knowledge regarding the genetic basis for T2DM and whether there is a unique genetic basis underlying GDM.

R.M. Watanabe
Department of Preventive Medicine, Keck School of Medicine University of Southern California, 1540 Alcazar Street, CHP-220, Los Angeles, CA 90089-9011, USA
e-mail: rwatanab@usc.edu

C. Kim and A. Ferrara (eds.), *Gestational Diabetes During and After Pregnancy*,
DOI: 10.1007/978-1-84882-120-0_13,

13.2 Genetics of T2DM

13.2.1 State of Knowledge Prior to 2007

Over 25 genome-wide linkage scans for T2DM[4] and countless candidate gene studies had been performed between 1976 and 2006. There were numerous successes related to autosomal dominant forms of diabetes,[5] altered forms of insulin,[6–9] and rare forms of diabetes like maternally inherited diabetes and deafness.[10] However, by 2006 peroxisome proliferator-activated receptor γ (*PPARG*[11, 12]), potassium inwardly-rectifying channel, subfamily J, member 11 (*KCNJ11*[13]), and transcription factor 7-like 2 (*TCF7L2*[14]) were the only "accepted" T2DM susceptibility genes. Other genes, such as calpain 10 (*CAPN10*[15]), protein tyrosine phosphatase 1B (*PTPN1*[16]), and hepatocyte nuclear factor-4α (*HNF4A*[17–19]) showed evidence of association with T2DM, but most of these were not consistently replicated across study populations, raising some question as to their validity as T2DM susceptibility genes. Unfortunately, the inability to identify diabetes genes simply reflected the nightmare originally described by Dr. Neel and the reality that the technology and methods of the time would not allow for identification of small gene effects.

In 1996, Risch and Merikangas suggested that complex disease susceptibility genes could be identified by genotyping a number of single nucleotide polymorphisms (SNP) in each gene across the human genome[20] and performing association analysis. However, the ability to genotype the requisite number of SNPs in a sufficiently large sample was not feasible at that time. Also, many recognized that the framework proposed by Risch and Merikangas was gene-centric and did not take into account the possibility of regulatory elements outside the coding region of genes or intronic SNPs that might result in alternative splice forms of the gene.

However, three milestones altered the genomics landscape. The Human Genome Project (http://genome.ucsc.edu), an effort to decode our DNA, released the first draft of the human genome in 2000.[21] The HapMap Project (http://www.hapmap.org), an effort to identify genetic differences across human populations, has to-date identified over six million common SNPs across the human genome.[22, 23] Finally, improved technology now allows for genotyping of hundreds of thousands of SNPs in thousands of individuals in a span of weeks.

13.2.2 State of Knowledge After 2006: Genome-Wide Association

Results from the first genome-wide association (GWA) study for T2DM appeared in February 2007[24] and was based on ~400,000 SNPs genotyped in approximately 2,800 T2DM cases and controls with promising associations in this first stage followed-up in a larger sample of ~5,500 cases and controls. This 2-stage approach was employed to reduce study cost, while maintaining statistical power close to what would have been achieved if all subjects had been genotyped for all SNPs.[25] The analysis identified five regions of the genome showing evidence of association with T2DM that survived stringent statistical criteria that accounted for the large number of tests performed (Table 13.1). Among the loci identified was *TCF7L2*, which acted as a positive control in this study and provided added confidence these loci were indeed T2DM susceptibility genes. Another was a nonsynonymous variant in the solute carrier family 30 (zinc transporter), member 8 (*SLC30A8*) encoding the zinc transporter regulating zinc concentration in insulin secretory vesicles of the β-cell. There were two regions of extended linkage disequilibrium harboring multiple genes. One region included hematopoietically expressed homeobox (*HHEX*), insulin-degrading enzyme (*IDE*), and kinesin family member 11 (*KIF11*), all of which could be logically tied to the biology underlying T2DM. The second region included exostoses (multiple) 2 (*EXT2*) and aristaless-like homeobox 4

Table 13.1 Current type 2 diabetes susceptibility genes and their reported effect sizes

Chromosome	SNP	Gene region	Description	Reported odds ratio	References
1	rs10923931	*NOTCH1*	Intronic	1.13	97
2	rs7578597	*THADA*	Nonsynonymous	1.15	97
3	rs4607103	*ADAMTS9*	Upstream from the gene	1.09	97
3	rs4402960	*IGF2BP2*	Intronic	1.14	26–28
3	rs1801282	*PPARG*	Nonsynonymous	0.79	12
4	rs10010131	*WFS1*	Intronic	0.90	98
6	rs7754840	*CDKAL1*	Intronic	1.12	26–28
7	rs864745	*JAZF1*	Intronic	1.10	97
8	rs13266634	*SLC30A8*	Nonsynonymous	1.18	24
9	rs10811661	*CDKN2A/2B*	Upstream from the genes	1.20	26–28
10	rs12779790	*CDC123-CAMK1D*	Intergenic	1.11	97
10	rs7903146	*TCF7L2*	Intronic	1.37	14
10	rs1111875	*HHEX-IDE-KIF11*	Downstream from the genes	1.19	24
11	rs7480010	- - -	Intergenic	1.14	24
11	rs5219	*KCNJ11*	Nonsynonymous	1.23	13
11	rs3740878	*EXT2*	Intronic	1.26	24
11	rs2237892	*KCNQ1*	Intronic	1.49	99, 100
11	rs10830963	*MTNR1B*	Intronic	1.09	41
12	rs7961581	*TSPAN8-LGR5*	Intergenic	1.09	97
16	rs8050136	*FTO*	Intronic	1.17	26–28
17	rs757210	*HNF1B*	Intronic	1.13	101

(*ALX4*), which although less obvious candidates, nonetheless have plausible biologic ties to T2DM. Interestingly, the final SNP was in a region on chromosome 11 that did not harbor any known human genes; a so-called "gene desert," which raised interesting questions regarding human genome architecture. This study demonstrated that large-scale anonymous interrogation of the human genome by association could indeed identify susceptibility genes for a complex disease.

This initial success was immediately followed in April 2007 by a series of three GWA studies that collaborated to improve the power of their individual studies by performing a meta-analysis.[26–28] These groups replicated some of the findings by the original GWA study, such as *TCF7L2*, *SLC30A8*, the *HHEX* region, and even the intragenic region on chromosome 11, but also identified additional new loci (Table 13.1). This meta-analysis approach has become the current standard for GWA studies and as of this writing, 21 T2DM susceptibility genes have been identified (Table 13.1).

13.2.3 T2DM-Related Quantitative Traits

A general rule of thumb in statistics is that analysis of a continuous variable will be statistically more powerful than an analysis that categorizes the continuous variable. For a variety of reasons, this maxim may not fully extend to the analysis of disease-related quantitative traits. For example, as one progresses toward disease both the disease process and disease treatment could significantly alter one tail of the trait distribution. However, in principle the analysis of such traits could provide additional insights into the genetic architecture underlying a complex disease. Many groups have begun to apply GWA to search for genes underlying variation in disease-related quantitative traits, hypothesizing that a gene regulating variability in a trait may also be a disease susceptibility variant. To date, genes underlying height,[29,30] lipids,[31,32] anthropometrics,[33–37] and fasting glucose[38–41] have been identified.

One obvious trait to examine with respect to diabetes is fasting glucose. Among the first loci to be identified as regulating fasting glucose concentrations was a promoter variant in glucokinase (*GCK*) first reported in the mid to late 1990s[42,43] and subsequently confirmed in a large meta-analysis in 2005 by Weedon et al.[44,45] This promoter variant appears to contribute to mild hyperglycemia and does not contribute to risk for T2DM, consistent with observations regarding coding variants in *GCK* and MODY2.[46,47] Interestingly, this variant also appears to be associated with birth weight,[44,45] suggesting implications for fetal development. Recent results from the Meta-Analysis of Glucose and Insulin-related traits Consortium (MAGIC) have shown that variation in *GCK* is associated with both fasting glucose levels and risk for type 2 diabetes (Dupuis et al., *Nat Genet.* 2010;42:105-116 (PMID 20081858).

A recent GWA meta-analysis of fasting glucose reported association with glucose-6-phosphatase, catalytic unit 2 (*G6PC2*[38,48]), which was replicated in a separate study.[39] This association was interesting in that *G6PC2* appeared to only be associated with fasting glucose and showed no evidence of association with T2DM.[38,39] Most recently, a large GWA-based meta-analysis by the Meta-Analysis of Glucose and Insulin-related traits Consortium (MAGIC) reported that melatonin receptor-1B (*MTNR1B*) was associated with fasting glucose,[41] but in contrast to *G6PC2*, also showed evidence for association with T2DM.[41] These observations were independently reported by Bouatia-Naji et al.[40] Overall, these results suggest that there may be genes that only contribute to the day-to-day regulation of fasting glucose levels, while others may also contribute to susceptibility to T2DM.

MAGIC also demonstrated that *MTNR1B* was associated with insulin secretion and β-cell function.[49] These results demonstrate that while there may be an initial association between a genetic variant and specific quantitative trait, the primary effect of the gene may be elsewhere in the biologic pathway. Therefore, it is important to examine the association with other traits to best characterize the specific biology underlying the gene. A second example is the fat and obesity associated (*FTO*) gene, which was initially identified as being associated with T2DM,[26–28] but has subsequently been shown to be primarily associated with body mass index and body fat.[33, 50]

It is also noteworthy that like T2DM susceptibility genes, genetic variants underlying quantitative traits typically have very small effect sizes. For example, *G6PC2* and *MTNR1B* each independently have a per allele effect of ~0.07 mM, accounting for a very small proportion of the variation in fasting glucose.[38–41] The fact that only a small proportion of the variation in these traits is accounted for by genes suggests additional loci for this and other traits.

13.3 Genetics of GDM

13.3.1 Heritability of GDM

Despite successful identification of genes associated with T2DM and T2DM-related traits, surprisingly there has been relatively little research in the area of GDM genetics. This may partly reflect the fact that the study of GDM genetics is fraught with difficulties. An essential first step in genetics research has been the determination of evidence for a genetic basis for the disease, typically achieved through assessment of heritability or familial clustering. However, performing such studies in a prospective fashion is hindered by, among other things, identification of multiple GDM cases in a single family. Similarly, retrospective studies are hampered by the evolution of the clinical definition of GDM and the fact that definitions differ (Chap. 1.2).[51–55] Furthermore, screening for GDM in the United States has not been routine until the 1990s, leading to possible ascertainment bias. There are also difficulties in ascertaining sufficient numbers of GDM cases, given its relatively low prevalence. Finally, many existing cohort studies typically lack DNA samples and resampling for DNA is either not possible or a Herculean task.

No published studies have estimated familiality with GDM. There has been only one unpublished attempt to estimate familiality of GDM. Williams and colleagues used the state-wide medical record system in the state of Washington to link sisters diagnosed with GDM and estimated the sibling GDM risk ratio to be 1.75 (Michelle Williams, personal communication), suggesting some evidence for a genetic basis for GDM. Although the risk ratio of 1.75 is likely an underestimate of the true sibling risk ratio, it does provide some evidence for familiality of GDM and suggests the genetic basis for GDM may fall within the range of T2DM.[56]

There have been studies examining whether GDM clusters with type 1 diabetes mellitus or T2DM. Dorner et al showed that offspring with type 1 diabetes whose mothers had GDM showed increased familial aggregation of diabetes on the maternal side compared with the paternal side.[57] There is also evidence for clustering of impaired glucose tolerance and T2DM in parents of a woman with GDM[58] and evidence for higher prevalence of T2DM specifically in mothers of women with GDM.[59] Kim and colleagues examined the association between family history of diabetes and history of GDM in the National Health and Nutrition Examination Survey and also found that sibling history of diabetes increased the odds of GDM (Catherine Kim, personal communication). Thus, there exists evidence of a link between both autoimmune and nonautoimmune forms of diabetes and GDM. The fact that GDM clusters with both autoimmune and nonautoimmune forms of diabetes suggests a potential overlap in genetic susceptibility among these various forms of the disease.

13.3.2 Candidate Gene Studies

Candidate genes related to both autoimmune and nonautoimmune forms of GDM have been assessed in a variety of cohorts[60–69] and candidate genes in GDM are also reviewed by Robitaille and Grant.[70] It appears that many of the candidate gene associations reported with modest evidence of association are likely to represent under-powered studies. However, the reader is cautioned to carefully evaluate results for genetic studies based on the sample collected and the analyses performed. The fact that a study does not achieve a certain, somewhat arbitrary, level of statistical significance, or is not of a sample size approaching that of a GWA should not be grounds for outright dismissal. For example, gene association studies are essentially signal-to-noise ratio problems. While one solution to this problem is to increase sample size to rise above the "noise," another approach is selective sample collection to reduce the "noise." Both can yield equally valid results.

One candidate gene of particular interest for GDM is *GCK*.[62,71–74] Although the frequency of *GCK* variants among GDM patients is low,[71] the important contribution of *GCK* variation to risk for GDM can be observed in MODY2 families, where a large proportion of female members present with GDM.[72] Saker et al speculated that because *GCK* variants typically result in subclinical hyperglycemia,[47,75] the frequency of *GCK* variants may be higher and only detectable upon pregnancy.[72] Their speculation was supported by Ellard et al who estimated that the prevalence of *GCK* variants may be as high as 80% in a small subset of women selected using stringent criteria.[74]

The BetaGene study is unique among studies examining candidate genes for GDM in that it is studying Mexican American families of probands with or without a diagnosis of GDM and has focused on T2DM-related quantitative traits, rather than GDM *per se*.[76–78] Another unique aspect of BetaGene is the examination of whether the association between a gene and trait is modified by adiposity. For example, the study found that *TCF7L2* was associated with both GDM and with insulin secretion and β-cell function.[76] However, the association between *TCF7L2* and insulin secretion and β-cell function differed by the subject's level of body fat. Similar observations were made for the association between insulin-like growth factor 2 mRNA binding protein 2 (*IGF2BP2*) and insulin sensitivity.[78] These are among the first observations to suggest that the effect of genes may be modified by other factors, like adiposity. The BetaGene investigators have also examined gene–gene interactions,[77] another critical component of the genetic architecture of complex diseases.

13.3.3 Genes for GDM?

The question of GDM genes is closely tied to the debate surrounding whether GDM represents a unique disease state, or whether pregnancy results in metabolic derangements revealing individuals already on a trajectory towards T2DM. If T2DM susceptibility variants are also associated with GDM, from a purely genetic perspective it would be difficult to argue a unique genetic predisposition for GDM. This does not take into account the possibility of unique environmental exposures related to pregnancy that may interact with genes to alter disease risk or may affect pregnancy outcomes.

One group has recently assessed a subset of T2DM susceptibility loci for association with GDM.[79] They selected a case–control set of 238 women with a history of GDM and 2,446 normal glucose tolerant women from the population-based Inter99 cohort[80] and eleven T2DM susceptibility loci were tested for association with GDM. Among the 11 T2DM genes tested, all but 1 showed estimated odds ratios >1.0 and among these loci 4 (*TCF7L2*, *CDKAL1*, *TCF2*, and *FTO*) showed nominal evidence for association with GDM. While not all 11 loci were associated with T2DM, a highly significant additive effect of all 11 loci on risk for GDM (OR = 1.18; $p = 3.2 \times 10^{-6}$) was found, suggesting that the genetic basis for GDM and T2DM may, in fact, be the same.

13.4 What Does the Future Hold?

The new GWA era means it is now likely possible to identify large GDM case–control samples and perform GWA studies to identify susceptibility genes for GDM. The unanswered question of whether GDM *per se* has a genetic basis may also be directly addressed using the GWA framework, by incorporating carefully selected samples of T2DM cases as a secondary contrast group into the study design. Also, it should be possible to begin to understand how gene variants in the mother and fetus interact in terms of pregnancy outcomes, an area that has received very little attention.[81,82]

Should GDM have unique genetic susceptibility loci, this information could be critical in developing new interventional strategies to not just treat GDM, but also prevent progression to T2DM, which appears to occur in a large proportion of GDM cases.[83,84]

Three important cautionary notes arise. First, one should not directly correlate the relatively small odds ratios associated with these gene variants in terms of risk for T2DM or GDM and their relative importance in terms of disease biology. A common misconception is that with such small odds ratios, these gene variants are not likely to be playing a large role in disease pathogenesis and are therefore clinically irrelevant. However, one cannot deny the important role *PPARG* plays in terms of T2DM treatment[85–87] and possibly prevention[88–90] via thiazolidinedione therapy. Similarly, *KCNJ11* is another important therapeutic target of the sulfonylurea class of medications.[87, 91–93] Yet, the odds ratio for T2DM risk associated with *PPARG* is ~1.2 and for *KCNJ11* is ~1.1.

Second, it is insufficient to simply know that a genetic variant is associated with a disease or disease-related trait. The relative role played by any gene in terms of disease pathogenesis requires additional molecular and physiologic study. This is exemplified by the role of *PPARG* and *KCNJ11* in terms of diabetes therapy and the interactions with adiposity observed in the BetaGene study.

Finally, knowledge of the genes underlying disease will not be useful in predicting future disease until the biologic effect of genes is well understood. Several studies have already attempted to determine if gene variants can be used to "predict" T2DM[94–96] or GDM.[79] Each of these analyses shows that gene variants alone do not predict T2DM nor do they significantly improve predictability over traditional clinical predictors. Rather, genetic information should be leveraged to improve clinical care through development of new pharmacologic agents or interventional strategies.

Our knowledge of the genetics underlying both T2DM and GDM will continue to improve over the next several years. At the time of this writing, I am aware of at least an additional eight genes related to T2DM or T2DM-related traits that will soon be appearing in the literature. "Next generation" sequencing methods allow for sequencing of the genome of a single individual in a relatively short time and at relatively low cost and will likely introduce yet another wave of genetic discoveries. Already this technology is being applied in the 1,000 Genomes Project (http://www.1000genomes.org), which has set a goal to completely sequence the genomes of 2,000 individuals selected from around the world.

Pharmacogenetics is likely to be an area that will significantly impact clinical care as we learn more about the relationship between genetic variation and drug responses. Also, genetic findings are raising interest in specific areas of diabetes research. For example, the *MTNR1B* findings have increased interest in studies of circadian rhythms and sleep disorders and their relation to diabetes and obesity; an area many clinicians have not considered a part of their interventional arsenal. Our own BetaGene study is now looking at the possible effect of genetic variation on longitudinal change in T2DM-related traits, based on our finding of interactions with adiposity.[76, 78] In the end, as we learn more about the intricacies of the genetic architecture underlying GDM and T2DM, it is easy to envision a time, in the not too distant future, when genetic information will be used for so-called "personalized medicine."

Acknowledgments I would like to thank my colleagues on the FUSION and BetaGene studies and in MAGIC, who have made many of the contributions discussed in this chapter. RMW was or is supported as principle investigator or coinvestigator on grants from the American Diabetes Association (05-RA-140), National Institutes of Health (DK69922, DK62370, and DK61628), and Merck & Co.

References

1. Morton NE, Collins A. Toward positional cloning with SNPs. *Curr Opin Mol Ther*. 2002;4: 259-264.
2. Collins FS. Identifying human disease genes by positional cloning. *Harvey Lect*. 1991;86: 149-164.

3. Neel JV. Diabetes mellitus – a geneticist's nightmare. In: Creutzfeldt W, Kobberling J, Neel JV, eds. *The Genetics of Diabetes*. New York: Springer; 1976:1-11.
4. McCarthy MI. Growing evidence for diabetes susceptibility genes from genome scan data. *Curr Diab Rep*. 2003;3:159-167.
5. Fajans SS, Bell GI, Polonsky KS. Molecular mechanisms and clinical pathophysiology of maturity onset diabetes of the young. *N Engl J Med*. 2001;345:971-980.
6. Keefer LM, Piron MA, De MP, et al. Impaired negative cooperativity of the semisynthetic analogues human [LeuB24]- and [LeuB25]-insulins. *Biochem Biophys Res Commun*. 1981;100:1229-1236.
7. Kwok SC, Steiner DF, Rubenstein AH, et al. Identification of a point mutation in the human insulin gene giving rise to a structurally abnormal insulin (insulin Chicago). *Diabetes*. 1983;32:872-875.
8. Nanjo K, Sanke T, Kondo M, et al. Mutant insulin syndrome: identification of two families with [LeuA3]insulin and determination of its biological activity. *Trans Assoc Am Physicians*. 1986;99:132-142.
9. Nanjo K, Miyano M, Kondo M, et al. Insulin Wakayama: familial mutant insulin syndrome in Japan. *Diabetologia*. 1987;30:87-92.
10. Kadowaki T, Kadowaki H, Mori Y. A subtype of diabetes mellitus associated with a mutation of mitochondrial DNA. *N Engl J Med*. 1994;330:962-966.
11. Deeb SS, Fajas L, Nemoto M, et al. A Pro12Ala substitution in PPARγ2 associated with decreased receptor activity, lower body mass index and improved insulin sensitivity. *Nat Genet*. 1998;20:284-287.
12. Altshuler D, Hirschhorn JN, Klannemark M, et al. The common PPARγ Pro12Ala polymorphism is associated with decreased risk of type 2 diabetes. *Nat Genet*. 2000;26:76-80.
13. Gloyn AL, Weedon MN, Owen KR, et al. Large-scale association studies of variants in genes encoding the pancreatic β-cell K_{ATP} channel subunits Kir6.2 (KCNJ11) and SUR1 (ABCC8) confirm that the KCNJ11 E23K variant is associated with type 2 diabetes. *Diabetes*. 2003;52:568-572.
14. Grant SF, Thorleifsson G, Reynisdottir I, et al. Variant of transcription factor 7-like 2 (TCF7L2) gene confers risk of type 2 diabetes. *Nat Genet*. 2006;38:320-323.
15. Horikawa Y, Oda N, Cox NJ, et al. Genetic variation in the gene encoding calpain-10 is associated with type 2 diabetes mellitus. *Nat Genet*. 2000;26:163-175.
16. Bento JL, Palmer ND, Mychaleckyj JC, et al. Association of protein tyrosine phosphatase 1B gene polymorphisms with type 2 diabetes. *Diabetes*. 2004;53:3007-3012.
17. Silander K, Mohlke KL, Scott LJ, et al. Genetic variation near the hepatocyte nuclear factor-4α gene predicts susceptibility to type 2 diabetes. *Diabetes*. 2004;53:1141-1149.
18. Love-Gregory LD, Wasson J, Ma J, et al. A common polymorphism in the upstream promoter region of the hepatocyte nuclear factor-4alpha gene on chromosome 20q is associated with type 2 diabetes and appears to contribute to the evidence for linkage in an Ashkenazi Jewish population. *Diabetes*. 2004;53:1134-1140.
19. Johansson S, Raeder H, Eide SA, et al. Studies in 3, 523 Norwegians and meta-analysis in 11, 571 subjects indicate that variants in the hepatocyte nuclear factor 4 alpha (HNF4A) P2 region are associated with type 2 diabetes in Scandanavians. *Diabetes*. 2007;56:3112-3117.
20. Risch N, Merikangas K. The future of genetic studies of complex human diseases. *Science*. 1996;273:1516-1517.
21. International Human Genome Mapping Consortium. A physical map of the human genome. *Nature*. 2001;409:934-941.
22. The International HapMap Consortium. The international HapMap project. *Nature*. 2003;426: 789-796.
23. The International HapMap Consortium. A haplotype map of the human genome. *Nature*. 2005;437:1299-1320.

24. Sladek R, Rocheleau G, Rung J, et al. A genome-wide association study identified novel risk loci for type 2 diabetes. *Nature*. 2007;445:881-885.
25. Skol AD, Scott LJ, Abecasis GR, et al. Joint analysis is more efficient than replication-based analysis for two-stage genome-wide association studies. *Nat Genet*. 2006;38:209-213.
26. Diabetes Genetics Initiative of Broad Institute of Harvard and MIT LUaNIfBR. Genome-wide association analysis identifies loci for type 2 diabetes and triglyceride levels. *Science*. 2007;316:1331-1336.
27. Scott LJ, Mohlke KL, Bonnycastle LL, et al. A genome-wide association study of type 2 diabetes in Finns detects multiple susceptibility variants. *Science*. 2007;316:1341-1345.
28. Zeggini E, Weedon MN, Lindgren CM, et al. Replication of genome-wide association signals in U.K. samples reveals risk loci for type 2 diabetes. *Science*. 2007;316:1336-1341.
29. Sanna S, Jackson AU, Nagaraja R, et al. Common variants in the GDF5-UQCC region are associated with variation in human height. *Nat Genet*. 2008;40:198-203.
30. Weedon MN, Lango H, Lindgren CM, et al. Genome-wide association analysis identifies 20 loci that influence adult height. *Nat Genet*. 2008;40:575-583.
31. Willer CJ, Sanna S, Jackson AU, et al. Newly identified loci that influence lipid concentrations and risk of coronary artery disease. *Nat Genet*. 2008;40:161-169.
32. Kathiresan S, Willer CJ, Peloso GM, et al. Common variants at 30 loci contribute to polygenic dyslipidemia. *Nat Genet*. 2009;41:56-65.
33. Frayling TM, Timpson NJ, Weedon MN, et al. A common variant in the *FTO* gene is associated with body mass index and predisposes to childhood and adult obesity. *Science*. 2007;316:889-894.
34. Scuteri A, Sanna S, Chen W-M, et al. Genome-wide asociation scan shows genetic variants in the FTO gene are associated with obesity-related traits. *PLoS Genet*. 2007;3:1200-1210.
35. Loos RJ, Lindgren CM, Li S, et al. Common variants near MC4R are associated with fat mass, weight and risk of obesity. *Nat Genet*. 2008;40:768-775.
36. Chambers JC, Elliott P, Zabaneh D, et al. Common genetic variation near MC4R is associated with waist circumference and insulin resistance. *Nat Genet*. 2008;40:716-718.
37. Thorleifsson G, Walters GB, Gudbjartsson DF, et al. Genome-wide association yields new sequence variants at seven loci that associate with measures of obesity. *Nat Genet*. 2009;41:18-24.
38. Chen W-M, Erdos MR, Jackson AU, et al. Variations in the *G6PC2/ABCB11* genomic region are associated with fasting glucose levels. *J Clin Invest*. 2008;118:2609-2628.
39. Bouatia-Naji N, Rocheleau G, Van Lommel L, et al. A polymorphism within the G6PC2 gene is associated with fasting plasma glucose levels. *Science*. 2008;320:1085-1088.
40. Bouatia-Naji N, Bonnefond A, Cavalcanti-Proenca C, et al. A variant near MTNR1B is associated with increased fasting plasma glucose levels and type 2 diabetes risk. *Nat Genet*. 2009;41:89-94.
41. Prokopenko I, Langenberg C, Florez JC, et al. Variants in MTNR1B influence fasting glucose levels. *Nat Genet*. 2009;41:77-81.
42. Stone LM, Kahn SE, Deeb SS, et al. Glucokinase gene variations in Japanese-Americans with a family history of NIDDM. *Diabetes Care*. 1994;17:1480-1483.
43. Stone LM, Kahn SE, Fujimoto WY, et al. A variation at position -30 of the β-cell glucokinase gene promoter is associated with reduced β-cell function in middle-aged Japanese-American men. *Diabetes*. 1996;45:428.
44. Weedon MN, Frayling TM, Shields B, et al. Genetic regulation of birth weight and fasting glucose by a common polymorphism in the islet promoter of the glucokinase gene. *Diabetes*. 2005;54:576-581.
45. Weedon MN, Clark VJ, Qian Y, et al. A common haplotype of the glucokinase gene alters fasting glucose and birth weight: Association in six studies and population-genetics analyses. *Am J Hum Genet*. 2006;79:991-1001.

46. Froguel Ph, Zouali H, Vionnet N, et al. Familial hyperglycemia due to mutations in glucokinase. *N Engl J Med*. 1993;328:697-702.
47. Hattersley AT. Maturity-onset diabetes of the young: clinical heterogeneity explained by genetic heterogeneity. *Diabet Med*. 1998;15:15-24.
48. Chen WM, Jackson AU, Scuteri A, et al. Genome-wide association scans in cohorts from Sardinia and Finland identify a locus for fasting glucose levels. [Abstract Program Number 259]. Presented at the annual meeting of the American Society of Human Genetics, October 2007, San Diego, CA. http://www.ashg.org/cgi-bin/ashg07s/ashg07?author=watanabe&sort=ptimes&sbutton=Detail&absno=11220&sid=462012
49. Lyssenko V, Nagorny CL, Erdos MR, et al. Common variant in MTNR1B associated with increased risk of type 2 diabetes and impaired early insulin secretion. *Nat Genet*. 2009;41:82-88.
50. Dina C, Meyre D, Gallina S, et al. Variation in *FTO* contributes to childhood obesity and severe adult obesity. *Nat Genet*. 2007;39:724-726.
51. National Diabetes Data Group. Classification and diagnosis of diabetes mellitus and other categories of glucose intolerance. *Diabetes*. 1979;28:1039-1057.
52. World Health Organization: Diabetes Mellitus: Report of a WHO Study Group, 1985.
53. The Expert Committee on the Diagnosis and Classification of Diabetes Mellitus. Report of the expert committee on the diagnosis and classification of diabetes mellitus. *Diabetes Care*. 1997;20:1183-1197.
54. World Health Organization: Definition, diagnosis and classification of diabetes mellitus and its complications. Report of a WHO Consultation, 1999.
55. Metzger BE. Summary and recommendation of the Third International Workshop-Conference on Gestational Diabetes Mellitus. *Diabetes*. 1991;40:197-201.
56. Rich SS. Mapping genes in diabetes. *Diabetes*. 1990;39:1315-1319.
57. Dorner G, Plagemann A, Reinagel H. Familial diabetes aggregation in type I diabetics: Gestational diabetes an apparent risk factor for increased diabetes susceptibility in the offspring. *Exp Clin Endocrinol*. 1987;89:84-90.
58. McLellan JA, Barrow BA, Levy JC, et al. Prevalence of diabetes mellitus and impaired glucose tolerance in parents of women with gestational diabetes. *Diabetologia*. 1995;38:693-698.
59. Martin AO, Simpson JL, Ober C, et al. Frequency of diabetes mellitus in mothers of probands with gestational diabetes: Possible maternal influence on the predisposition to gestational diabetes. *Am J Obstet Gynecol*. 1985;151:471-475.
60. Freinkel N, Metzger BE, Phelps RL, et al. Gestational diabetes mellitus: a syndrome with phenotypic and genotypic heterogeneity. *Horm Metab Res*. 1986;18:427-439.
61. Ober C, Xiang KS, Thisted RA, et al. Increased risk for gestational diabetes mellitus associated with insulin receptor and insulin-like growth factor II restriction fragment length polymorphisms. *Genet Epidemiol*. 1989;6:559-569.
62. Chiu KC, Go RC, Aoki M, et al. Glucokinase gene in gestational diabetes mellitus: population association study and molecular scanning. *Diabetologia*. 1994;37:104-110.
63. Festa A, Krugluger W, Shnawa N, et al. Trp64Arg polymorphismof the β3-adrenergic receptor gene in pregnancy: Association with mild gestational diabetes mellitus. *J Clin Endocrinol Metab*. 1999;84:1695-1699.
64. Rissanen J, Mykkänen L, Markkanen A, et al. Sulfonylurea receptor 1 gene variants are associated with gestational diabetes and type 2 diabetes but not with altered secretion of insulin. *Diabetes Care*. 2000;23:70-73.
65. Chen Y, Liao WX, Roy AC, et al. Mitochondrial gene mutations in gestational diabetes mellitus. *Diabetes Res Clin Pract*. 2000;48:29-35.
66. Aggarwal P, Gill-Randall R, Wheatley T, et al. Identification of mtDNA mutation in a pedigree with gestational diabetes, deafness, Wolff-Parkinson-White syndrome and placenta accreta. *Hum Hered*. 2001;51:114-116.

67. Megia A, Gallart L, Fernandez-Real JM, et al. Mannose-binding lectin gene polymorphisms are associated with gestational diabetes mellitus. *J Clin Endocrinol Metab.* 2004;89: 5081-5087.
68. Lauenborg J, Damm P, Ek J, et al. Studies of the ADA/VAL98 polymorphism of the hepatocyte nuclear factor-1α gene and the relationship to β-cell function during an OGTT in glucose-tolerant women with and without previous gestational diabetes mellitus. *Diabet Med.* 2004;21:1310-1315.
69. Weng J, Ekelund M, Lehto M, et al. Screening for MODY mutations, GAD antibodies, and type 1 diabetes-associated HLA genotypes in women with gestational diabetes mellitus. *Diabetes Care.* 2002;25:68-71.
70. Robitaille J, Grant AM. The genetics of gestational diabetes mellitus: evidence for relationship with type 2 diabetes mellitus. *Genet Med.* 2008;10:240-250.
71. Stoffel M, Bell KL, Blackburn CL, et al. Identification of glucokinase mutations in subjects with gestational diabetes mellitus. *Diabetes.* 1993;42:937-940.
72. Saker PJ, Hattersley AT, Barrow B, et al. High prevalence of a missense mutation of the glucokinase gene in gestational diabetic patients due to a founder-effect in a local population. *Diabetologia.* 1996;39:1325-1328.
73. Allan CJ, Argyropoulos G, Bowker M, et al. Gestational diabetes mellitus and gene mutations which affect insulin secretion. *Diabetes Res Clin Pract.* 1997;36:135-141.
74. Ellard S, Beards F, Allen LI, et al. A high prevalence of glucokinase mutations in gestational diabetic subjects selected by clinical criteria. *Diabetologia.* 2000;43:250-253.
75. Page RC, Hattersley AT, Levy JC, et al. Clinical characteristics of subjects with a missense mutation in glucokinase. *Diabet Med.* 1995;12:209-217.
76. Watanabe RM, Allayee H, Xiang AH, et al. Transcription factor 7-like 2 (*TCF7L2*) is associated with gestational diabetes mellitus and interacts with adiposity to alter insulin secretion in Mexican Americans. *Diabetes.* 2007;56:1481-1485.
77. Black MH, Fingerlin TE, Allayee H, et al. Evidence of interaction between peroxisome proliferator-activated receptor-γ2 and hepatocyte nuclear factor-4α contributing to variation in insulin sensitivity in Mexican Americans. *Diabetes.* 2008;57:1048-1056.
78. Li X, Allayee H, Xiang AH, et al. Variation in *IGF2BP2* interacts with adiposity to alter insulin sensitivity in Mexican Americans. *Obesity.* 2009;17:729-736.
79. Lauenborg J, Grarup N, Damm P, et al. Common type 2 diabetes risk gene variants asociated with gestational diabetes. *J Clin Endocrinol Metab.* 2009;94:145-150.
80. Glümer C, Jørgensen T, Borch-Johnsen K, et al. Prevalences of diabetes and impaired glucose regulation in a Danish population: the Inter99 study. *Diabetes Care.* 2003;26:2335-2340.
81. Singh R, Pearson ER, Clark PM, et al. The long-term impact on offspring of exposure to hyperglycaemia in utero due to maternal glucokinase gene mutations. *Diabetologia.* 2007;50:620-624.
82. Pearson ER, Boj SF, Steele AM, et al. Macrosomia and hyperinsulinaemic hypoglycaemia in patients with heterozygous mutations in the HNF4A gene. *PLoS Med.* 2007;4:e118.
83. Kjos SL, Peters RK, Xiang A, et al. Predicting future diabetes in Latino women with gestational diabetes. *Diabetes.* 1995;44:586-591.
84. Kim C, Newton KM, Knopp RH. Gestational diabetes and the incidence of type 2 diabetes. *Diabetes Care.* 2002;25:1862-1868.
85. Schwartz S, Raskin P, Fonseca V, et al. Effect of troglitazone in insulin-treated patients with type II diabetes mellitus. *N Engl J Med.* 1998;338:861-866.
86. Baba S. Pioglitazone: a review of Japanese clinical studies. *Curr Med Res Opion.* 2001;17: 166-189.
87. Kahn SE, Haffner SM, Heise MA, et al. Glycemic durability of rosiglitazone, metformin, or glyburide monotherapy. *N Engl J Med.* 2006;355:2427-2443.

88. Buchanan TA, Xiang AH, Peters RK, et al. Preservation of pancreatic β-cell function and prevention of type 2 diabetes by pharmacological treatment of insulin resistance in high-risk hispanic women. *Diabetes*. 2002;51:2796-2803.
89. Xiang AH, Peters RK, Kjos SL, et al. Effect of pioglitazone on pancreatic β-cell function and diabetes risk in Hispanic women with prior gestational diabetes. *Diabetes*. 2006;55:517-522.
90. The DREAM Trial Investigators. Effect of rosiglitazone on the frequency of diabetes in patients with impaired glucose tolerance or impaired fasting glucose: a randomised controlled trial. *Lancet*. 2006;368:1096-1105.
91. Minuk HL, Vranic M, Marliss EB, et al. Glucoregulatory and metabolic response to exercise in obese noninsulin-dependent diabetes. *Am J Physiol*. 1981;240:E458-E464.
92. Prigeon RL, Jacobson RK, Porte D Jr, et al. Effect of sulfonylurea withdrawal on proinsulin levels, B cell function, and glucose disposal in subjects with noninsulin-dependent diabetes mellitus. *J Clin Endocrinol Metab*. 1996;81:3295-3298.
93. Shapiro ET, Van Cauter E, Tillil H, et al. Glyburide enhances the responsiveness of the β-cell to glucose by does not correct the abnormal patterns of insulin secretion in noninsulin-dependent diabetes mellitus. *J Clin Endocrinol Metab*. 1989;69:571-576.
94. Balkau B, Lange C, Fezeu L, et al. Predicting diabetes: clinical, biological, and genetic approaches: data from the Epidemiological Study on the Insulin Resistance Syndrome (DESIR). *Diabetes Care*. 2008;31:2056-2061.
95. van HM, Dehghan A, Witteman JC, et al. Predicting type 2 diabetes based on polymorphisms from genome-wide association studies: a population-based study. *Diabetes*. 2008;57:3122-3128.
96. Lango H, Palmer CN, Morris AD, et al. Assessing the combined impact of 18 common genetic variants of modest effect sizes on type 2 diabetes risk. *Diabetes*. 2008;57:3129-3135.
97. Zeggini E, Scott LJ, Saxena R, et al. Meta-analysis of genome-wide association data and large-scale replication identifies additional susceptibility loci for type 2 diabetes. *Nat Genet*. 2008;40:638-645.
98. Sandhu MS, Weedon MN, Fawcett KA, et al. Common variants in WFS1 confer risk of type 2 diabetes. *Nat Genet*. 2007;39:951-953.
99. Yasuda K, Miyake K, Horikawa Y, et al. Variants in KCNQ1 are associated with susceptibility to type 2 diabetes mellitus. *Nat Genet*. 2008;40:1092-1097.
100. Unoki H, Takahashi A, Kawaguchi T, et al. SNPs in KCNQ1 are associated with susceptibility to type 2 diabetes in East Asian and European populations. *Nat Genet*. 2008;40:1098-1102.
101. Winckler W, Weedon MN, Graham RR, et al. Evaluation of common variants in the six known maturity-onset diabetes of the young (MODY) genes for association with type 2 diabetes. *Diabetes*. 2007;56:685-693.

Section V

Comorbidities of GDM

Maternal Obesity and Epidemiological Review of Pregnancy Complications

14

Wanda K. Nicholson

14.1 Introduction

Both the developed world and developing countries are experiencing a rapid increase in the prevalence of adult obesity (body mass index or BMI ≥ 30 kg/m^2). Globally, a 50% increase in obesity was reported from 1995 to 2000. Estimates from the International Obesity Task Force (IOTF) (http://www.iotf.org/intro/global.htm) indicate that over 300 million adults are obese and another 1 billion are overweight worldwide. Obesity in the United States has reached epidemic proportions, with an estimated 33% of women of all ages classified as obese.[1] Data from the National Health and Nutrition Examination Survey (1999–2004) indicate that among *nonpregnant* women aged 20–39 years, approximately 25% are overweight, 28% are obese and 6% are considered extremely obese.[1,2] About one-third (29%) of childbearing women aged 20–39 years are obese and 8% are extremely obese. With the increase in sedentary lifestyles and caloric intake in the United States, the number of overweight and obese adults is projected to rise even further over the coming decades. As such, the effect of obesity on maternal and neonatal outcomes[3] is destined to become one of the biggest challenges for clinicians providing perinatal care in the twenty-first century. This chapter provides an epidemiologic review of the evidence on the effect of maternal obesity on pregnancy complications. Where possible, potential mechanistic pathways underlying the effect of obesity on each complication is presented. We include maternal and fetal complications that are specific to the prenatal period.

14.2 Defining Overweight and Obesity

The three primary measures of obesity include ideal body weight, absolute body weight, and BMI. BMI, defined as weight in kilograms per height in meters squared (kg/m^2), is the

W.K. Nicholson
Department of Obstetrics and Gynecology, Centre for Women's Health Research,
University of North Carolina at Chapel Hill, Chapel Hill, MD, USA
e-mail: wkichol@med.unc.edu

C. Kim and A. Ferrara (eds.), *Gestational Diabetes During and After Pregnancy*,
DOI: 10.1007/978-1-84882-120-0_14,

Table 14.1 Categories of body mass index (BMI) for adults, 20 years and older

Weight category	BMI (kg/m^2)
Underweight	<18.5
Normal weight	18.5–24.9
Overweight	25.0–29.9
Obesity	30.0–39.9
Extreme obesity	≥40

From data of the World Health Organization[4]

most commonly used measure of obesity. It is used to estimate adiposity because of its strong correlation with fat mass. BMI is limited, however, in that it does not account for differences that may exist in fat mass by sex, age, or race/ethnicity. But for most patients, BMI is a reliable and easily usable tool to assess obesity. Clinicians can access an on-line BMI calculator for use in clinical practice at the National Heart Lung and Blood Institute website (http://www.nhlbisupport.com/bmi/).

The 1998 Clinical Guidelines on the Identification, Evaluation and Treatment of Overweight and Obesity in Adults accepts the following weight classifications for adults aged 20 years and older: underweight is defined as a BMI < 18.5 kg/m^2, normal weight is a BMI 18.5–24.9 kg/m^2, overweight is a BMI 25.0–29.9 kg/m^2 and obesity is a BMI ≥ 30 kg/m^2. The World Health Organization (WHO), National Institutes of Health (NIH) and the IOTF recommend these same threshold values in clinical practice and epidemiologic studies.[4] (Table 14.1) Several early studies have used BMI values for overweight and obesity that vary from those outlined above, making it difficult to draw meaningful conclusions across studies and populations. Recent analyses, however, have consistently used the categories advocated by the NIH and IOTF.

14.3 Obesity and Childbearing

Childbearing has been considered by many as one of the most important factors contributing to the development of long term obesity.[5–8] Most of the weight gain with childbearing is thought to occur with the first pregnancy.[6,7] In addition to being heavier at the time of conception, women are gaining more weight during pregnancy. One in five American women gains more than 40 pounds during pregnancy and most will retain about 40% of the weight.[9] Racial and ethnic subgroups of women are at greater risk for excessive gestational weight gain and gestational diabetes mellitus (GDM) compared with their white counterparts.[10] In a cross-sectional analysis,[11] obese African-American women had a higher likelihood of cesarean delivery (odds ratio [OR] 1.40, 95% confidence interval [CI] 1.24–1.58) and low birth weight infants (OR 1.94, 95% CI 1.57–2.40) compared to white women. Single status and high parity are associated with higher risks of weight retention, particularly among minority women.[12] Rural residence has also been linked to greater risk of obesity in women.[13,14] Living in nonmetropolitan areas may be related to greater postpartum weight retention.[15,16]

Despite the rising prevalence of obesity in childbearing women and the disproportionate number of minority women affected by obesity, there is no national source of data on obesity trends during pregnancy. The Pregnancy Risk Assessment Monitoring System (PRAMS), a population-based surveillance project supported by the Centers for Disease Control and Prevention (CDC) and state health departments, examines trends in pre-pregnancy obesity in 39 states. The Behavioral Risk Factor Surveillance System (BRFSS) is a viable source of robust regional estimates but is limited in the ability to provide national trends.

14.4 Obesity in the Nondiabetic Parturient

It is well known that pregnancy involves some degree of insulin resistance. There is a 40–50% increase in the level of insulin resistance during pregnancy and insulin resistance increases as pregnancy progresses. The influence of overweight and obesity on maternal and fetal health is thought to mirror, in some respects, the mechanisms of gestational and overt diabetes. Obesity was first acknowledged as a risk factor for pregnancy more than 50 years ago.[17] Recent evidence from the Hyperglycemia and Adverse Pregnancy Outcome (HAPO) Study[18] strongly suggest that varying degrees of hyperglycemia less than definitive GDM affect fetal development and newborn adiposity. Similar to the range of complications in obese, nonpregnant adults, maternal obesity is associated with higher risk of hypertensive disorders, development of gestational and type 2 diabetes mellitus and thrombo-embolic disease. Also, there can be difficulties with antenatal ultrasound assessment of the fetus in women with obesity. Operative complications include an increase in the likelihood of cesarean delivery, postoperative wound infection, endometritis, and anesthetic complications, including intubation and epidural placement. Newborn complications include congenital malformations, specifically neural tube defects and stillbirths.

14.5 Maternal Complications

14.5.1 Gestational Diabetes Mellitus

The etiology of GDM and the various risk factors related to the development of GDM are covered in detail in other chapters. In this section, we provide a summary of the association of maternal overweight and obesity with GDM. The prevalence of GDM ranges between 3 and 15%, depending on the diagnostic testing used, race/ethnicity of the population, and family history of type 2 diabetes. With the increase in maternal obesity, however, there has been a parallel increase in the prevalence of GDM.[19–21] Multiple investigations[22–26] have shown a higher likelihood of GDM with increasing weight, height, and BMI. The associations between obesity, hypertension, and insulin resistance in type 2 diabetes are also well recognized. However, obesity is thought to be an independent risk factor for developing GDM. Obesity has been estimated to be associated with a 20% increased risk of GDM.[27] Ramos[25] found a twofold increase in GDM among overweight women (OR 2.0; 95% CI 1.8–2.2). Bianco[22] reported a threefold increase in GDM among obese women compared with normal weight women. Further, the likelihood of GDM appears to increase substantially with increasing maternal BMI, indicating a dose–response relationship. A meta-analysis of 20 studies[23] reported a pooled relative risk estimate for the likelihood of developing GDM of 2.14 (95% CI 1.8, 2.5), 3.56 (95% CI 3.1, 4.2), and 8.6 (95% CI 5.1, 16) among overweight, obese, and severely obese women, respectively, compared with normal weight women (Fig. 14.1a–c). These investigations can inform the development of clinical interventions to reduce pre-pregnancy BMI and the development of GDM.

14.5.2 Hypertensive Disorders

Maternal obesity is associated with an increased risk of hypertensive disorders of pregnancy, including chronic hypertension, preeclampsia (gestational proteinuric hypertension), and gestational hypertension. Maternal obesity with the accompanying presence of hypertriglyceridemia, hyperglycemia, and insulin resistance is thought to put the expectant mother at risk for hypertension and preeclampsia. Chronic hypertension may occur prior to conception or elevations in blood pressure may be identified for the first time during pregnancy. Hemodynamic alterations in arterial blood pressure, hemo-concentration, and cardiac function that occur more commonly in the nonpregnant obese woman also occur commonly in the obese parturient.

Findings from several large, population-based cohort studies support the association of maternal BMI with development of preeclampsia.[22,28–44] The risk of pregnancy-induced hypertension or preeclampsia is substantially greater if the mother is overweight or obese in the pregravid or early pregnancy period.[30,45] Underlying mechanisms likely include the influence of elements of the metabolic syndrome, including obesity, hypertension, insulin resistance, and hyperlipidemia, on placental endothelial dysfunction. Therefore, well-designed studies examining the relation of obesity with preeclampsia account for potential confounders, including diabetes, chronic hypertension, and parity.[22,30–35,37] Sebire et al[33] retrospectively analyzed maternal BMI at entry into prenatal care and the development of preeclampsia in 127,213 pregnancies in northwest England. Women were categorized as normal weight, moderately obese, and very obese. Compared with normal weight women (BMI 20–24.9 kg/m^2), women who were moderately obese (BMI 25–29.9 kg/m^2) and very obese (BMI $\geq$ 30 kg/m^2) had a 1.4 (1.28–1.60) and 2.14 (1.85–2.47) times higher likelihood of preeclampsia, respectively. Women at higher BMI levels were more likely to report a history of hypertension and diabetes prior to pregnancy. However, adjustment for demographic characteristics, parity, and prior history of hypertension or diabetes did not attenuate the magnitude of association between obese women and preeclampsia. Baeten et al,[31] in a U.S. cohort, reported higher likelihood of preeclampsia (OR 3.3; 95% CI 3.0–3.7) among women with BMI $\geq$ 30 kg/m^2 compared with women with BMI < 20 kg/m^2, after adjustment for maternal demographics, smoking status, and gestational weight gain. Among 15,262 women

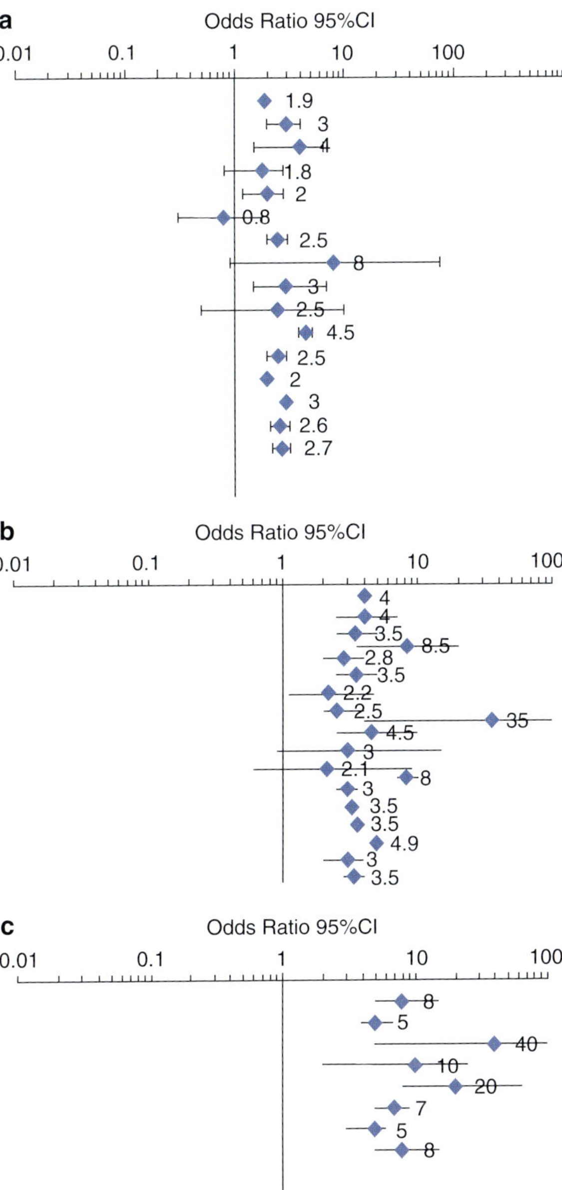

Fig. 14.1 (**a**) Maternal overweight and likelihood of GDM (**b**) Maternal obesity (BMI ≥ 30 kg/m^2) and likelihood of GDM. (**c**) Severe maternal obesity and likelihood of GDM. (Modified from Chu et. al.[23])

from the Nurses' Health Study, Thadhani et al reported a greater likelihood of preeclampsia among women with BMI ≥ 30 kg/m^2 compared with women with BMI 21–22.9 kg/m^2 after adjusting for parity, diabetes, family history of hypertension, and cholesterol level. In most studies, the relation between BMI and preeclampsia increased with each BMI category, suggesting a dose–response relationship. A recent meta-analysis reported that the likelihood of preeclampsia doubled for each 5–7 kg/m^2 increase in BMI.[46]

While it is likely that the observed association between pre-pregnancy BMI and preeclampsia is confounded by the presence of chronic hypertension, diabetes, and hyperlipidemia, the relation between BMI and preeclampsia has remained essentially unchanged after adjustment for these factors in multiple studies. Consistent with other studies of maternal obesity, pre-pregnancy BMI was based on self-reported pre-pregnancy height and weight. Also, there is heterogeneity in the BMI categories used in individual studies. Such variations make it difficult to compare results across studies or to derive a pooled estimate of the risk of preeclampsia. However, despite heterogeneity in BMI categories or potential bias in self-reported measures, there is a large body of epidemiologic studies with consistent results with multivariate adjustment for confounders.

14.5.3 Cesarean Delivery

Numerous studies report a positive association between maternal obesity and cesarean delivery.[28, 47–49] The biological pathway through which obesity affects labor is not completely understood.[50, 51] Some investigators have hypothesized that obesity results in a soft tissue dystocia, where maternal pelvic soft tissue narrows the birth canal and increases the risk of failure of infant descent.[47, 52, 53] Other studies suggest that the increased risk of cesarean is related to differences in labor progression or response to oxytocin in obese women compared with normal weight women.[54] Obesity can also affect the risk of cesarean delivery through the increase in comorbidities, particularly GDM and hypertension.[55,56]

Because of the higher prevalence of GDM in obese women, it is important to determine whether obesity increases the risk of cesarean delivery independent of GDM or whether the effect of obesity is mediated through a higher prevalence of GDM in obese women. Multiple studies consistently report a higher likelihood of cesarean delivery among obese women. Several studies have been conducted among women without GDM.[49, 52,57–59] For example, Jensen et al[49] reported a 1.8 times higher likelihood of cesarean (OR 1.8; 95% CI 1.6–2.2) among obese women without GDM compared to normal weight women. Two studies among obese women with GDM reported higher cesarean delivery among obese women with GDM.[60,61] Among seven studies[25, 28, 33, 47, 50, 60, 62, 63] that controlled for GDM, maternal obesity was associated with a 1.2–4.0 higher likelihood of cesarean delivery among obese women vs. normal weight women. Similar findings have been reported for overweight and severely obese women. A meta-analysis[64] of 20 studies reported pooled estimates for the likelihood of cesarean delivery by BMI categories. The likelihood of cesarean delivery was 1.46 (95% CI 1.34–1.60), 2.05 (95% CI 1.86–2.27), and 2.89 (95% CI 2.28–3.79) higher, respectively, among overweight, obese, and severely obese women compared with normal weight women (Table 14.2).

Table 14.2 Pooled estimates for cesarean delivery by BMI status from meta-analysis by Chu et al[64]

Comparison groups	Number of studies	Odds ratio	95% Confidence interval
Overweight vs. normal	23	1.46	1.34–1.60
Obese vs. normal	29	2.05	1.86–2.27
Severely obese vs. normal	7	2.89	2.28–3.79

14.5.4 Preterm Delivery

The relationship of obesity to spontaneous preterm labor and delivery is still being investigated. Multiple investigations have been conducted. Several studies report a small, but positive association; others report no relation between maternal BMI and spontaneous preterm labor. In the Primary Preterm Prevention Study, obese women were less likely to have spontaneous preterm birth than were normal weight women (6.2 vs. 11.2%).[65] Conversely, studies do show an association between maternal obesity and indicated preterm birth, particularly in deliveries occurring prior to 32 weeks gestation. In most instances, these deliveries occur in response to hypertension, preeclampsia, or conditions involving poor fetal growth or well-being.

14.5.5 Thrombo-Embolic Events

Pregnancy is a hypercoagulable state. Obesity further increases the risk of thrombosis by promoting venous stasis, increasing blood viscosity and promoting activation of the coagulation cascade. Women are at highest risk at term and there is an increased risk with cesarean delivery.[66, 67] Roberts reported a substantial increase in the odds of deep vein thrombosis (DVT) in overweight and obese women in a prospective study of 14,000 parturients in Nova Scotia even after adjustment for other risk factors. Obese women were 1.9 times more likely to have a DVT (OR 1.9; 1.1–3.9) compared with normal weight women. Severely obese women (BMI $\geq$40 kg/m^2) were 4 times more likely to experience a DVT (OR 4.3; 95% CI 1.2–14.84) relative to normal weight women. Thrombo-embolism is the leading cause of maternal death in pregnancy in developed countries. It is possible that the incidence will increase with increasing maternal obesity. Suggested medical interventions for obese women include the use of pneumatic compression stockings during antenatal hospitalizations as well as labor, cesarean delivery, and postpartum recuperation. Clinicians should encourage ambulation and consider heparin prophylaxis in obese women with prolonged antenatal or postpartum hospitalizations.

14.5.6 Other Maternal Complications

The obese parturient is at risk for several additional complications including wound infection and anesthesia complications. Intubation can be more difficult. The placement of epidural anesthesia can be complicated by difficulty in identifying landmarks. Anatomical distortion can sometimes lead to a higher rate of epidural failure in obese women. Also, because the onset of labor and need for cesarean delivery is unpredictable, obese patients are at increased risk of aspiration due to elevations in gastric residual volume and lower gastric pH.[68]

Several small studies have examined wound infection in obese women. In a cohort of 239 women, Wall et al[69] reported higher rates of infection in obese women (BMI greater than 35 kg/m^2) who had a vertical compared to transverse skin incision (34.6 vs. 9.4%). Wolfe and associates[70] reported no relation between the type of skin incision and postoperative infection in 107 obese women. Houston and Raynor[71] examined the use of the supraumbilical midline skin incision with a fundal uterine incision and breech extraction of the fetus compared with low transverse skin incision. The supraumbilical approach provided less operative time and better wound healing, presumably due to a lesser amount of adipose tissue involved in creating the incision.

Additional studies, ideally prospective and with standard measures of BMI, are needed to provide better data on the incidence of wound infection in women who are overweight or obese. Despite the paucity of large cohort studies, the postoperative morbidity experienced by obese women with wound infection is substantial and greatly influences perinatal cost of care.

14.6 Fetal Complications

14.6.1 Stillbirths

Although there has been a decline in the rate of stillbirths in the United States, stillbirths are not a rare event, with nearly seven stillbirths occurring per 1,000 deliveries (live and stillbirths). Data from the CDC show that there were over 27,000 stillbirths in the year 2000.[72] Several epidemiologic studies have reported an increased risk of stillbirth among women who are obese, compared with normal weight women, but the exact mechanism is not completely understood. GDM and hypertensive disease are known risk factors for stillbirths and are more prevalent among obese women. It is also possible that obese women have undiagnosed GDM or some degree of glucose intolerance that adversely affects the developing fetus.

Pre-pregnancy BMI and fetal death were examined in the Danish National Birth Cohort among 54,505 pregnant women. Overweight women had a two times higher risk of stillbirth compared with normal weight women.[73] Overweight women also experienced a higher risk after 40 weeks gestation (2.9; 95% CI 1.1–7.7). Obese women had a 2.4 times higher risk of stillbirth compared with normal weight women. In a large British study of 325,395 women, overweight and obesity were still associated with fetal death after adjustment for complications of pregnancy (OR 1.1; 95% CI 0.9–1.2) and (OR 1.4; 95% CI 1.1–1.7), respectively.[33] Further, Cnattingius et al[74] reported an increase in the likelihood of fetal death among obese nulliparous women in Sweden. In a prospective study of over 167,000 women, pregnancies among overweight and obese nulliparous women had a 3.2 (95% CI 1.6–6.2) and 4.3 (95% CI 2.0–9.3) higher odds of fetal death relative to their normal weight counterparts. Among parous women, only obese women had a significant increase in the risk of late fetal death (OR 2.0; 1.2–3.3). Finally, Salihu[75] reported that obese mothers were about 40% more likely to experience stillbirth than were nonobese women, after adjustment for demographics and clinical risk factors (HR 1.4; 95% CI 1.3–1.5). Further, there was a dose-dependent relationship between classifications of obesity and stillbirth (P for trend

<0.01). For a balanced review, it is important to summarize investigations which reported no association between maternal BMI and stillbirths. Djrolo reported no association between maternal overweight (OR 0.5; 95% 0.15, 1.5) or obesity (0.6; 0.18, 2.0) and stillbirth among a cohort of 323 women. A strength of this study is the use of BMI categories recommended by the World Health Organization (WHO) and Institute of Medicine (IOM), but the analysis is likely limited by sample size and insufficient power, as evidenced by the wide CIs, to detect a meaningful association.

14.6.2 Neural Tube Defects

Neither the presence nor magnitude of association between maternal obesity and neural tube defects (NTDs) has been definitively established. Multiple studies have suggested that maternal obesity without diabetes is associated with an increased risk of delivering an infant with a birth defect,[76, 77] particularly NTDs.[78] Neural tube defects are caused by a failure of neural tube closure 3–4 weeks after conception.[79] While the majority of studies have shown an increased risk of NTDs with maternal obesity, other research has shown no association. Also, the magnitude of risk associated with obesity has varied widely, ranging from essentially no risk to a threefold increase in risk. The mechanisms underlying the relation of obesity with NTD are not completely understood. The risk of congenital anomalies is known to be higher among infants of women with diabetes. Therefore, one possible explanation is that obese women have some degree of underlying insulin resistance and higher circulating glucose levels which may also place their infants at risk. Other theories include a reduction in the amount of folic acid that crosses the placenta due to insufficient maternal absorption, chronic hypoxia, and increased circulating levels of triglycerides, uric acid, estrogen, and insulin.[76, 80]

Waller et al[80] were the first to report an increased risk of NTDs (both anencephaly and spina bifida) in the offspring of obese women (OR 1.8; 95% CI 1.01–3.19), and especially spina bifida (2.6; 1.5–4.5). Subsequent studies reported similar results.[81–84] Even after adjustment for ethnicity, maternal age, education, and socioeconomic status, Watkins et al[76] reported that each 1 kg/m^2 increase in BMI was associated with a 7% increase in the likelihood of having an infant with a NTD. In a recent multi-site, population-based study, Waller et al[77] reported adjusted ORs for risk of spina bifida and anencephaly. Obese women had a two times greater risk of spina bifida compared with normal weight women (OR 2.10; 95% 1.62–2.71). There was no increased risk reported in overweight compared with normal weight women.

Little or no association between maternal overweight and NTDs has been reported.[80, 85–87] Hendricks reported an OR of 0.99 (95% CI 0.58, 1.58). Among 499 cases and 534 controls, Waller reported no association (OR 0.92; 95% CI 0.55, 1.55), between maternal overweight status and NTDs. Moore conducted a cohort study of 100 women and found no association between overweight and NTDs. Two studies[84, 88] reported a higher likelihood of NTD (OR 1.91; 95% CI 1.20, 3.04) and (OR 1.61; 95% CI 1.27, 2.05), respectively. A recent meta-analysis[89] summarized the findings from 12 (4 cohort and 8 case–control) studies. Using a random effects model, they reported a pooled unadjusted estimate of 1.70 (95% CI 1.34–2.15) for obese women and 1.22 (95% CI 0.99–1.49) for overweight women when compared with normal weight women.

The variability in individual studies of NTDs are due, in part, to differences in study design, including the definitions used for overweight and obesity, variation in the definition of NTDs, and the use of self-reported or measured maternal height and weight. Table 14.3 summarizes the characteristics of several studies included in this review. Only three of the studies used the standard definitions of overweight and obesity recommended by the IOM and the WHO. Five studies[80, 83, 85, 88, 90] used threshold values for overweight and obesity

Table 14.3 Characteristics of select studies of maternal obesity and neural tube defects (NTDs)[76–79]

References	Study design/data sources	Source of maternal weight and height	Definitions	NTDs included
Anderson et al[82]	Case–control, Birth defects surveillance system	Self-reported	Normal:18.5–24.9 kg/m^2 Overweight: 25–29.9 kg/m^2 Obese: 30–39.9 kg/m^2 Severely obese: ≥40 kg/m^2	Anencephaly, spina bifida
Feldman et al[91]	Retrospective cohort	Retrieved from database	Normal: 100–140 lbs Overweight: 141–180 lbs Obese: 181–260 lbs Severely obese: 261–300 lbs	Did not specify NTDs
Hendricks et al[86]	Case–control, Birth defects surveillance system	Self-reported	Normal:18.5–24.9 kg/m^2 Overweight: 25–29.9 kg/m^2 Obese: ≥30 kg/m^2	Anencephaly, spina bifida, encephalocele
Kallen[90]	Retrospective cohort	National birth registry	Normal:19.8–26 kg/m^2 Overweight: 26.1–29 kg/m^2 Obese: >29 kg/m^2	Anencephaly, spina bifida
Mikhail et al, 2005	Case–control, Perinatal database and clinical records	Weight and height abstracted from patient records to derive calculated BMI	Normal: <27 kg/m^2 Overweight: ≥27 kg/m^2	NTDs
Moore et al[85]	Prospective cohort from screening women in 100 obstetrical clinics	Measured	Normal: <25 kg/m^2 Overweight: 25–27.9 kg/m^2 Obese: ≥28 kg/m^2	Did not specify type of NTDs

Table 14.3 (continued)

References	Study design/data sources	Source of maternal weight and height	Definitions	NTDs included
Ray et al[81]	Retrospective cohort from screening women during antenatal visits and discharge database	Retrieved from database	Normal: 52–64.1 kg Overweight: 64.2–85.6 kg Obese: >85.6 kg	Spina bifida, anencephaly
Shaw et al[88]	Case–control, Birth defects surveillance system	Self-reported	Normal: 19–27 kg/m^2 Overweight: 28–30 kg/m^2 Obese: 31–37 kg/m^2 Severely obese: ≥38 kg/m^2	Anencephaly, spina bifida cystic, craniorachischisis, iniencephaly
Waller et al[80]	Case–control, Perinatal database and genetic records	Self-reported	Normal: 19–27 kg/m^2 Overweight: 28–30 kg/m^2 Obese: 31–37 kg/m^2 Severely obese: ≥38 kg/m^2	Anencephaly, spina bifida, encephalocele
Watkins et al[83]	Case–control, Birth defects surveillance system	Retrieved from birth certificates	Normal: 19.9–26 kg/m^2 Overweight: 26.1–29 kg/m^2 Obese: >29 kg/m^2	Anencephaly, spina bifida
Watkins et al[76]	Case–control, Birth defects surveillance system	Self-reported	Normal: 18.5–24.9 kg/m^2 Overweight: 25–29.9 kg/m^2 Obese: ≥30 kg/m^2	Anencephaly, spina bifida, encephalocele
Werler et al[84]	Case–control, Surveillance program based on tertiary and birth hospitals	Self-reported	Normal: 50–69 kg Overweight: 70–89 kg Obese: 90–109 kg Severely obese: ≥110 kg	Anencephaly, spina bifida, encephalocele

that were similar to the standard definitions. Three studies used weight alone (in kilograms or pounds) to designate normal, overweight, and obese women.[81,84,91] While these investigations contribute important, relevant information, the results are somewhat difficult to compare due to heterogeneity in the categorizations of overweight and obesity. Several studies included all types of NTDs, whereas other studies focused on the two most common types of defects, which include anencephaly and spina bifida. Finally, it is possible that some women were misclassified as overweight or obese due to the use of self-reported maternal height and weight. Validity studies suggest that reproductive-age women tend to underestimate weight and overestimate height.[92] If so, the association between maternal obesity and NTDs would most likely be underestimated, and therefore, would not substantially modify the results of published studies. Overall, maternal obesity is associated with an increased risk of NTDs, although the absolute increase is likely small.

14.7 Fetal Ultrasound Assessment

Obstetrical ultrasound is a primary tool in the identification of congenital anomalies, such as NTDs and in the evaluation of fetal growth and well-being. Maternal obesity can limit the accuracy of prenatal ultrasound and can therefore increase the likelihood of an undetected fetal structural abnormality. Hendler et al[93] reported suboptimal rates of visualization of the fetal cardiac structures by 43% in the babies of obese women. Wolfe and associates[94] conducted a prospective study of 1,622 ultrasounds performed in the second and third trimesters of pregnancy. The average gestational age at the time of ultrasound was 25 weeks. Each ultrasound was reviewed and classified as visualized or suboptimally visualized. Among women with BMI in the 97th percentile, visualization was decreased to 63%. Visualization of all organ systems was decreased by 14.5% in women with BMI greater than the 90th percentile compared with women with normal BMI.

Several studies have investigated the best portion of the maternal abdomen on which to conduct ultrasound and investigated optimal timing of second trimester anatomical ultrasound. Rosenberg[95] conducted a small study assessing ultrasound images through the umbilicus, the thinnest section of the abdominal wall. He reported that 18 of 19 previously incomplete cardiac surveys were possible with the transumbilical approach. Optimal timing for performing second-trimester anatomical scans in obese women is reported to be at 18–20 weeks gestation based on a prospective study by Lantz.[96]

14.8 Conclusions

Rates of obesity are increasing across populations. Women of childbearing age are among those affected. Maternal obesity can affect not only the health of the mother, but also the well-being of her children.[97] The underlying cause of this epidemic is multifactorial, including caloric intake, physical activity and potential familial and genetic components. The perinatal period is an important time frame during which to critically address obesity, particularly in the glucose-tolerant parturient who is still at risk for multiple complications, mirroring many of those that occur among glucose-intolerant women. There is a large and consistent body of literature supporting an association between maternal obesity and GDM, hypertensive disorders, cesarean delivery, NTDs, and stillbirths. Further mechanistic studies are necessary to better understand the effect of obesity on development of NTDs and the occurrence of stillbirth. Additional longitudinal studies are needed to further explore the relation of maternal obesity and spontaneous preterm delivery. While there are fewer large multicenter studies on maternal obesity and postoperative complications, multiple single site studies support a higher likelihood of anesthetic, wound, and thrombo-embolic events in this population. Further studies in these areas should focus on the implementation of operative interventions and postoperative care guidelines to reduce the incidence of these complications. Perhaps most importantly, evidence-based interventions to promote appropriate maternal weight in the preconception and interconception periods are paramount in addressing the maternal obesity epidemic and the associated pregnancy complications.

References

1. Ogden CL, Carroll MD, Curtin LR, McDowell MA, Tabak CJ, Flegal KM. Prevalence of overweight and obesity in the United States, 1999-2004. *JAMA*. 2006;295:1549-1555.
2. Ogden CL, Carroll MD, McDowell MA, Flegal KM. Obesity among adults in the United States–no statistically significant chance since 2003-2004. *NCHS Data Brief*. 2007;(1):1-8.
3. Hedderson MM, Weiss NS, Sacks DA, et al. Pregnancy weight gain and risk of neonatal complications: macrosomia, hypoglycemia, and hyperbilirubinemia. *Obstet Gynecol*. 2006;108: 1153-1161.
4. World Health Organization. *Physical Status: The Use and Interpretation of Anthropometry*. WHO Technical Report Series 854. Geneva, Switzerland: World Health Organization; 1995:1-42.
5. Bradley PJ. Conditions recalled to have been associated with weight gain in adulthood. *Appetite*. 1985;6:235-241.
6. Gunderson EP, Abrams B. Epidemiology of gestational weight gain and body weight changes after pregnancy. *Epidemiol Rev*. 2000;22:261-274.
7. Gunderson EP, Abrams B, Selvin S. The relative importance of gestational gain and maternal characteristics associated with the risk of becoming overweight after pregnancy. *Int J Obes Relat Metab Disord*. 2000;24:1660-1668.
8. Rossner S. Short communication: pregnancy, weight cycling and weight gain in obesity. *Int J Obes Relat Metab Disord*. 1992;16:145-147.
9. Institute of Medicine. Weight gain during pregnancy: reexamining the guidelines. www.iom.edu/pregnancyweightgain; 2009. Last accessioned 24.07.09.
10. Smith DE, Lewis CE, Caveny JL, Perkins LL, Burke GL, Bild DE. Longitudinal changes in adiposity associated with pregnancy. The CARDIA Study. Coronary Artery Risk Development in Young Adults Study. *JAMA*. 1994;271:1747-1751.
11. Nicholson WK, Fox HE, Cooper LA, Strobino D, Witter F, Powe NR. Maternal race, procedures, and infant birth weight in type 2 and gestational diabetes. *Obstet Gynecol*. 2006;108:626-634.
12. Lewis CE, Smith DE, Wallace DD, Williams OD, Bild DE, Jacobs DR Jr. Seven-year trends in body weight and associations with lifestyle and behavioral characteristics in black and white young adults: the CARDIA study. *Am J Public Health*. 1997;87:635-642.
13. Ewing R, Schmid T, Killingsworth R, Zlot A, Raudenbush S. Relationship between urban sprawl and physical activity, obesity, and morbidity. *Am J Health Promot*. 2003;18:47-57.
14. Sobal J, Troiano R, Frongillo E. Rural-urban differences in obesity. *Rural Sociol*. 1996;61: 289-305.
15. Duelberg SI. Preventive health behavior among black and white women in urban and rural areas. *Soc Sci Med*. 1992;34:191-198.
16. Scheonborn C, Barnes P. Leisure-time physical activity among adults: United States 1997-98. In: *Advanced Data from Vital and Health Statistics*. Hyattsville, MD: National Center for Health Statistics; 2002.

17. Galtier-Dereure F, Boegner C, Bringer J. Obesity and pregnancy: complications and cost. *Am J Clin Nutr*. 2000;71:1242S-1248S.
18. HAPO Study Cooperative Research Group. Hyperglycemia and Adverse Pregnancy Outcome (HAPO) Study: associations with neonatal anthropometrics. *Diabetes* 2009;58:453-459.
19. Dabelea D, Snell-Bergeon JK, Hartsfield CL, Bischoff KJ, Hamman RF, McDuffie RS. Increasing prevalence of gestational diabetes mellitus (GDM) over time and by birth cohort: Kaiser Permanente of Colorado GDM Screening Program. *Diabetes Care*. 2005;28:579-584,
20. Ferrara A, Kahn HS, Quesenberry CP, Riley C, Hedderson MM. An increase in the incidence of gestational diabetes mellitus: Northern California, 1991-2000. *Obstet Gynecol*. 2004;103: 526-533.
21. Thorpe LE, Berger D, Ellis JA, et al. Trends and racial/ethnic disparities in gestational diabetes among pregnant women in New York City, 1990-2001. *Am J Public Health*. 2005;95: 1536-1539.
22. Bianco AT, Smilen SW, Davis Y, Lopez S, Lapinski R, Lockwood CJ. Pregnancy outcome and weight gain recommendations for the morbidly obese woman. *Obstet Gynecol*. 1998;91:97-102.
23. Chu SY, Callaghan WM, Kim SY, et al. Maternal obesity and risk of gestational diabetes mellitus. *Diabetes Care*. 2007;30:2070-2076.
24. Hedderson MM, Williams MA, Holt VL, Weiss NS, Ferrara A. Body mass index and weight gain prior to pregnancy and risk of gestational diabetes mellitus. *Am J Obstet Gynecol*. 2008;198(409):e401-e407.
25. Ramos GA, Caughey AB. The interrelationship between ethnicity and obesity on obstetric outcomes. *Am J Obstet Gynecol*. 2005;193:1089-1093.
26. Rudra CB, Sorensen TK, Leisenring WM, Dashow E, Williams MA. Weight characteristics and height in relation to risk of gestational diabetes mellitus. *Am J Epidemiol*. 2007;165:302-308.
27. Gabbe SG, Gregory RP, Power ML, Williams SB, Schulkin J. Management of diabetes mellitus by obstetrician-gynecologists. *Obstet Gynecol*. 2004;103:1229-1234.
28. Edwards LE, Hellerstedt WL, Alton IR, Story M, Himes JH. Pregnancy complications and birth outcomes in obese and normal-weight women: effects of gestational weight change. *Obstet Gynecol*. 1996;87:389-394.
29. Ogunyemi D, Hullett S, Leeper J, Risk A. Prepregnancy body mass index, weight gain during pregnancy, and perinatal outcome in a rural black population. *J Matern Fetal Med*. 1998;7:190-193.
30. Sibai BM, Ewell M, Levine RJ, et al. Risk factors associated with preeclampsia in healthy nulliparous women. The Calcium for Preeclampsia Prevention (CPEP) Study Group. *Am J Obstet Gynecol*. 1997;177:1003-1010.
31. Baeten JM, Bukusi EA, Lambe M. Pregnancy complications and outcomes among overweight and obese nulliparous women. *Am J Public Health*. 2001;91:436-440.
32. Lee SK, Sobal J, Frongillo EA, Olson CM, Wolfe WS. Parity and body weight in the United States: differences by race and size of place of residence. *Obes Res*. 2005;13:1263-1269.
33. Sebire NJ, Jolly M, Harris JP, et al. Maternal obesity and pregnancy outcome: a study of 287, 213 pregnancies in London. *Int J Obes Relat Metab Disord*. 2001;25:1175-1182.
34. Conde-Agudelo A, Belizan JM. Risk factors for pre-eclampsia in a large cohort of Latin American and Carribean women. *Br J Obstet Gynecol*. 2000;107:75-83.
35. CS RHS, Lipworth L. Comparison of risk factors for preeclampsia and gestational hypertension in a population-based cohort study. *Am J Epidemiol*. 1998;147:1062-1070.
36. BG KM, Zondervan HA, Treffers PE. Risk factors for preeclampsia in nulliparous women in distinct ethnic groups: a prospective study. *Obstet Gynecol*. 1998;92:174-178.
37. SM TR, Hunter DJ, Manson JE, Solomon CG, Curhan GC. High body mass index and hypercholesterolemia. *Obstet Gynecol*. 1999;94:543-550.
38. Bowers D, Cohen WR. Obesity and related pregnancy complications in an inner-city clinic. *J Perinatol*. 1999;19:216-219.

39. VS SJD, Lerer T, Ingardia CJ, Wax JR, Curry JL. Obesity-related complications of pregnancy vary by race. *J Matern Fetal Med.* 2000;9:238-241.
40. Conde-Agudelo A, Belizan JM. Risk factors for pre-eclampsia in a large cohort of Latin American and Caribbean women. *BJOG.* 2000;107:75-83.
41. Knuist M, Bonsel GJ, Zondervan HA, Treffers PE. Risk factors for preeclampsia in nulliparous women in distinct ethnic groups: a prospective cohort study. *Obstet Gynecol.* 1998;92: 174-178.
42. Ros HS, Cnattingius S, Lipworth L. Comparison of risk factors for preeclampsia and gestational hypertension in a population-based cohort study. *Am J Epidemiol.* 1998;147:1062-1070.
43. Steinfeld JD, Valentine S, Lerer T, Ingardia CJ, Wax JR, Curry SL. Obesity-related complications of pregnancy vary by race. *J Matern Fetal Med.* 2000;9:238-241.
44. Thadhani R, Stampfer MJ, Hunter DJ, Manson JE, Solomon CG, Curhan GC. High body mass index and hypercholesterolemia: risk of hypertensive disorders of pregnancy. *Obstet Gynecol.* 1999;94:543-550.
45. Sibai BM, Gordon T, Thom E, et al. Risk factors for preeclampsia in healthy nulliparous women: a prospective multicenter study. The National Institute of Child Health and Human Development Network of Maternal-Fetal Medicine Units. *Am J Obstet Gynecol.* 1995;172:642-648.
46. O'Brien T, Ray J, Chan W. Maternal body mass index and the risk of preeclampsia: a systematic overview. *Epidemiology.* 2003;14:368-374.
47. Crane SS, Wojtowycz MA, Dye TD, Aubry RH, Artal R. Association between pre-pregnancy obesity and the risk of cesarean delivery. *Obstet Gynecol.* 1997;89:213-216.
48. Rosenberg TJ, Garbers S, Chavkin W, Chiasson MA. Prepregnancy weight and adverse perinatal outcomes in an ethnically diverse population. *Obstet Gynecol.* 2003;102:1022-1027.
49. DP JDM, Sorensen B, Molsted-Pederson L, Westergaard JG, Ovesen P, Beck-Nielsen H. Pregnancy outcome and prepregnancy body mass index in 2459 glucose-tolerant Danish women. *Am J Obstet Gynecol.* 2003;189:239-244.
50. Dietz PM, Callaghan WM, Morrow B, Cogswell ME. Population-based assessment of the risk of primary cesarean delivery due to excess prepregnancy weight among nulliparous women delivering term infants. *Matern Child Health J.* 2005;9:237-244.
51. American College of Obstetricians and Gynecologists. ACOG Committee. Opinion number 315 S, 2005. Obesity in pregnancy. *Obstet Gynecol.* 2005;106:671-675.
52. Kaiser PS, Kirby RS. Obesity as a risk factor for cesarean in a low-risk population. *Obstet Gynecol.* 2001;97:39-43.
53. Young TK, Woodmansee B. Factors that are associated with cesarean delivery in a large private practice: the importance of prepregnancy body mass index and weight gain. *Am J Obstet Gynecol.* 2002;187:312-318.
54. Vahratian A, Zhang J, Troendle JF, Savitz DA, Siega-Riz AM. Maternal prepregnancy overweight and obesity and the pattern of labor progression in term nulliparous women. *Obstet Gynecol.* 2004;104:943-951.
55. H-HB YX, Zhang H, Zhang C, Zhang Y, Zhang C. Women with impaired glucose intolerance during pregnancy have significantly poor pregnancy outcomes. *Diabetes Care.* 2002;25:1619-1624.
56. Greene MF, Solomon C. Gestational diabetes mellitus – time to treat. *NEJM.* 2005;352: 2544-2546.
57. Hamon C, Fanello S, Catala L, Parot E. Maternal obesity: effects on labor and delivery: excluding other diseases that might modify obstetrical management. *J Gynecol Obstet Biol Reprod (Paris).* 2005;34:109-114.
58. Kumari AS. Pregnancy outcome in women with morbid obesity. *Int J Gynaecol Obstet.* 2001;73:101-107.
59. Usha Kiran TS, Hemmadi S, Bethel J, Evans J. Outcome of pregnancy in a woman with an increased body mass index. *BJOG.* 2005;112:768-772.

60. Ray JG, Vermeulen MJ, Shapiro JL, Kenshole AB. Maternal and neonatal outcomes in pregestational and gestational diabetes mellitus, and the influence of maternal obesity and weight gain: the DEPOSIT study. Diabetes Endocrine Pregnancy Outcome Study in Toronto. *QJM*. 2001;94:347-356.
61. Philipson EH, Kalhan SC, Edelberg SC, Williams TG. Maternal obesity as a risk factor in gestational diabetes. *Am J Perinatol*. 1985;2:268-270.
62. Ehrenberg HM, Durnwald CP, Catalano P, Mercer BM. The influence of obesity and diabetes on the risk of cesarean delivery. *Am J Obstet Gynecol*. 2004;191:969-974.
63. Johnson JW, Longmate JA, Frentzen B. Excessive maternal weight and pregnancy outcome. *Am J Obstet Gynecol*. 1992;167:353-370; discussion 370-372.
64. Chu SY, Kim SY, Schmid CH, et al. Maternal obesity and risk of cesarean delivery: a meta-analysis. *Obes Rev*. 2007;8:385-394.
65. GR HI, Mercer BM. Association between maternal body mass index and spontaneous and indicated preterm birth. *Am J Obstet Gynecol*. 2005;192:882-886.
66. Castro LC, Avina RL. Maternal obesity and pregnancy outcomes. *Curr Opin Obstet Gynecol*. 2002;14:601-606.
67. Ramachenderan J, Bradford J, Mclean M. Maternal obesity and pregnancy complications: A review. *Aust N Z J Obstet Gynecol*. 2008;48:225-235.
68. Perlow JH, Morgan MA. Massive maternal obesity and perioperative cesarean morbidity. *Am J Obstet Gynecol*. 1994;170:560-565.
69. Wall PD, Deucy EE, Glantz JC, Pressman EK. Vertical skin incision and wound complications in the obese parturient. *Obstet Gynecol*. 2003;102:952-956.
70. Wolfe HM, Gross T, Sokol RJ. Determinants of morbidity in obese women delivered by cesarean. *Obstet Gynecol*. 1988;71:691-696.
71. Houston MC, Raynor BD. Postoperative morbidity in the morbidly obese parturient woman: supraumbilical and low transverse abdominal approaches. *Am J Obstet Gynecol*. 2000;182: 1033-1035.
72. Barfield W, Martin J, Hoyert D for the centres for disease control and prevention racial ethnic trends in fetal mortality: United States, 1990-2000. *MMWR Morb Mortal Wkly Rep*. 2004;53:529-532.
73. Nohr EA, Bech BH, Davies MJ, Frydenberg M, Henriksen TB, Olsen J. Prepregnancy obesity and fetal death: a study within the Danish National Birth Cohort. *Obstet Gynecol*. 2005;106:250-259.
74. Cnattingius S, Stephansson O. The epidemiology of stillbirth. *Semin Perinatol*. 2002;26:25-30.
75. Salihu HM, Dunlop AL, Hedayatzadeh M, Alio AP, Kirby RS, Alexander GR. Extreme obesity and risk of stillbirth among black and white gravidas. *Obstet Gynecol*. 2007;110:552-557.
76. Watkins ML, Rasmussen SA, Honein MA, Botto LD, Moore CA. Maternal obesity and risk for birth defects. *Pediatrics*. 2003;111:1152-1158.
77. Walker DK, Shaw GM, Rasmussen SA. Prepregnancy obesity as a risk factor for structural birth defects. *Arch Pediatr Adolesc Med*. 2007;161:745-750.
78. Stothard KJ, Tennant PW, Bell R, Rankin J. Maternal overweight and obesity and the risk of congenital anomalies: a systematic review and meta-analysis. *JAMA*. 2009;301:636-650.
79. MC BLD, Khoury MJ, Erickson JD. Neural-tube defects. *NEJM*. 1999;341:1509-1519.
80. Waller DK, Mills JL, Simpson JL. Are obese women at higher risk for producing malformed offspring? *Am J Obstet Gynecol*. 1994;170:541-548.
81. Ray JG, Wyatt PR, Vermeulen MJ, Meier C, Cole DE. Greater maternal weight and the ongoing risk of neural tube defects after folic acid flour fortification. *Obstet Gynecol*. 2005;105:261-265.
82. Anderson JL, Waller D, canfield MA, Shaw GM, Watkins ML, Werler MM. Maternal obesity, gestational diabetes and central nervous system birth defects. *Epidemiology*. 2005;16:87-92.
83. Watkins ML, Scanlon KS, Mulinare J, Khoury MJ. Is maternal obesity a risk factor for anencephaly and spina bifida? *Epidemiology*. 1996;7:507-512.
84. Werler MM, Louik C, Shaprio S, Mitchell AA. Prepregnant weight in relation to risk of neural tube defects. *JAMA*. 1996;275:1089-1092.

85. Moore LL, Singer MR, Bradlee ML, Rothman KJ, Milunsky A. A prospective study of the risk of congenital defects associated with maternal obesity and diabetes mellitus. *Epidemiology*. 2000;11:689-694.
86. Hendricks KA, Nuno OM, Suarez L, Larsen R. Effects of hyperinsulinemia and obesity on risk of neural tube defects among Mexican Americans. *Epidemiology*. 2001;12:630-635.
87. Mikhail LN, Walker CK, Mittendorf R. Association between obesity and fetal cardiac malformations in African American. *J Natl Med Assoc*. 2002;94:695-700.
88. Sahw GM, Velie EM, Schaffer D. Risk of neural tube defect-affected pregnancies among obese women. *JAMA*. 1996;275:1093-1096.
89. Rasmussen SA, Chu SY, Kim SY, Schmid CH, Lau J. Maternal obesity and risk of neural tube defects: a metaanalysis. *Am J Obstet Gynecol*. 2008;198:611-619.
90. Kallen K. Maternal smoking, body mass index, and neural tube defects. *Am J Epidemiol*. 1998;147:1103-1111.
91. Feldman B, Yaron Y, Critchfield G, et al. Distribution of neural tube defects as a function of maternal weight: no apparent correlation. *Fetal Diagn Ther*. 1999;14:185-189.
92. Nieto-Garcia FJ, Bush TL, Keyl PM. Body mass defnitions of obesity: sensitivity and specificity using self-reported weight and height. *Epidemiology*. 1990;1:146-152.
93. Hendler I, Blackwell SC, Bujold E, et al. Suboptimal second-trimester ultrasonographic visualization of the fetal heart in obese women: should we repeat the examination? *J Ultrasound Med*. 2005;24:1205-1209; quiz 1210-1211.
94. Wolfe HM, Sokol RJ, Martier SM, Zador IE. Maternal obesity: a potential source of error in sonographic prenatal diagnosis. *Obstet Gynecol*. 1990;76:339-342.
95. Rosenberg JC, Guzman ER, Vintzileos AM. Transumbilical placement of the vaginal probe in obese pregnant women. *Obstet Gynecol*. 1995;85:132-134.
96. Lantz ME, Chisholm CA. The preferred timing of second-trimester obstetric sonography based on maternal body mass index. *J Ultrasound Med*. 2004;23:1019-1022.
97. Hampton T. Maternal diabetes and obesity may have lifelong impact on health of offspring. *JAMA*. 2004;292:789-790.

Maternal Comorbidities During Gestational Diabetes Mellitus: Obstetrical Complications, Prematurity, and Delivery

15

Cristiane Guberman and Siri L. Kjos

15.1 Introduction

This chapter reviews obstetrical and delivery complications in the setting of gestational diabetes (GDM) e.g., preterm labor, the risk of shoulder dystocia, respiratory distress, shoulder dystocia, birth trauma, and cesarean delivery. We evaluate various approaches and interventions that may minimize undesirable outcomes.

15.2 Preterm Delivery

Preterm delivery, defined as delivery before 37 weeks of gestation, has increased by approximately one third over the last 25 years, to 12.8% of deliveries in 2006, with about three-quarters of these occurring between 34 and 36 weeks.[1] Preterm births can be categorized into spontaneous vs. indicated.[2] Indicated preterm births, accounting for ~25% of preterm births,[3] occur when a medical or obstetrical condition exists which creates an undue risk for the mother, the fetus, or both.

Is preterm delivery increased in women with GDM? Preeclampsia and hypertensive disease are the most common indications for pre-term delivery, accounting for approximately half of preterm births[3] and occur more frequently in women with GDM, as discussed in the chapter on hypertensive disorders during pregnancy. In a large case–control study, after adjustment for weight, age, ethnicity, and prenatal care, GDM was found to be significantly associated with an increased risk of hypertensive disorders compared to control women, including severe preeclampsia (odds ratio (OR) 1.5, 95% CI 1.1, 2.1), mild preeclampsia (OR 1.5, 95% CI 1.3, 1.8) and gestational hypertension (OR 1.4, 95% CI 1.2, 1.6).[4]

S.L. Kjos (✉)
Department of Obstetrics and Gynecology,
Harbor UCLA Medical Center, Torrance, CA 90509, USA
e-mail: skjos@obgyn.humc.edu

C. Kim and A. Ferrara (eds.), *Gestational Diabetes During and After Pregnancy*,
DOI: 10.1007/978-1-84882-120-0_15, © Springer-Verlag London Limited 2010

The association between GDM and eclampsia, a rare complication of preeclampsia, was not significant (OR 1.3, 95% CI 0.5, 3.2). The recent Hyperglycemia and Pregnancy Outcomes (HAPO) observational study, with blinded glucose tolerance testing in over 25,000 women with normal to mild GDM, found a significant relationship between increasing glucose levels and preeclampsia.[5] Hypertensive disorders of pregnancy can also induce obstetrical complications, e.g., intrauterine growth restriction or abruption, which by themselves require preterm delivery. Indicated deliveries in diabetic women due to poor glycemic control or renal disease are less commonly seen in pregnancies complicated by GDM.

Spontaneous preterm birth occurs in the absence of maternal or fetal conditions prompting delivery and accounts for approximately 75% of preterm birth.[3] Spontaneous preterm birth does not appear to be increased in women with GDM. In a controlled study examining 550 consecutive deliveries in women with intensively managed GDM, the rate of preterm delivery was 6.2% compared with 6.5% in controls.[6] In the blinded observational HAPO study there was a small, but significant positive association between increased 1- and 2-h postglucose challenge levels and preterm delivery before 37 weeks.[5] The accompanying trial did not differentiate between spontaneous and indicated preterm birth. GDM may not be a risk factor in spontaneous preterm birth, possibly because GDM women have increased frequency of prenatal visits and monitoring along with a low incidence of maternal underweight, itself a risk factor for spontaneous pre-term birth.[7]

15.3 Term Delivery

Obstetrical complications relating to delivery at term include stillbirth, shoulder dystocia, birth trauma, and cesarean delivery. Women with GDM often have coexisting morbidities such as older maternal age, higher parity, hypertension, obesity, and a history of a prior large-for-gestational age (LGA) infant, stillbirth, or cesarean delivery, all of which are independently associated with increased obstetric complications.[8] Many of these same factors are indications for early and second trimester GDM screening.[9] When addressing obstetrical complications, it is important to try to assess the independent contributions of the diagnosis and treatment of GDM above the woman's baseline risk factors for newborn and maternal morbidity.

When and how should women with GDM be delivered? The question of when and by which route a woman whose pregnancy is complicated by GDM should be delivered needs to evaluate each risk factor and their interactions. It may be safer to pursue expectant management with the fetus remaining in-utero. Expectant management also increases the risk of stillbirth, continued accelerated growth, and a LGA infant. In turn, LGA infants have greater risk of shoulder dystocia, birth trauma, labor induction, and cesarean delivery. The alternative option to schedule delivery at near term or early term can increase newborn complications such as respiratory distress, transient tachypnea of the newborn (TTN), or jaundice. While evidence-based guidelines are lacking, it is unlikely that one clear answer will emerge, as one must consider the individual comorbidities, glycemic control, obstetrical history, and the patient's own desires. The major risks associated with GDM will be considered independently to assist the practitioner to develop an individualized delivery plan to minimize risk.

Risk of stillbirth: Historically, women with pre-existing diabetes have been induced near term or prior to their estimated due date to avoid intrauterine fetal demise (IUFD). The pathophysiology of diabetes-associated IUFD is well documented in pregnant women with type 1 and type 2 diabetes, and is related to fetal hyperglycemia, hyperinsulinemia, and acidosis.[10, 11] In 1973, O'Sullivan et al[12] observed that women with untreated GDM had a fourfold increase in stillbirth, which initiated the strategy of euglycemic treatment goals for women with GDM – similar to treatment of women with pregestational diabetes – using insulin therapy and induction of labor at or near term to avoid stillbirth. Since the 1980s, the ability to achieve normal glucose levels with self-monitoring of blood glucose and insulin therapy and the advent of weekly or bi-weekly antepartum fetal testing has reduced the diabetic stillbirth rate to rates near those in pregnancies of healthy women.[13] Both of these management strategies developed concurrently, and largely without randomized trials, and both have become the standard of care in diabetic pregnancies.[15]

The most common antepartum fetal surveillance is the twice weekly nonstress test (NST) employing continuous external fetal heart rate monitoring coupled with evaluation of amniotic fluid volume (AFI), summing four quadrants of amniotic fluid measured by ultrasound. When such tests are equivocal, more complex tests such as the biophysical profile, contraction stress, or Doppler evaluation of the umbilical artery can be undertaken. When the fetal heart rate pattern during the NST demonstrates spontaneous accelerations, and moderate variability and absent decelerations, fetal hypoxia can be excluded. Conversely, when the fetal heart rate variability is moderate to absent, decelerations are present, or amniotic fluid volume is reduced, fetal hypoxia cannot be excluded.[14] Women with mild GDM generally do not start testing until term (37–38 weeks); women requiring medical therapy or having other high risk factors, e.g., prior stillbirth or hypertension, begin testing at 32–34 weeks.[15] Several large series[16–20] following this strategy have demonstrated excellent perinatal outcomes with a low false-negative results, i.e., in-utero demise within days of a normal test. These strategies have also prompted delivery prior to the onset of labor when testing was nonreassuring or suspicious for fetal jeopardy in approximately 9–13% of tested pregnancies.[17,21] It is unlikely that randomized controlled trials will ever be done to validate the need for antepartum testing in women with GDM or diabetes. Such a trial would require an enormous cohort, as stillbirth is an extremely rare event, with one study reporting a rate 1.4 per 1,000 births in a tested population consisting primarily of GDM.[17] Despite the lack of rigorous study, the widespread acceptance and excellent perinatal outcome associated with antepartum testing have established it as a *de facto* standard of practice.

The Fifth International Workshop Conference on GDM[10] recognized that there was insufficient data to make evidence-based recommendations for intensive antepartum fetal monitoring, or whether any monitoring method was superior in women with GDM. They did endorse maternal self-monitoring of fetal movements, or "daily kick counts," during the last 8–10 weeks of pregnancy, with any reduction in the perception of fetal movements requiring immediate medical evaluation. This recommendation was a change from the prior conference recommendations, which endorsed intensive antepartum surveillance.[21] This change in view has come from the low stillbirth rates in women with GDM who meet glycemic targets with medical nutritional therapy and physical activity regimens alone, and in whom fetal growth is appropriate for gestational age. For women with more severe GDM, they recommended that the method and frequency of fetal surveillance should be guided by the severity of maternal hyperglycemia or the presence of other adverse risk factors.

Risk of respiratory distress syndrome and transient tachypnea of the newborn: Elective delivery in late preterm or early term infants, as previously advocated in diabetic women to reduce stillbirth risk, has been associated with an increase in both respiratory distress syndrome (RDS)[22] and TTN. Delayed biochemical lung maturation in offspring of diabetic gestations[23] has been associated with fetal hyperinsulinemia[24] and hyperglycemia[25] in clinical and animal studies.[26,27] Fetal lung maturity can be determined by the measurement of surfactant in the amniotic fluid and has proved to be a useful adjunct in decreasing the risk of neonatal respiratory distress.[28–30] Current obstetrical practices, including accurate pregnancy dating, delaying delivery until term, and achieving euglycemic control have virtually eliminated neonatal respiratory distress (<1%) in the infant of the diabetic mother and makes any randomized controlled trial unlikely. In a historically controlled prospective trial, 1,585 term diabetic women (primarily with GDM) with reliable dating criteria were prospectively enrolled to undergo delivery without amniocentesis documentation of fetal lung maturation.[31] In women with GDM, the incidence of RDS (0.8% vs. 0.8%) and TTN (1.3% vs.0.8%) was similar to rates in term historical controls that had undergone amniocentesis prior to delivery. Cesarean delivery was the only independent predictor of RDS (adjusted RR 2.21, 95% CI, 2.04–2.27). The Fifth International Workshop Conference on GDM did not recommend assessment of fetal lung maturation after 38 weeks of gestation in reliably dated and well-controlled patients; if delivery is indicated at an earlier gestational age for maternal or fetal indications, delivery should be effected without regard to lung maturity testing.[10]

Whenever possible, elective cesarean delivery in all pregnancies should be delayed until 39 completed weeks of gestation if possible.[32] Cesarean delivery of infants delivered near term and early term, at gestational ages of 34, 35, 36, and 37 weeks was associated with progessively decreasing risk of requiring supplemental oxygen (ORs: 18.67, 8.76, 4.95, and 2.04 respectively) or ventilatory assistance (ORs 19.8, 9.04, 5.24, and 2.35 respectively) compared with cesarean deliveries at 38–40 weeks.[33] Furthermore, in term infants there was an increase in risk for each week a cesarean delivery occurred before 39 completed weeks: the OR for RDS at 37 completed weeks compared with 38 completed weeks was 1.74; for 38 weeks compared with 39 weeks the OR was 2.4.[34] Elective cesarean without labor compared with cesarean after labor was also associated with increased risk of RDS (35.5/10,000, vs. 12.2/1,000, OR 2.9). In another study, a randomized trial examining the administration of antenatal corticosteroids to normal term infants (37–41 weeks, $n=942$) undergoing elective cesarean deliveries compared with placebo controls found a significant reduction in RDS (0.002% vs. 0.11%, RR 0.21) and TTN (0.021% vs. 0.041%, RR 0.54) with antenatal corticosteroids.[35] The authors conclude that when considering an elective cesarean delivery at term, the increased risk of admission with respiratory distress should be considered and discussed with the mother. The 50% reduction in respiratory distress achieved by antenatal steroids is similar to delaying cesarean delivery until 39 completed weeks of gestation. These studies reinforce the American College of Obstetricians and Gynecologists (ACOG) recommendation to perform elective cesarean deliveries after 39 completed weeks in all women. Antenatal steroid therapy for threatened preterm labor is recommended before 34 completed weeks and should not be withheld from women with GDM.[36] It is likely that increased glucose monitoring and additional or increased insulin therapy may be required during the 48-h course of therapy in more severe GDM.

Risk of shoulder dystocia and infant birth trauma. Shoulder dystocia is defined as the need for additional obstetrical maneuvers to effect delivery of the shoulders when gentle downward traction on the fetal head fails.[37] The risk for shoulder dystocia increases with increasing birth weights in both diabetic and nondiabetic pregnancies. Nesbitt et al examined 1992 birth data from California by birth weight categories by diabetic (primarily GDM) and nondiabetic pregnancies and by spontaneous and operative vaginal deliveries.[38] The rates of shoulder dystocia were higher in diabetic women compared with nondiabetic women for each 250 g increase in birth weight for spontaneous deliveries. For birth weights categories starting at 3,500, 3,750, 4,000, 4,250, 4,500, and 4,750 g the respective rates were 3.0, 5.8, 8.4, 12.3, 19.9, and 23.5%. These rates were further increased with operative vaginal deliveries: 4.0, 8.5, 12.2, 16.7, 27.3, and 34.8%, respectively. The increased risk of shoulder dystocia in infants of similar birth weights born to diabetic vs. nondiabetic mothers is likely related to the increased truncal obesity,[39] larger shoulder diameter[40] in infants of diabetic mothers, and higher rates of maternal obesity.[41] Several studies have evaluated use of ultrasound prior to delivery to assist in the prediction of birth weight and shoulder dystocia. In order to assess whether ultrasound was possibly being more accurate than clinical estimates in obese diabetic women, Sacks[42] reviewed the predictive ability of ultrasound examination to identify macrosomic birth weights (4,000–4,500 g). While studies demonstrated that 71–82% of expected fetal weights (EFWs) were within 10% of actual birth weights, the sensitivity (68–80%), specificity (78–96%), and negative predictive value (81–87%) were limited. Combining the ultrasound EFW (>4,000 g) with clinical risk factors for macrosomia and excess amniotic fluid volume may improve the weight prediction.[43] Similarly studies have attempted to use various ultrasound methods to predict shoulder dystocia, all with limited accuracy.[44] One recent and simple method found that positive difference (≥2.6 cm) between the abdominal diameter and biparietal diameter was associated with shoulder dystocia in almost 40% of diabetic women.[45] Despite many studies, the occurrence of a shoulder dystocia remains an unpredictable emergency more common in diabetic women.[40,46] The obstetrician and delivery staff should consider and be ready to institute a preplanned sequence of maneuvers to release the shoulder.

Birth trauma to the infant, e.g., fracture of the humerus or clavicle, brachial plexus palsy, or facial palsy is more likely to occur during a difficult delivery complicated by shoulder dystocia. Rates of 20–40% have been reported in series examining cases of shoulder dystocia women with diabetes. The most serious injury is brachial plexus injury, which occurs infrequently with shoulder dystocia, ranging from 4 to 13% percent.[41,44,47–49] Most cases of brachial plexus palsy resolve spontaneously in early infancy, and of the remaining 5–7%, three-quarters will achieve the restoration of upper arm function when surgical correction is undertaken within the first year of life.[50] Interestingly, large population surveys have found that only one quarter to almost one half of brachial palsy cases are associated with identified shoulder dystocias during delivery.[51–53] Brachial plexus injuries have also occurred with cesarean deliveries.[54]

Should cesarean delivery be offered to prevent shoulder dystocia when macrosomia is suspected in diabetic women? To date, there are no randomized controlled trials that compare trial of labor with primary cesarean delivery in diabetic women with estimated fetal weights (EFW) 4,000–4,500 g. ACOG does not recommend primary cesarean delivery unless the EFW >4,500 g in diabetic women[40] while other published opinions select thresholds from 4,000 to 4,500 g.[58, 59] One controlled study evaluated a protocol of cesarean delivery for ultrasound EFW ≥4,250 g and labor induction for LGA growth (>90th percentile at 38 weeks).[55] Following these guidelines, 11% of the diabetic population underwent cesarean section or induction for macrosomia, and the rate of shoulder dystocia was decreased significantly (1.5%) compared with historical controls 3 years earlier (2.8%). In a similar study, a 3-fold decrease in risk of shoulder dystocia supported the policy of offering cesarean delivery for diabetic women in whom the EFW was 4,250 g or more.[56] This approach may lower perinatal morbidity at the expense of the mother whose risk of cesarean delivery increases at least twofold.[57-59] The increased operative risk has persisted despite improved glycemic control and normalized growth of infants. One randomized controlled trial in women with diet-controlled GDM targeted pregnancies at high risk for LGA infants by abdominal circumference measurements ≥75th percentile for gestational age. Aggressive insulin therapy with lower glycemic targets compared with diet therapy alone was successful in reducing the LGA rate (13% vs. 45%) but resulted in a paradoxical increase in cesarean delivery (43% vs. 17%).[60] Similarly in the Toronto Tri-Hospital study, women with identified and treated GDM were compared with women with blinded testing of glucose tolerance. Those with GDM had a twofold increased risk of cesarean delivery after adjustment for multiple risk factors.[61] The women with treated GDM had a lower rate (10.5%) of macrosomia but a higher rate (34%) of cesarean delivery, compared with women with untreated borderline GDM, who had a 29% macrosomia rate with a 30% cesarean rate. Macrosomia was found to be a risk factor for cesarean delivery in the untreated borderline GDM group, but was found to have no impact on risk of cesarean delivery in women with known, treated GDM. The authors suggest that the diagnosis of GDM in and of itself may lower the obstetrician's threshold for cesarean delivery.

15.4 Should Women with GDM be Managed Expectantly or Induced?

Currently there is no evidence-based guideline for timing and route of delivery to minimize both maternal and neonatal complications in GDM pregnancies. A single best strategy has proved elusive, in large part due to the many variables which must be considered, i.e., the fetal condition, estimated fetal weight, prior maternal history of macrosomia, shoulder dystocia, or cesarean delivery, severity and control of diabetes, coexisting disease, the estimated chance of successful labor induction, and the personal biases of both the woman and her doctor. While historical factors such as prior cesarean deliveries and prepregnancy weight are not modifiable after conception, many risk factors have been minimized by today's obstetrical care, notably fetal overgrowth and risk of stillbirth. Logically, as these two factors are normalized, one should be able to allow pregnancies with GDM to await spontaneous labor.

In nondiabetic women with ultrasound EFW >4,000 g, randomization to induction vs. elective cesarean delivery reduced neither primary cesarean rates nor neonatal morbidity.[62] The only randomized controlled trial in women with well-controlled insulin treated diabetes (93% with GDM) without evidence of macrosomia and in good control, evaluated the effect of expectant management vs. active labor induction on cesarean delivery and neonatal morbidity.[63] Expectant management increased the gestational age of delivery by 1 week without a significant reduction in cesarean delivery (31% vs. 25%, respectively). However, all indices of fetal growth, whether birth weight, macrosomia or LGA infants, were significantly increased with expectant management. Even when gestational age at delivery and maternal weight were controlled the birth weight was significantly increased with expectant management, suggesting that a subset of infants continue to have accelerated growth in-utero, and further prolongation of gestation magnifies this growth. Almost half (49%) of those randomize to expectant management subsequently underwent delivery before spontaneous labor for either obstetrical or medical indications. The low threshold for intervention demonstrated by obstetricians in this study may be similar to the low threshold for cesarean delivery demonstrated in other studies.[61–64]

A Cochrane database review of this topic[64] concluded that the policy of induction of labor at 38 weeks of gestation in diabetic mothers treated with insulin was associated with the reduction in birth weight above 4,000 g and above the 90th percentile. That intervention did not increase risk of cesarean section and neonatal morbidity remained the same on the two groups. This suggested that there might be a little advantage in delaying delivery beyond 38–39 weeks and induction of labor might be a reasonable option, but more trials are necessary with a larger sample size to evaluate elective delivery in these women. The Fifth International Workshop Conference on GDM also noted that some studies suggest that delivery past 38 weeks can lead to an increase in the rate of LGA infants without reducing the rate of cesarean deliveries.[10] They also state that there is no data supporting delivery prior to 38 weeks gestation in the absence of objective evidence of maternal or fetal compromise. Nor is there any data to indicate whether there is greater risk of perinatal morbidity/mortality in infants of women with well-controlled GDM if pregnancy is allowed to proceed past 40 weeks gestation. Increasingly, the best strategy to minimize both maternal and newborn morbidity appears to normalize maternal glucose and normalize fetal growth, avoiding LGA and disproportionate growth.

The risk of cesarean delivery: As discussed, women with GDM have an approximate twofold increased risk of cesarean delivery after adjusting for confounding factors including maternal age, body mass index, and birth weight.[65,66] When practitioners are blinded to glucose results, both the Toronto Tri-Hospital[65] and HAPO studies[5] found a linear increased risk of cesarean delivery and increased birth weight or LGA rate with untreated increasing levels of glucose. In addition to the risk associated with GDM *per se*, these women often have other independent risk factors for cesarean delivery. A retrospective analysis of 5,735 women with gestational and pregestational diabetes found 11 independent predictors of cesarean delivery.[67] Eight of these were not modifiable: prior cesarean delivery (RR 5.34), no prior live birth (RR 3.17), no prior vaginal delivery (RR 2.28), prior stillbirth (RR 1.71), maternal age ≥35 years (RR 1.53), requiring insulin during pregnancy (RR 1.53), highest fasting plasma glucose before therapy (RR 1.04), and preeclampsia/hypertension (RR 2.56). The remaining three were potentially modifiable: labor induction (RR 3.32), birth weight (RR 1.12 per 250g) and predelivery body mass index (BMI) (RR 1.03 per kg/m^2). In summary, studies examining protocols to reduce cesarean delivery will need to address these multiple predictors to lower morbidity.

Obesity (BMI ≥30 kg/m^2) is common in women with GDM and in and of itself markedly increases the maternal perinatal morbidity, i.e., the risk of cesarean delivery, anesthesia risk and time, wound infection and dehiscence, postpartum fever, postpartum hemorrhage and postpartum deep venous thrombophlebitis (DVT).[68,69] No prospective trials evaluate how best to decrease these morbidities. Some authors recommend a vertical skin incision over a low transverse incision for better exposure, while others believe vertical incisions are more painful, have slower recovery, and a higher incidence of evisceration. One retrospective study examining postoperative complications in women with BMI >35 kg/m^2 undergoing primary cesarean found a higher rate of wound complications (34.6% vs. 9.4%) with vertical vs. transverse skin incisions.[70] Data is equally conflicting regarding the closure of the subcutaneous tissue or use of subcutaneous drains. One randomized controlled trial in obese women undergoing cesarean section found subcutaneous suture or drainage decreased the incidence of postoperative wound complications when subcutaneous tissue exceeded 2 cm.[71] In contrast, the ACOG Committee Opinion suggesting subcutaneous closure may increase the risk of wound disruption.[72] Lastly, postpartum obese women should receive DVT prophylaxis including early ambulation and compression stockings. The data is incomplete as to whether postoperative heparin therapy is appropriate for the obese parturient.

15.5 Summary

Over the last 30 years, technological and patient care developments, in glucose monitoring and insulin administration, ultrasound evaluation of fetal growth and weight, antepartum fetal surveillance, evaluation of fetal lung maturation, labor induction, and cesarean delivery have contributed to a reduction in perinatal morbidity for women with GDM and their newborns. As many of these factors developed simultaneously, e.g., improved glycemic control and antepartum surveillance, it is difficult to assess the independent contribution of each. The historical risks of stillbirth and RDS are now rare in pregnancies complicated by GDM, and increasingly permit spontaneous delivery at term. Today, it is possible to normalize maternal glucose levels through the use of self blood glucose monitoring, medical nutritional therapy and medical therapy. The best way to decrease risks of shoulder dystocia and cesarean delivery is to reduce the risk of LGA infants. New strategies, demonstrated in RCTs, use ultrasound to monitor fetal growth, to modify glycemic targets have been shown to significantly reduce LGA and SGA growth.[73] Similarly, new recommendations for maternal weight gain may reduce both the risk of GDM and LGA infants and maternal cesarean rates and postoperative complications. In the near future, new international diagnostic criteria[5] for GDM will be based on maternal and newborn morbidity. New developments, and the continued push for evaluation of evidence-based care protocols will decrease obstetrical complications in women with GDM and their offspring.

References

1. Hamilton BE, Martin JA, Sutton PD, et al. Births: final data for 2005. *Natl Vital Stat Rep.* 2007;56(6):4.
2. Meis P, Michielutte R, Peters T, et al. Factor associated with preterm birth in Cardiff, Wales. *Am J Obstet Gynecol.* 1995;173:597-602.

3. Meis P, Goldenber R, Mercer B, et al. The Preterm Prediction Study: risk factors for indicated preterm births. *Am J Obstet Gynecol.* 1998;178:562-567.
4. Bryson CL, Loannou GN, Rulyak SJ, Critchlow C. Association between gestational diabetes and pregnancy-induced hypertension. *Am J Epidemiol.* 2003;158:1148-1153.
5. Metzger BE, The HAPO Study Cooperative Research Group. Hyperglycemia and adverse pregnancy outcomes. *N Eng J Med.* 2008;358:1991-2002.
6. Bar-hava I, Barnhard Y, Scarpelli SA, Orvieto R, Ben-Rafael DMY. Gestational diabetes and preterm labour: is glycaemic control a contributing factor? *Eur J Obstet Gynecol Reprod Biol.* 1997;93:111-114.
7. Mercer B, Goldenber RI, Das A, et al. The Preterm Prediction Study: a clinical risk assessment system. *Am J Obstet Gynecol.* 1996;174:1885-1895.
8. Johnson TRB, Gregory KD, Niebyl JR. Preconception and prenatal care: part of the continuum. In: Gabbe SG, Niebyl JR, Simpson JL. 5th ed. *Obstetrics Normal and Problem Pregnancies*. Philidelphia, PA: Elsevier; 111-137.
9. Metzger BE, Buchanan TA, Coustan DR, et al. Summary and Recommendation of the Fifth International Workshop Conference on Gestational Diabetes Mellitus. *Diabetes Care.* 2007;30(suppl 2):S251-S260.
10. Mimouni F, Miodovnik M, Siddiqui TA, Khoury J, Tsang RC. Perinatal asphyxia in infants of insulin-dependent diabetic women. *J Pediatr.* 1988;113:345-353.
11. Dudley DJ. Diabetic-associated stillbirth: incidence, pathophysiology and prevention. *Clin Perinatol.* 2007;34:611-616.
12. O'Sullivan JB, Charles D, Mahan C, Dandrow RV. Gestational diabetes and perinatal mortality rate. *Am J Obstet Gynecol.* 1973;116:901-904.
13. Landon MB, Catalano PM, Gabbe SG. Diabetes mellitus complicating pregnancy. In: Gabbe SG, Niebyl JR, Simpson JL. 5th ed. *Obstetrics Normal and Problem Pregnancies*. Philidelphia, PA: Elsevier; 2007:976-1010.
14. American College of Obstetrician and Gynecologists. Antepartum Fetal Surveillance. Clinical management guidelines for obstetrician-gynecologists. ACOG Practice Bulletin. #9. *Int J Gynaecol Obstet.* 2000;68:175-185.
15. Lagrew DC, Pircon RA, Towers CV, Dorchester W, Freeman RK. Antepartum fetal surveillance in patients with diabetes: when to start? *Am J Obstet Gynecol.* 1993;168:1820-1826.
16. Kjos SL, Leung A, Henry OA, Victor MR, Paul RH, Medearis AL. Antepartum surveillance in diabetic pregnancies: predictors of fetal distress. *Am Jo Obstet Gynecol.* 1995;173:1532-1539.
17. Girz BA, Divon MY, Merkatz IR. Sudden fetal death in women with well-controlled intensively montiored gestational diabetes. *J Perinatol.* 1992;12:229-233.
18. Landon MB, Gabbe SG. Antepartum fetal surveillance in gestational diabetes mellitus. *Diabetes*. 1985;34:50-54.
19. Landon MB, Gabbe SG. Fetal surveillance in the pregnancy complicated by diabetes mellitus. *Clin Obstet Gynecol.* 1991;34:535-543.
20. Johnson JM, Lange IR, Harman CR, et al. Biophysical profile scoring in the management of the diabetic pregnancy. *Obstet Gynecol.* 1988;72:841-846.
21. Metzger BE, Coustan DR, The Organizing Committee. Summary and Recommendations of the fourth international workshop-conference on gestational diabetes mellitus. *Diabetes Care.* 1998;21(suppl 2):161-167.
22. Robert MF, Neff RK, Hubbel JP, Tauesch HW, Avery ME. Association between maternal diabetes and the respiratory distress syndrome in the newborn. *N Engl J Med.* 1976;284: 357-360.
23. Gluck L, Kulovich MV. Lecithin/sphingomyelin ratios in amniotic fluid in normal and abnormal pregnancies. *Am J Obstet Gynecol.* 1973;115:339-379.
24. Warburton D, Lew C, Platzker A. Primary hyperinsulinemia reduces surface active material flux in tracheal fluid of fetal lambs. *Pediatr Res.* 1981;15:1422-1429.

25. Karlsson K, Kjellmer I. The outcome of diabetic pregnancies in relationship to the mother's blood sugar level. *Am J Obstet Gynecol.* 1972;112:213-220.
26. Lawrence S, Warshaw J, Nielson HC. Delayed lung maturation in the macrosomic offspring of genetically determined diabetic (db/+) mic. *Pediatr Res.* 1989;25:173-179.
27. Bourbon JR, Pignol B, Marin L, et al. Maturation of fetal lung rat in diabetic pregnancies of graduated severity. *Diabetes.* 1985;43:734-743.
28. Gabbe S, Lownsohn R, Mestman J, Freeman RK, Gobelsmann U. Lecithin spingomyelin ratio in pregnancies complicated by diabetes mellitus. *Am J Obstet Gynecol.* 1977;128:757-785.
29. Farrel P, Engle M, Curet L, et al. Saturated phospholipids in amniotic fluid of normal and diabetic pregnancies. *Obstet Gynecol.* 1984;64:77-86.
30. Kjos SL, Walther F, Montoro M, et al. Prevalence and etiology of respiratory distress in infants of diabetic mothers: predictive value of fetal lung maturation testing. *Am J Obstet Gynecol.* 1990;163:898-903.
31. Kjos SL, Berkowitz KM, Kung B. Prospective delivery of reliably dated term infants of diabetic mothers without determination of fetal lung maturity: comparison to historical control. *J Mat-Fetal Neonat Med.* 2002;12:1-5.
32. American College of Obstetrician and Gynecologists. Fetal lung maturity. Clinical management guidelines for obstetrician-gynecologists. ACOG Practice Bulletin #97. *Obstet Gynecol.* 2008;112:717-726.
33. Escobar GJ, Clark GJD. Short-term outcomes of infants born at 35 and 36 weeks gestation: We need to ask more questions. *Semin Perinatol.* 2006;30:28-33.
34. Rennie MJJ, JM MPJ. Neonatal respiratory morbidity and mode of delivery at term: influence of timing of elective caesarean section. *Br J Obstet Gynaecol.* 1995;102:101-106.
35. Stutchfield P, Whitaker R, Russell I, Antenatal Steroids for Term Elective Caesarean Section (ASTECS Research Team). Antenatal betamethasone and incidence of neonatal respiratory distress after elective caesarean section: pragmatic randomized trial. *BMJ.* 2005;331:662-668.
36. American College of Obstetrician and Gynecologists. Committee on Obstetric Practice: antenatal corticosteroid therapy for fetal maturation. ACOG Committee Opinion. *Obstet Gynecol.* 2002;99:871-873.
37. American College of Obstetrician and Gynecologists. Shoulder Dystocia. Clinical management guidelines for obstetrician-gynecologists. ACOG Practice Bulletin #40. *Obstet Gynecol.* 2002;100:1045-1049.
38. Nesbitt TS, Gilbert WM, Herrshen B. Shoulder dystocia and associated risk factors with macrosomic infants born in California. *Am J Obstet Gynecol.* 1998;179:476-480.
39. Catalano PM, Thomas AJ, Huston LP, Fung CM. Effect of maternal metabolism on fetal growth and body compostion. *Diabetes Care.* 1998;21(suppl 2)B85-B90.
40. MacFarand MB, Trylovich CG, Langer O. Anthropometric differences in macrosomia infants of diabetic and nondiabetic mothers. *J Matern-Fetal Med.* 1998;7:292-295.
41. Acker DB, Sachs BP, Friedman EA. Risk factors for shoulder dystocia in the average-weight infant. *Obstet Gynecol.* 1985;67:614-618.
42. Sacks DA, Sacks A. Estimateing fetal weight in the management of macrosomia. *Obstet Gynecol Surv.* 2000;55:229-239.
43. Hackmon R, Borstein E, Ferber A, Horani J, O'Reilly-Green CP, Divon MY. Combined analysis with amniotic fluid index and estimated fetal weight for prediction of severe macrosomia at birth. *Am J Obstet Gynecol.* 2007;196:333.e1-333.e4.
44. Landon MB, Sonek J, Foy P, Hamilton L, Gabbe S. Sonographic measurement of fetal humeral soft tissue thickness in pregnancy complicated by GDM. *Diabetes.* 1991;40(suppl 2):66-70.
45. Miller RS, Devine PC, Johnson EB. Sonographic fetal asymmetry predicts shoulder dystocia. *J Ultrasound Med.* 2007;26:1523-1528.
46. Gherman RB, Chauhan S, Ouzounian JG, Lerner H, Gonik B, Goodwin TM. Shoulder dystociaL the unpreventable obstetric emergency with empric management guidelines. *Am J Obstet Gynecol.* 2006;195:657-672.

47. Metha SH, Blackwell SC, Bujold E, Solol RJ. What factors are associated with neonatal injury following shoulder dystocia? *J Perinatol.* 2006;26:85-88.
48. Ecker JL, Greenberg JA, Norwitz ER, Nadel AS, Repke JT. Birthweight as a predictor of brachial plexus injury. *Obstet Gynecol.* 1997;89:643-647.
49. Mollberg M, Hagverg H, Bager B, Kilja H, Ladfors L. High birth weight and shoulder dystocia. The strongest risk factors for obstetrical brachial plexus palsy in a Swedish population–based study. *Acta Obstet Gynecol Scand.* 2005;84:654-659.
50. Dumont CE, Forin V, Asfazadourian H, et al. Function of the upper limb after surgery for obstetric brachial plexus palsy. *J Bone Joint Surg Br.* 2001;83:894-900.
51. Gregory KD, Henry OA, Ramicone E, Chan LS, Platt LD. Maternal and infant complications in high and normal weight infants by method of delivery. *Obstet Gynecol.* 1998;2:507-513.
52. Gilbert WM, Nesbitt TS, Danielsen B. Associated factors in 1611 cases of brachial plexus injury. *Obstet Gynecol.* 1999;93:536-540.
53. Graham EM, Forouzan I, Morgan MA. A retrospective analysis of Erb's palsy cases and their relation to birth weight and trauma during delivery. *J Perinat Med.* 1981;9:286-292.
54. Gherman RB, Ouzounian JG, Satin AJ, Goodwin TM, Phelan JP. A comparison of shoulder dystocia-associated transient and permanent brachial plexus palsies. *Obstet Gynecol.* 2003;102:544-548.
55. Conway DL, Langer O. Elective delivery of infants with macrosomia in diabetic women: reduced shoulder dystocia versus increase cesarean delivery. *Am J Obstet Gynecol.* 1998;178:922-925.
56. Mullin P, Gherman R, et al. The relationship of shoulder dystocia to estimated fetal weight. Presented at the 68th annual meeting of the Pacific Coast Obstetrical and Gynecological society, Ashland,OR; 2001.
57. Placek PJ, Taffel SM. Recent patterns in cesarean delivery in the United States. Recent patterns in cesarean delivery in the United States. *Gynecol Clin North Am.* 1988;15:607-627.
58. Landon MB, Gabbe SG, Sachs SL. Management of diabetes mellitus and pregnancy: a survery of obstetriacians and maternal-fetal specialists. *Obstet Gynecol.* 1990;75:635-640.
59. Drury IM, Stronge JM, Foley ME, MacDonald DW. Pregnancy in the diabetic patient: timing and mode of delivery. *Obstet Gynecol.* 1983;62:279-282.
60. Buchanan TA, Kjos SL, Montoro MN, et al. Use of fetal ultrasound to select metabolic therapy for pregnancies complicated by mild gestational diabetes. *Diabetes Care.* 1994;17:275-283.
61. Naylor CD, Sermer M, Chen E, Sykora K. Cesarean delivery in relation to birthweight and gestational glucose tolerance: pathophysiology or practice style. *JAMA.* 1996;265:1165-1170.
62. Gonnen O, Rosen DJ, Dolfin Z, Tepper R, Markov S, Fejgin MD. Induction of labor versus expectant management in macrosomia. A randomized study. *Obstet Gynecol.* 1997;89:913-917.
63. Kjos SL, Henry OA, Montoro M, Buchanan TA, Mestman JH. Insulin-requiring diabetes in pregnancy: a randomized trial of active induction of labor and expectant management. *Am J Obstet Gynecol.* 1993;169:611-615.
64. Boulvain M, Stan CM, Irion O. Elective delivery in diabetic pregnant women. Issue 4, 2009. Cochrane Database of Systematic Reviews. Art. No.: CD001997.
65. Ray JG, et al. Maternal and neonatal outcomes in pregestational and gestational diabetes mellitus, and the influence of maternal obesity and weight gain: the DEPOSIT study. Diabetes Endocrine Pregnancy Outcome Study in Toronto. *Q J Med.* 1994;2001:347-356.
66. Blackwell SC et al. Why are cesarean delivery rates so high in diabetic pregnancies? *J Perinat Med.* 2000;28:316-320.
67. Sl K, Berkowitz K, Xiang A. Independent predictors of Cesarean delivery in women with diabetes. *J Maternal-Fetal Neonatal Med.* 2004;15:61-67.
68. Catalano PM. Management of obesity in pregnancy. *Am J Obstet Gynecol.* 2007;109: 419-433.
69. Sebire NJ, Jolly M, Harris JP, et al. Maternal obesity and pregnancy outcome: a study of 287, 213 pregnancies in London. *Int J Obes Relat Metab Disord.* 2001;25:1175-1182.

70. Wall PD, et al. Vertical skin incision and wound complications in the obese parturient. *Obstet Gynecol.* 2003;102(5 pt1):952-956.
71. Allaire AD, Fisch J, McMahon MJ. Subcutaneous drain vs. suture in obese women undergoing cesarean delivery. A prospective, randomized trial. *J Reprod Med.* 2000;45:327-331.
72. American College of Obstetrician and Gynecologists. Committee on Obstetric Practice: Obesity in Pregnancy. ACOG Committee Opinion No 315. *Obstet Gynecol.* 2005;106: 671-675.
73. Kjos SL, Schaefer-Graf UM. Modified therapy for gestational diabetes using high-risk and low-risk fetal abdominal circumference growth to select strict versus relaxed maternal glycemic targets. *Diabetes Care.* 2007;30(suppl 2):S200-S205.

The Diabetic Intrauterine Environment: Short and Long-Term Consequences

16

Dana Dabelea

16.1 Introduction

Diabetes during pregnancy is a growing problem worldwide. Type 2 diabetes is increasing at an alarming rate[1] and is occurring in younger individuals more often than previously,[2] resulting in more women being diagnosed with type 2 diabetes during their reproductive years. In addition, gestational diabetes (GDM) has also been shown to be increasing among all racial/ethnic groups in several studies in the United States.[3, 4] The observed increase probably reflects the well-documented obesity epidemic.[5]

The hypothesis of fetal over-nutrition or fuel mediated teratogenesis proposed in the 1950s by Pederson[6] postulates that intrauterine exposure of the fetus of women with diabetes in pregnancy to hyperglycemia causes permanent fetal changes, leading to malformations, greater birth weight, and an increased risk of developing type 2 diabetes and obesity in later life. In the 1980s this hypothesis was broadened to include the possibility that other fuels, such as free fatty acids (FFA), ketone bodies, and amino acids also increased fetal growth.[7] More recently, it has been suggested that fetal over-nutrition may also occur in nondiabetic but obese pregnancies.[8] The notion that inadequate "nutrition" at critical periods of development in fetal life is a key determinant of childhood and adult health has important implications.[9–11] Animal studies have demonstrated that the metabolic imprinting caused by the diabetic intrauterine environment can be transmitted across generations.[12, 13] It has been suggested that a "vicious cycle" results, explaining at least in part the increases in type 2 and GDM seen over the past several decades.

This chapter reviews the evidence on the effect of intrauterine over-nutrition on fetal growth, metabolic imprinting, and offspring risk of obesity and type 2 diabetes later in life. Possible mechanisms for these effects are reviewed, and the clinical and public health implications are discussed.

D. Dabelea
Department of Epidemiology, Colorado School of Public Health,
University of Colorado Denver, 13001 East 17th Avenue, Campus Box B-119,
Aurora, CO 80045, USA
e-mail: Dana.Dabelea@ucdenver.edu

C. Kim and A. Ferrara (eds.), *Gestational Diabetes During and After Pregnancy*,
DOI: 10.1007/978-1-84882-120-0_16,

16.2 Intrauterine Over-Nutrition and Fetal Growth

Fetal over-nutrition has generally been inferred indirectly from measures such as maternal prepregnancy weight, height, weight gain during pregnancy, and infant birth weight. Maternal metabolism has seldom been assessed and most studies to date have focused on maternal hyperglycemia and diabetes.

16.2.1 Maternal Diabetes and Obesity and Fetal Growth

Infants of diabetic mothers display excess fetal growth, often resulting in large-for-gestational age (LGA) or macrosomia,[14,15] consequently increasing the risk for cesarean delivery and traumatic birth injury.[15]

It is thought that excessive fetal growth and other metabolic changes related to intrauterine exposure to diabetes can lead to increased adiposity in the offspring. There is evidence that increased adiposity is present at birth in infants of mothers with GDM. Catalano et al[16] studied a group of 195 infants born to mothers with GDM and 220 infants of mothers with normal glucose tolerance, and found that fat mass, but not birth weight or fat-free mass, was 20% higher in the infants exposed to diabetes *in utero*. Maternal fasting glucose level measured during the oral glucose tolerance test was the strongest correlate of infant adiposity, further supporting the hypothesis that the degree of hyperglycemia determines the metabolic effect on the neonate. The results of this study suggest that, even in the absence of LGA or macrosomia, the exposure to the diabetic intrauterine milieu causes alterations in fetal growth patterns that likely predispose these infants to overweight and obesity later in life.

Much less is known about whether and how fetal programming is driven by exposure *in utero* to maternal obesity in the absence of diabetes. Maternal height and "frame size," regarded as markers of lifelong nutritional status, are important determinants of fetal growth.[17] Birth weight was shown to increase linearly with increasing prepregnancy body mass index (BMI) and with increasing weight gain during pregnancy.[18, 19] Vohr et al found that maternal prepregnancy weight, and weight gain during pregnancy were significant predictors not only of macrosomia, but also of neonatal adiposity (based on skinfold assessment) among both infants of mothers with GDM and control infants.[20] Moreover, these patterns of adiposity present at birth persisted at age 1 year.[21] More recently, increased maternal pregravid weight and estimated insulin resistance were shown to explain most of the variance in birth weight (48%) and fat mass at birth (46%).[22] In a Canadian study[23] mother's prepregnancy weight, weight gain during pregnancy, and parity were stronger correlates of birth weight percentile than plasma glucose levels.

Since maternal obesity during pregnancy is a state of insulin resistance,[24] it can be hypothesized that, during gestation, obese women make available increased amounts of nutrients to the fetus, resulting in increased fetal growth, especially in adipose tissue. In support of this hypothesis, Brown et al[25] have described independent associations between maternal waist/hip ratio and infant's birth weight and ponderal index. Maternal central obesity was shown to be associated with metabolic changes that may influence fetal growth, including insulin resistance, hyperinsulinemia, dyslipidemia, and elevated blood glucose levels.[26] Insulin, which is influenced by maternal nutritional and metabolic status, is an important regulator of fetal growth.[27] Maternal insulin resistance and hyperinsulinemia in pregnancies complicated by obesity and diabetes may increase the transfer of nutrients from mother to offspring in order to meet maximal (although not optimal) fetal requirements, even at the expense of maternal health.[17]

16.2.2 Maternal Glucose Supply and Fetal Growth

Maternal hyperglycemia, extreme enough to be recognized as GDM, is a clear risk factor for macrosomia. However, most macrosomic infants are not born to mothers diagnosed with GDM, but to mothers with obesity without recognized glucose intolerance.[28–30] Health care providers disagree about several aspects of GDM, including criteria for diagnosis, associated perinatal and maternal morbidity and optimal therapeutic strategies.[31–36] The current approach in the United States consists of determining plasma glucose levels 1 h after a 50-g oral glucose load in a nonfasting state at 24–28 weeks' gestation, followed by a diagnostic 3-h 100-g glucose load only in women with an abnormal screening test. However, women with lesser degrees of glucose intolerance, who exhibit an abnormal glucose screening test but do not meet diagnostic criteria for GDM may also be at risk for delivering a macrosomic infant.[37,38]

Several recent studies suggest that the relation between glycemia during pregnancy and infant body size is linear. A retrospective study conducted on 143 infants of nondiabetic mothers in Rhode Island showed a linear relationship between the 50-g glucose screen and infant BMI (r=0.24, p=0.007).[20] Similarly, in a different study of 6,854 consecutive pregnant women screened for GDM, increasing glucose concentration at screening was associated with higher prevalence of macrosomia.[39] In a large community-based study in Mysore, South India, maternal fasting glucose at 30-weeks of gestation was positively associated with infant birth weight (79 g increase per 1 mmol/L higher glucose), ponderal index, and head circumference even among mothers who did not fulfill the Carpenter-Coustan criteria for GDM diagnosis.[40] There were similar findings in a study of 917 nondiabetic women in Scotland, in which birth weight, length, head circumference, and skinfolds were positively related to maternal fasting plasma glucose concentrations measured in the third trimester of pregnancy.[41]

Since maternal fuel supply across a population is a continuum, the relationship between glycemia and offspring size at birth should be present across the entire distribution of maternal glucose concentrations. As discussed in the chapter by Steering Committee for the Hyperglycemia and Adverse Pregnancy Outcomes (HAPO) study, HAPO was a major international effort including over 20,000 pregnant women that specifically tested and confirmed the hypothesis that maternal glucose levels during pregnancy show a linear association with adverse pregnancy outcomes (including birth weight), thus indicating the need to reconsider current GDM diagnostic criteria.[42] In HAPO, an increase in the fasting glucose levels at 24–32 weeks of gestation of 1 SD (30.9 mg/dL) was associated with 1.38-fold higher odds (95% CI=1.32–1.44) for neonatal macrosomia (birth weight above the 90th percentile) and 1.55-fold higher odds (95% CI = 1.47–1.64) for neonatal hyperinsulinemia (cord blood C-peptide above the 90th percentile).

The timing of excessive nutrient delivery to the fetus may also be a critical component in the fetal accretion of fat. Among women with pre-existing diabetes, suboptimal glycemic control in the first trimester of pregnancy is a stronger predictor of neonatal macrosomia than is suboptimal control in the third trimester.[43] There is also evidence that glucose transfer by placental GLUT 1 transporters may be programmed early in pregnancy.[44–46] Aberrancies of glucose metabolism in GDM women have only been examined in the late second and third trimester of pregnancy. There are, in fact, no studies that examine whether hyperglycemia occurs early in obese pregnant women. Such early nutrient excess could possibly program placental transfer of substrates much sooner than previously appreciated.

16.2.3 Maternal Lipid Supply and Fetal Growth

Although unrecognized maternal hyperglycemia is likely to be an important contributor to excess fetal growth, especially in obese pregnancies, descriptive evidence suggests that alterations in maternal lipid metabolism[47] may also be an important mechanism and contribute substantially to "fuel mediated teratogenesis."[7]

FFA and triglycerides have been shown to be increased in mothers of obese neonates,[48] and due to the limited de novo lipogenic capacity of the fetus, most precursors for fetal fat accretion are supplied by transplacental transfer of maternal substrates derived from lipids.[47, 48] In the late second trimester, coincident with the increasing insulin resistance of pregnancy, women shift from fat storage to accelerated lipolysis so that FFA and glycerol can be used for maternal energy needs, sparing glucose as a fuel for the fetus. However, nonesterified fatty acids can be transferred across the placenta, which may occur directly, or secondarily, by hydrolysis of triglycerides.

Evidence exists that excess maternal obesity may increase lipid availability, modulate delivery of lipid substrates to the fetus, and be an important determinant of excess fetal growth. In a study of pregnant Italian women with various degrees of glucose intolerance, presence of the metabolic syndrome in mid-pregnancy predicted neonatal macrosomia independent of glucose tolerance status.[49] Other authors found an association between maternal serum triglyceride levels at 24–32 weeks of gestation and macrosomia among nondiabetic women with positive screening tests,[50–52] independent of maternal prepregnancy BMI, weight gain during pregnancy, and mid-pregnancy plasma glucose levels.[51] These observations suggest that maternal triglyceride concentrations in mid-pregnancy may have important predictive value for fetal overgrowth in nondiabetic pregnancies; however, these findings may be limited to women with positive diabetic screening tests. Increased available lipid substrate due to hydrolysis of maternal triglycerides may be used directly as an energy source for the fetus.[53] Alternatively, triglycerides may be used for maternal fat oxidation and glycerol production for maternal gluconeogenesis, preserving glucose for preferential use by the fetal-placental unit.[47]

16.2.4
Maternal Insulin Resistance and Inflammation and Fetal Growth

Human pregnancy is an insulin-resistant condition,[54] which facilitates the transfer of nutrients from mother to fetus.[55] The insulin resistance of normal pregnancy that occurs in the second and third trimester is thought to be mediated by placental hormones and is a physiological adaptation that ensures that maternal glucose is adequately delivered to the fetus.[56] In early pregnancy, peripheral sensitivity to insulin and glucose is similar to pregravid levels but may already be high if the woman is very obese.[55,57–59] Recent data suggest that the degree to which insulin resistance is present in late gestation is primarily dependent on pregravid obesity and only secondarily mediated through placental hormones.[60] With increased insulin resistance, glucose uptake and suppression of hepatic glucose production are decreased resulting in increased circulating concentrations of fuels and increased fuel availability to the fetus.

Although there is abundant evidence concerning the effects of obesity on metabolic pathways in nonpregnant individuals, such information is sparse with respect to pregnancy. In nonpregnant subjects, obesity is a recognized state of low-grade inflammation.[61, 62] Limited data suggest that similar inflammatory implications of obesity may exist during pregnancy. In a recent study of 47 normoglycemic pregnant women, Ramsay et al[63] demonstrated microvascular endothelial dysfunction, metabolic abnormalities (fasting hyperinsulinemia, hypertriglyceridemia and low HDL-cholesterol), and low-grade inflammation (elevated C-reactive protein (CRP) and interleukin-6 (IL-6)), in obese vs. lean pregnant women. These comprehensive data demonstrate that, as in nonpregnant obese individuals, obesity in pregnancy is associated not only with marked hyperinsulinemia (without necessarily glucose dysregulation) and dyslipidemia, but also impaired endothelial function, higher blood pressure, and inflammatory up-regulation. In a different study of 180 pregnant women, higher maternal CRP levels correlated strongly with prepregnancy maternal obesity, but not with GDM presence.[61] These data suggest a model in which prepregnant obesity mediates a state of mild systemic inflammation present throughout pregnancy, with possible metabolic consequences, including greater insulin resistance and glucose intolerance in late gestation. Such a state may also have fetal programming implications, as suggested by several lines of evidence.[64] For example, altered maternal vascular function may dysregulate nutrient flow to the fetus[65] A proinflammatory state may be associated with future cardiovascular disease in the offspring.[66] Rats injected with IL-6 throughout pregnancy had offspring with greater body fat and increased insulin resistance.[67] Of note, the dysregulation of several metabolic pathways by pregestational obesity described above may be independent of maternal fuels, including maternal diabetes.

16.3
Long-Term Consequences of Intrauterine Exposure to Maternal Diabetes and Obesity

The infant of the diabetic mother eventually becomes the child, the adolescent, and the adult offspring of the diabetic mother. The legacy of the diabetic intrauterine environment, acquired during gestation, cannot be ignored. It is widely recognized now that the effects of the diabetic intrauterine environment extend beyond those apparent at birth.[68] Importantly, these effects are independent of birth weight,[24, 69, 70] and appear to be similar regardless of mother's type of diabetes.[71,72]

16.3.1 Childhood Growth and Risk for Obesity

The role of exposure to diabetes *in utero* on infant and childhood growth, later obesity, and type 2 diabetes has been prospectively examined in two studies: the Pima Indian Study and the Diabetes in Pregnancy Study at Northwestern University in Chicago. The offspring of Pima Indian women with pre-existent type 2 diabetes and GDM were larger for gestational age at birth, and, at every age, they were heavier for height than the offspring of prediabetic or nondiabetic women.[73–75] Even in normal birth weight offspring of diabetic pregnancies, childhood obesity was still more common than among offspring of nondiabetic pregnancies.[69]

Researchers at The Diabetes in Pregnancy Center at Northwestern University have reported excessive growth in offspring of women with diabetes during pregnancy.[76] By age 8 years the children were, on average, 30% heavier than expected for their height. In this study, amniotic fluid insulin was collected at 32–38 weeks of gestation. At the age of 6 years there was a significant positive association between the amniotic fluid insulin and childhood obesity, as estimated by the symmetry index. The insulin concentrations in 6-year-old children who had a symmetry index of less than 1.0 (86.1 pmol/L) or between 1.0 and 1.2 (69.9 pmol/L) were only half of what was measured in the more obese children with a symmetry index greater than 1.2 (140.5 pmol/L, $p<0.05$ for each comparison). Thus, a direct correlation between an objective measure of the altered diabetic intrauterine environment and the degree of obesity in children and adolescents was demonstrated in this study.

Not all studies have shown as clear an association between exposure to GDM and childhood adiposity. Gillman et al[77] reported on obesity and overweight among 9–14-year-old offspring of mothers with GDM, with all data collected by questionnaire. In this study, exposure to GDM while *in utero* was also associated with a 40% increased odds of being overweight as an adolescent; however these odds were attenuated when further adjustments were made for birth weight (odds ratio 1.3, 95% confidence interval 0.9–1.9) and maternal BMI (odds ratio 1.2, 95% confidence interval 0.8–1.7). While these results suggest that any increase in childhood obesity associated with prenatal exposure to gestational diabetes is not independent of birth weight and maternal obesity, there are important limitations to this study. All data were collected by questionnaire, and self-reported weight may be inaccurate. In addition, only about half of the mothers with children agreed to have the study contact their children, and of the eligible children only 68% of the girls and 58% of the boys completed the questionnaires, for an overall response rate of approximately 34%.

Similarly, In a retrospective chart review study, Whitaker et al found no difference in overweight (≥85th percentile for weight) for children ages 5–10 according to maternal GDM status.[78] The inconsistency in these results may be partly explained by differences in exposure prevalence across populations studied, as the Pima Indians are a population with extremely high rates of obesity and diabetes, including during pregnancy. Further studies are needed to evaluate the effect of intrauterine diabetes exposure on fetal and childhood growth among different ethnic groups.

16.3.2 Abnormal Glucose Tolerance and Risk for Type 2 Diabetes

For more than 30 years, Pima Indian women have had routine oral glucose tolerance tests approximately every 2 years as well as during pregnancy.[75] Women who had diabetes before or during pregnancy were termed diabetic mothers; those who developed diabetes only after pregnancy were termed prediabetic mothers. By age 5–9 and 10–14 years, type 2 diabetes was present almost exclusively among the offspring of diabetic women. In all age groups there was significantly more diabetes in the offspring of diabetic women than in those of prediabetic and nondiabetic women, and there were much smaller differences in diabetes prevalence between offspring of prediabetic and nondiabetic women.[79]

The comparison between offspring of diabetic and prediabetic women is an attempt to control for any potential confounding effect of a genetic predisposition to obesity and diabetes on the relationship between exposure to the maternal diabetic environment and obesity and diabetes in the offspring. The ideal way to approach this question is to examine sibling pairs in which one sibling is born before and one is born after the onset of their mother's diabetes.[80] Using this design, the prevalence of type 2 diabetes was compared in Pima Indian siblings born before and after their mother developed diabetes.[80] There were 19 nuclear families with sibling pairs ($n=28$ pairs) discordant for both type 2 diabetes and exposure to a pregnancy complicated by diabetes. In 21 of the 28 sib-pairs, the sibling who developed type 2 diabetes was born after the mother's diagnosis of diabetes and in only 7 of the 28 pairs was the sibling with type 2 diabetes born before (odds ratio 3.0, $p<0.01$). In contrast, among 84 siblings and 39 sib-pairs from 24 families of diabetic fathers, the risk for type 2 diabetes was similar in the sib-pairs born before and after father's diagnosis of diabetes. Since siblings born before and after a diabetic pregnancy are believed to carry a similar risk of inheriting the same susceptibility genes, the excess risk associated with maternal diabetes likely reflects the effect of intrauterine exposure associated with or directly due to hyperglycemia and/or other fuel alterations of a diabetic pregnancy.

Recently, the SEARCH Case–Control Study provided novel evidence that intrauterine exposure to maternal diabetes and obesity are important determinants of type 2 diabetes in youth of other racial/ethnic groups (non-Hispanic white, Hispanic and African American). In this study, youth with type 2 diabetes were more likely to have been exposed to maternal diabetes or obesity *in utero* than were nondiabetic controls ($p<0.0001$ for each). After adjusting for offspring age, sex and race/ethnicity, exposure to maternal diabetes (OR=5.7; 95% CI=2.4–13.4) and exposure to maternal prepregnancy obesity (2.8; 95% CI=1.5–5.2) were independently associated with type 2 diabetes in the offspring. Adjustment for other perinatal and socio-economic factors did not alter these associations.[81]

16.3.3 Insulin Resistance, Secretion, and Cardiovascular Abnormalities

Several studies performed in newborns of diabetic mothers have shown an enhanced insulin secretion to a glycemic stimulus.[82] Consistent with these findings, Van Assche[83] and Heding[84] described hyperplasia of the beta cells in newborns of diabetic mothers. Conversely, impaired insulin secretion has also been proposed as a possible mechanism. Among Pima Indian adults the acute insulin response to infused glucose was 40% lower in individuals whose mothers had diabetes during pregnancy than in those whose mothers developed diabetes after the birth of the subject.[85]

Animal studies have shown that exposure to diabetes *in utero* can induce cardiovascular dysfunction in adult offspring.[86] Few human studies have examined cardiovascular risk factors in offspring of diabetic pregnancies. By 10–14 years, offspring of diabetic pregnancies enrolled in the Diabetes in Pregnancy follow-up study at Northwestern University had significantly higher systolic and mean arterial blood pressure than offspring of nondiabetic pregnancies.[76] Higher concentrations of markers of endothelial dysfunction (ICAM-1, VCAM-1, E-selectin), as well as increased cholesterol-to-HDL ratio were reported among offspring of mothers with type 1 diabetes compared with offspring of nondiabetic pregnancies, independent of current BMI.[87] Recently, the Pima Indian investigators have shown that, independent of adiposity, 7–11-year-old offspring exposed to maternal diabetes during pregnancy have significantly higher systolic blood pressure than offspring of mothers who did not develop type 2 diabetes until after the index pregnancy.[88] These data suggest that *in utero* exposure to diabetes confers risks for the development of cardiovascular disease later in life that are independent of adiposity and may be in addition to genetic predisposition to diabetes or cardiovascular disease.

16.4 Clinical and Public Health Implications

The hypothesis of fuel-mediated teratogenesis suggests that excess fetal growth caused by maternal fuel abnormalities also results in adult disease in the offspring, and so interventions to reduce the transmission of obesity, cardiovascular disease, and type 2 diabetes would logically focus on normalizing maternal metabolism and fuel delivery to the infant.

There is evidence that hyperglycemia increases fetal growth and also may induce other metabolic changes which are associated with adult chronic disease. However, there is little information available regarding the optimal level of glycemic control needed to prevent metabolic changes in the offspring. Intensive treatment in women with GDM reduced birth weight and incidence of macrosomia in infants born to mothers who participated in the intervention compared to women who received routine care.[89] However, more evidence is needed to determine optimal glucose levels during pregnancy that would prevent long-term metabolic disturbances in the offspring.

While excess glucose stimulates fetal insulin production and results in increased fetal growth and adiposity, fetal growth appears to be increased even in nondiabetic obese pregnancies. It is therefore likely that, in addition to hyperglycemia, alterations in other maternal fuels or derangement in placental transport of fuels are also involved in fetal overgrowth. In addition, maternal obesity and weight gain during pregnancy contribute to fetal overgrowth, and adjustment for maternal obesity attenuates some of the effect of exposure to intrauterine diabetes on obesity and type 2 diabetes risk in the offspring.

There is also a need to evaluate the effects of exposure to maternal hyperglycemia and obesity on fetal growth, adiposity and insulin resistance in an ethnically diverse population. For example, biologic mechanisms may differ across racial/ethnic groups – either absolutely or relatively. In addition, the prevalence of different risk factors will likely differ by racial/ethnic group, such that even if the mechanisms are similar, the attributable fractions for specific risk factors will differ according to race/ethnicity, and this may drive strategies for prevention.

Much more information is needed to determine the most effective strategies to address the risk of chronic metabolic diseases in the infant of the diabetic mother. However, it is increasingly clear that public health efforts to prevent type 2 diabetes should focus on not only adult lifestyle risk factors such as obesity and sedentary lifestyle, but also on prenatal exposure to diabetes and obesity *in utero*. Reduced obesity in women of reproductive age and prevention of excessive weight gain during pregnancy may not only lessen the risk of GDM in the mother, but will likely also reduce the risk of excess fetal growth, future obesity and type 2 diabetes in the offspring.

References

1. Hussain A, Claussen B, Ramachandran A, Williams R. Prevention of type 2 diabetes: a review. *Diabetes Res Clin Pract*. 2007;76:317-326.
2. Dabelea D, Pettitt DJ, Jones KL, Arslanian SA. Type 2 diabetes mellitus in minority children and adolescents. An emerging problem. *Endocrinol Metab Clin North Am*. 1999;28(9):709-729.
3. Dabelea D, Snell-Bergeon JK, Hartsfield CL, Bischoff KJ, Hamman RF, McDuffie RS. Increasing prevalence of gestational diabetes mellitus (GDM) over time and by birth cohort: Kaiser Permanente of Colorado GDM Screening Program. *Diab Care*. 2005;28:579-584.
4. Ferrarra A, Kahn HS, Quesenberry CP, Riley C, Hedderson MM. An increase in the incidence of gestational diabetes mellitus: Northern California, 1991–2000. *Obstet Gynecol*. 2004; 103:526-533.
5. Sobngwi E, Boudou P, Mauvais-Jarvis F. Effect of a diabetic environment in utero on predisposition to type 2 diabetes. *Lancet*. 2003;361:1861-1865.
6. Pedersen J. Weight and lenght at birth in infants of diabetic mothers. *Acta Endocrinol*. 1954;16:330-342.
7. Freinkel N. Banting Lecture 1980. Of pregnancy and progeny. *Diabetes*. 1980;29:1023-1035.
8. Whitaker RC, Dietz WH. Role of the prenatal environment in the development of obesity. *J Pediatr*. 1998;132:768-776.
9. Barker DJ, Fall CH. Fetal and infant origins of cardiovascular disease. *Arch Dis Child*. 1993;68:797-799.
10. Barker DJ, Gluckman PD, Godfrey KM, Harding JE, Owens JA, Robinson JS. Fetal nutrition and cardiovascular disease in adult life [see comments]. *Lancet*. 1993;341:938-941.
11. Barker DJ. In utero programming of chronic disease. *Clin Sci (Colch)*. 1998;95:115-128.

12. Aerts L, Sodoyez-Goffaux F, Sodoyez JC, Malaisse WJ, Van Assche FA. The diabetic intra-uterine milieu has a long-lasting effect on insulin secretion by B cells and on insulin uptake by target tissues. *Am J Obstet Gynecol.* 1988;159:1287-1292.
13. Gauguier D, Nelson I, Bernard C. Higher maternal than paternal inheritance of diabetes in GK rats. *Diabetes.* 1994;43:220-224.
14. Lampl M, Jeanty P. Exposure to maternal diabetes is associated with altered fetal growth patterns: A hypothesis regarding metabolic allocation to growth under hyperglycemic-hypoxemic conditions. *Am J Hum Biol.* 2004;6:237-263.
15. Jansson T, Cetin I, Powell TL. Placental transport and metabolism in fetal overgrowth — a workshop report. *Placenta.* 2006;27(suppl A):S109-S113.
16. Catalano PM, Thomas A, Huston-Presley L, Amini SB. Increased fetal adiposity: a very sensitive marker of abnormal in utero development. *Am J Obstet Gynecol.* 2003;189:1698-1704.
17. Perry IJ, Lumey LH. In: Kuh D, Ben-Shlomo Y, eds. *A Life Course Approach to Chronic Disease Epidemiology.* Oxford: Oxford University Press; 2004:345.
18. Luke B. Nutritional influences on fetal growth. *Clin Obstet Gynecol.* 1994;37:538-549.
19. Abrams BF, Berman CA. Nutrition during pregnancy and lactation. *Prim Care.* 1993;20:585-597.
20. Vohr BR, McGarvey ST, Coll CG. Effects of maternal gestational diabetes and adiposity on neonatal adiposity and blood pressure. *Diabetes Care.* 1995;18:467-475.
21. Vohr BR, McGarvey ST. Growth patterns of large-for-gestational-age and appropriate-for-gestational-age infants of gestational diabetic mothers and control mothers at age 1 year. *Diabetes Care.* 1997;20:1066-1072.
22. Catalano PM, Kirwan JP. Maternal factors that determine neonatal size and body fat. *Curr Diab Rep.* 2001;1:71-77.
23. Ouzilleau C, Roy MA, Leblanc L, Carpentier A, Maheux P. An observational study comparing 2-hour 75-g oral glucose tolerance with fasting plasma glucose in pregnant women: both poorly predictive of birth weight. *CMAJ.* 2003;168:403-409.
24. Catalano PM, Kirwan JP, Haugel-de Mouzon S, King J. Gestational diabetes and insulin resistance: role in short- and long-term implications for mother and fetus. *J Nutr.* 2003; 133:1674S–1683S.
25. Brown JE, Potter JD, Jacobs DR Jr. Maternal waist-to-hip ratio as a predictor of newborn size: results of the Diana Project. *Epidemiology.* 1996;7:62-66.
26. McKeigue PM, Pierpoint T, Ferrie JE, Marmot MG. Relationship of glucose intolerance and hyperinsulinaemia to body fat pattern in South Asians and Europeans. *Diabetologia.* 1992; 35:785-791.
27. Fowden AL. The role of insulin in prenatal growth. *J Dev Physiol.* 1989;12:173-182.
28. Langer O, Conway DL. Level of glycemia and perinatal outcome in pregestational diabetes. *J Matern Fetal Med.* 2000;9:35-41.
29. Langer O. Fetal macrosomia: etiologic factors. *Clin Obstet Gynecol.* 2000;43:283-297.
30. Langer O, Yogev Y, Most O, Xenakis EM. Gestational diabetes: the consequences of not treating. *Am J Obstet Gynecol.* 2005;192:989-997.
31. Ratner RE. Clinical review 47: gestational diabetes mellitus: after three international workshops do we know how to diagnose and manage it yet? *J Clin Endocrinol Metab.* 1993;77:1-4.
32. Jarrett RJ. Gestational diabetes: a non-entity? *Brit Med J.* 1993;306:37-38.
33. Buchanan TA, Kjos SL. Gestational diabetes: risk or myth? *J Clin Endocrinol Metab.* 1999;84:1854-1857.
34. Kjos SL, Buchanan TA. Gestational diabetes mellitus. *N Engl J Med.* 1999;341:1749-1756.
35. Dornhorst A, Chan SP. The elusive diagnosis of gestational diabetes. *Diabet Med.* 1998; 15:7-10.
36. Ferrara A, Hedderson MM, Quesenberry CP, Selby JV. Prevalence of gestational diabetes mellitus detected by the national diabetes data group or the carpenter and coustan plasma glucose thresholds. *Diabetes Care.* 2002;25:1625-1630.

37. Sermer M, Naylor CD, Gare DJ. Impact of increasing carbohydrate intolerance on maternal-fetal outcomes in 3637 women without gestational diabetes. The Toronto Tri-Hospital Gestational Diabetes Project. *Am J Obstet Gynecol.* 1995;173:146-156.
38. Leikin EL, Jenkins JH, Pomerantz GA, Klein L. Abnormal glucose screening tests in pregnancy: a risk factor for fetal macrosomia. *Obstet Gynecol.* 1987;69:570-573.
39. Yogev Y, Langer O, Xenakis EM, Rosenn B. The association between glucose challenge test, obesity and pregnancy outcome in 6390 non-diabetic women. *J Matern Fetal Neonatal Med.* 2005;17:29-34.
40. Hill JC, Krishnaveni GV, Annamma I, Leary SD, Fall CH. Glucose tolerance in pregnancy in South India: relationships to neonatal anthropometry. *Acta Obstet Gynecol Scand.* 2005;84:159-165.
41. Farmer G, Russell G, Hamilton-Nicol DR. The influence of maternal glucose metabolism on fetal growth, development and morbidity in 917 singleton pregnancies in nondiabetic women. *Diabetologia.* 1988;31:134-141.
42. The HAPOStudy Cooperative Research Group. Hyperglycemia and adverse pregnancy outcomes. *New Engl J Med.* 2008;358:1991-2002.
43. Rey E, Attie C, Bonin A. The effects of first-trimester diabetes control on the incidence of macrosomia. *Am J Obstet Gynecol.* 1999;181:202-206.
44. Illsley NP. Glucose transporters in the human placenta. *Placenta.* 2000;21:14-22.
45. Illsley NP. Placental glucose transport in diabetic pregnancy. *Clin Obstet Gynecol.* 2000;43:116-126.
46. Gaither K, Quraishi AN, Illsley NP. Diabetes alters the expression and activity of the human placental GLUT1 glucose transporter. *J Clin Endocrinol Metab.* 1999;84:695-701.
47. Butte NF. Carbohydrate and lipid metabolism in pregnancy: normal compared with gestational diabetes mellitus. *Am J Clin Nutr.* 2000;71:1256S-1261S.
48. Di Cianni G, Miccoli R, Volpe L. Maternal triglyceride levels and newborn weight in pregnant women with normal glucose tolerance. *Diabet Med.* 2005;22:21-25.
49. Bo S, Menato G, Gallo ML. Mild gestational hyperglycemia, the metabolic syndrome and adverse neonatal outcomes. *Acta Obstet Gynecol Scand.* 2004;83:335-340.
50. Nolan CJ, Proietto J. The feto-placental glucose steal phenomenon is a major cause of maternal metabolic adaptation during late pregnancy in the rat. *Diabetologia.* 1994;37:976-984.
51. Kitajima M, Oka S, Yasuhi I, Fukuda M, Rii Y, Ishimaru T. Maternal serum triglyceride at 24–32 weeks' gestation and newborn weight in nondiabetic women with positive diabetic screens. *Obstet Gynecol.* 2001;97:776-780.
52. Knopp RH, Magee MS, Walden CE, Bonet B, Benedetti TJ. Prediction of infant birth weight by GDM screening tests. Importance of plasma triglyceride. *Diabetes Care.* 1992;15:1605-1613.
53. Peterson CM, Jovanovic-Peterson L, Mills JL. The Diabetes in Early Pregnancy Study: changes in cholesterol, triglycerides, body weight, and blood pressure. The National Institute of Child Health and Human Development–the Diabetes in Early Pregnancy Study. *Am J Obstet Gynecol.* 1992;166:513-518.
54. Catalano PM, Vargo KM, Bernstein IM, Amini SB. Incidence and risk factors associated with abnormal postpartum glucose tolerance in women with gestational diabetes. *Am J Obstet Gynecol.* 1991;165:914-919.
55. Cousins L. Insulin sensitivity in pregnancy. *Diabetes.* 1991;40(suppl 2):39-43.
56. Barbour LA. New concepts in insulin resistance of pregnancy and gestational diabetes: long-term implications for mother and offspring. *J Obstet Gynaecol.* 2003;23:545-549.
57. Catalano PM, Tyzbir ED, Wolfe RR, Roman NM, Amini SB, Sims EA. Longitudinal changes in basal hepatic glucose production and suppression during insulin infusion in normal pregnant women. *Am J Obstet Gynecol.* 1992;167:913-919.
58. Catalano PM, Tyzbir ED, Wolfe RR. Carbohydrate metabolism during pregnancy in control subjects and women with gestational diabetes. *Am J Physiol.* 1993;264:E60-E67.
59. Catalano PM, Tyzbir ED, Roman NM, Amini SB, Sims EA. Longitudinal changes in insulin release and insulin resistance in nonobese pregnant women. *Am J Obstet Gynecol.* 1991;165:1667-1672.

60. Kirwan JP, Hauguel-De MS, Lepercq J. TNF-alpha is a predictor of insulin resistance in human pregnancy. *Diabetes*. 2002;51:2207-2213.
61. Ford ES. Body mass index, diabetes, and C-reactive protein among U.S. adults. *Diabetes Care*. 1999;22:1971-1977.
62. Yudkin JS. Abnormalities of coagulation and fibrinolysis in insulin resistance. Evidence for a common antecedent? *Diab Care*. 1999;22(suppl 3):C25-C30.
63. Ramsay JE, Ferrell WR, Crawford L, Wallace AM, Greer IA, Sattar N. Maternal obesity is associated with dysregulation of metabolic, vascular, and inflammatory pathways. *J Clin Endocrinol Metab*. 2002;87:4231-4237.
64. Retnakaran R, Hanley AJ, Raif N, Connelly PW, Sermer M, Zinman B. C-reactive protein and gestational diabetes: the central role of maternal obesity. *J Clin Endocrinol Metab*. 2003; 88:3507-3512.
65. Ramsay JE, Stewart F, Greer IA, Sattar N. Microvascular dysfunction: a link between pre-eclampsia and maternal coronary heart disease. *BJOG*. 2003;110:1029-1031.
66. Forsen T, Eriksson JG, Tuomilehto J, Teramo K, Osmond C, Barker DJ. Mother's weight in pregnancy and coronary heart disease in a cohort of Finnish men: follow up study. *Brit Med J*. 1997;315:837-840.
67. Dahlgreen J, Nilsson C, Jennische E, et al. Prenatal cytokine exposure results in obesity and gender-specific programming. *Am J Physiol Endocrinol Metab*. 2001;281:E326–E334.
68. Pettitt DJ, Knowler WC. Diabetes and obesity in the Pima Indians: a crossgenerational vicious cycle. *J Obesity Weight Regul*. 1988;7:61-65.
69. Pettitt DJ, Knowler WC, Bennett PH, Aleck KA, Baird HR. Obesity in offspring of diabetic Pima Indian women despite normal birth weight. *Diabetes Care*. 1987;10:76-80.
70. Harder T, Kohlhoff R, Dorner G, Rohde W, Plagemann A. Perinatal 'programming' of insulin resistance in childhood: critical impact of neonatal insulin and low birth weight in a risk population. *Diabet Med*. 2001;18:634-639.
71. Silverman BL, Metzger BE, Cho NH, Loeb CA. Impaired glucose tolerance in adolescent offspring of diabetic mothers: Relationship to fetal hyperinsulinism. *Diabetes Care*. 1995; 18:611-617.
72. Weiss PA, Scholz HS, Haas J, Tamussino KF, Seissler J, Borkenstein MH. Long-term follow-up of infants of mothers with type 1 diabetes: evidence for hereditary and nonhereditary transmission of diabetes and precursors. *Diabetes Care*. 2000;23:905-911.
73. Pettitt DJ, Nelson RG, Saad MF, Bennett PH, Knowler WC. Diabetes and obesity in the offspring of Pima Indian women with diabetes during pregnancy. *Diabetes Care*. 1993;16:310-314.
74. Pettitt DJ, Baird HR, Aleck KA, Bennett PH, Knowler WC. Excessive obesity in offspring of Pima Indian women with diabetes during pregnancy. *New Engl J Med*. 1983;308:242-245.
75. Pettitt DJ, Bennett PH, Knowler WC, Baird HR, Aleck KA. Gestational diabetes mellitus and impaired glucose tolerance during pregnancy. *Long-term effects on obesity and glucose tolerance in the offspring Diabetes*. 1985;34(suppl 2):119-122.
76. Silverman BL, Rizzo T, Green OC. Long-term prospective evaluation of offspring of diabetic mothers. *Diabetes*. 1991;40(suppl 2):121-125.
77. Gillman MW, Rifas-Shiman S, Berkey CS, Field AE, Colditz GA. Maternal gestational diabetes, birth weight, and adolescent obesity. *Pediatrics*. 2003;111:e221-e226.
78. Whitaker RC, Pepe MS, Seidel KD, Wright JA, Knopp RH. Gestational diabetes and the risk of offspring obesity. *Pediatrics*. 1998;101:E 91-E 97.
79. Dabelea D, Pettitt DJ. Intrauterine diabetic environment confers risks for type 2 diabetes mellitus and obesity in the offspring, in addition to genetic susceptibility. *J Pediatr Endocrinol Metab*. 2001;14:1085-1091.
80. Dabelea D, Hanson RL, Lindsay RS. Intrauterine exposure to diabetes conveys risks for type 2 diabetes and obesity: a study of discordant sibships. *Diabetes*. 2000;49:2208-2211.

81. Dabelea D, Mayer-Davis EJ, Lamichhane AP. Association of intrauterine exposure to maternal diabetes and obesity with type 2 diabetes in youth: the SEARCH Case-Control Study. *Diab Care*. 2008;31:1422-1426.
82. Pildes RS, Hart RJ, Warrner R, Cornblath M. Plasma insulin response during oral glucose tolerance tests in newborns of normal and gestational diabetic mothers. *Pediatrics*. 1969;44:76-83.
83. Van Assche FA, Gepts W. The cytological composition of the foetal endocrine pancreas in normal and pathological conditions. *Diabetologia*. 1971;7:434-444.
84. Heding LG, Persson B, Stangenberg M. B-cell function in newborn infants of diabetic mothers. *Diabetologia*. 1980;19:427-432.
85. Gautier JF, Wilson C, Weyer C. Low acute insulin secretory responses in adult offspring of people with early onset type 2 diabetes. *Diabetes*. 2001;50:1828-1833.
86. Holemans K, Gerber RT, Meurrens K, De Clerck F, Poston L, Van Assche FA. Streptozotocin diabetes in the pregnant rat induces cardiovascular dysfunction in adult offspring. *Diabetologia*. 1999;42:81-89.
87. Manderson JG, Mullan B, Patterson CC, Hadden DR, Traub AI, McCance DR. Cardiovascular and metabolic abnormalities in the offspring of diabetic pregnancy. *Diabetologia*. 2002;45:991-996.
88. Bunt JC, Tataranni PA, Salbe AD. Intrauterine exposure to diabetes is a determinant of hemoglobin A(1)c and systolic blood pressure in pima Indian children. *J Clin Endocrinol Metab*. 2005;90:3225-3229.
89. Crowther CA, Hiller JE, Moss JR, McPhee AJ, Jeffries WS, Robinson JS. Effect of treatment of gestational diabetes mellitus on pregnancy outcomes. *N Engl J Med*. 2005;352:2477-2486.

Section VI

Management of GDM During Pregnancy

Exercise Recommendations in Women with Gestational Diabetes Mellitus

17

Raul Artal, Gerald S. Zavorsky, and Rosemary B. Catanzaro

17.1 Introduction

This chapter provides the physiological background of exercise prescription for pregnant patients affected by gestational diabetes mellitus (GDM) and type 2 diabetes. Also included is a review of the pertinent literature. The American College of Obstetricians and Gynecologists (ACOG) and the American Diabetes Association (ADA) have endorsed exercise as "a helpful adjunctive therapy" for GDM.[1,2] Exercise protocols for women with GDM or for GDM prevention are underutilized due to provider's reluctance to prescribe exercise as well as lack of patient compliance.

Pregnancy has been characterized as a diabetogenic event brought about by hormones with diabetogenic effects (estrogen, human placental lactogen also called human chorionic somatomammotropin (HPL), cortisol, and progesterone). The diabetogenic effects of these hormones lead to insulin resistance and increased insulin requirements. During pregnancy, catabolic stress hormones trigger an increase in metabolism with wide shifts between the fed and fasting states.[3] In pregnancy, fasting blood glucose is lower, but as a result, post-prandial gluconeogenesis causes glucose levels to increase. To modulate the increase in glucose levels, an increase in insulin secretion occurs throughout gestation. Despite counter-regulatory processes, patients with GDM experience increased fat storage and adipocyte hypertrophy and hyperplasia resulting in decreased insulin sensitivity. The impaired insulin sensitivity in patients with GDM results in decreased glucose uptake by muscles and splanchnic organs, whereas hepatic glucose production is enhanced.

While dietary strategies are a mainstay of treatment to optimize pregnancy outcomes, up to 39% of GDM women cannot be managed with diet alone.[4] Many of these patients will experience fasting or postprandial hyperglycemia, or both, despite dietary interventions. Although insulin corrects the hyperglycemia, it does not affect peripheral insulin

R. Artal (✉)
Department of Obstetrics, Gynecology and Women's Health,
Saint Louis University, St. Louis, MO, USA
e-mail: artalr@slu.edu

C. Kim and A. Ferrara (eds.), *Gestational Diabetes During and After Pregnancy*,
DOI: 10.1007/978-1-84882-120-0_17, © Springer-Verlag London Limited 2010

resistance. Thus, the logical intervention would be exercise, which will decrease insulin resistance.

Physical activity improves glucose tolerance through at least two mechanisms: (1) improved insulin sensitivity, primarily through insulin-stimulated muscle glucose uptake, which in turn is directly related to energy expenditure, and (2) insulin-independent mechanisms directly related to glucose transportation (GLUT4).

It is well established that regular exercise training improves insulin sensitivity and insulin-stimulated muscle glucose uptake in type 2 diabetes patients.[5] Insulin sensitivity is defined as the concentration of insulin required to cause 50% of its maximal effect on glucose transport.[6] Some of the purported mechanisms include training-induced enhancement of the insulin-mediated increase in muscle blood flow and glucose extraction from blood.[5] Insulin sensitivity is increased 12–48 h after a single exercise session in both healthy[7–11] and insulin resistant subjects,[9,12,13] but this effect is lost after 3–6 days of inactivity.[14–17] However, in well-trained subjects, a single bout of exercise can improve insulin sensitivity. In one study, eight well-trained subjects stopped training for 10 days.[18] The maximum rise in plasma insulin concentration in response to a 100-g oral glucose load was 100% higher after 10 days without exercise than when the subjects were exercising regularly. Despite the increased insulin levels, blood glucose concentrations were higher after 10 days without exercise. One bout of exercise after 11 days without exercise returned insulin binding and the insulin and glucose responses to an oral 100-g glucose load almost to the initial "trained" value. These results demonstrate that bouts of exercise play an important role in insulin sensitivity.[18]

Studies suggest that insulin sensitivity after a single bout of exercise is negatively related to energy expenditure. In one study,[11] 30 nonobese subjects exercised on a treadmill at 2.0 L/min (60% of aerobic capacity) for 30–120 min. It was demonstrated that the exercise-induced changes in homeostasis model assessment of insulin resistance (HOMA-IR) was negatively and curvilinearly correlated to energy expenditure ($r=-0.67$, $p=0.001$). HOMA-IR decreased by 30% compared to preexercise in subjects who expended more than 900 kcal during the exercise bout.[11]

Glucose uptake is also partially regulated via insulin-independent mechanisms involving a contraction-induced increase in the amount of GLUT4 isoform of the glucose transporter translocating from muscle cytosol to muscle cell membrane.[14,21,22] Muscle glucose uptake is affected by the size of the total muscle mass engaged in exercise,[23] the intensity of the work performed,[24] and the length of time the exercise is performed.[25] There is a significant negative relationship between muscle glycogen concentration in exercising muscle and glucose uptake in the same exercising muscle.[25] A large contracting skeletal muscle like the vastus lateralis can increases its glucose uptake by 11- to 20-fold (from rest) after 40 min of cycling exercise in which the whole body oxygen consumption is about 2–2.3 L/min.[25,26] Therefore, activation of large muscles, such as the quadriceps, can be particularly influential in glucose tolerance. Many exercise programs fail in achieving their objective, i.e., euglycemia, either because large muscle groups were not activated or because the duration and intensity of the exercise routine were too limited.[27,28]

The benefits of activity upon glucose tolerance have historically been outweighed by concerns regarding potential hypoglycemic effects upon the fetus. The insulin resistance that develops in pregnancy leads to higher than normal secretion of insulin to maintain euglycemia, essential for the development of the fetus. Glucose, considered the major metabolic substrate for growth and development of the fetus, is increasingly utilized in the second and third trimesters of pregnancy.[29] Hypoglycemia for extended periods of time, or when blood glucose is too tightly controlled, has been demonstrated to have a negative impact on the growth and development of the fetus.[30] Maternal fasting and/or starvation are conditions that can challenge the energy reserves, particularly glucose levels. Exercise can similarly challenge maternal glucose reserves with potentially deleterious effects to the fetus. Fasting and exercise lead to an increase in insulin secretion as well as free fatty acid and ketones; when either fasting or exercise is prolonged, there is a decrease in glucose levels.[14]

Although exercise and fasting share physiologic similarities, they represent different metabolic conditions. One major difference is the release of catecholamines during exercise, a response intended to stimulate gluconeogenesis. The predominant catecholamine released during exercise is norepinephrine, which has a stimulating effect on the uterus. This may result in regular uterine contractions or labor; thus, the recommendation for patients at risk for premature labor is not to engage in physical activity.[31] With the exclusion of these women, physical activity does not appear to have detrimental effects.[31–33] Relevant to an exercise protocol for diabetic patients, it was established by us that pregnant women can exercise continuously for 45 min at 55% of aerobic capacity (VO_2 max) before potentially experiencing hypoglycemia.[32]

17.2 Exercise Programs for GDM Treatment

Exercise has been reported as an adjunctive intervention in the management of GDM; however, studies are varied in intensity, frequency, and duration of the exercise prescription. Table 17.1 summarizes exercise studies using various frequencies, intensities, duration, and exercise prescriptions in women with GDM. In these studies, which range from 11 to 96 participants, the exercise intensities range from 50 to 70% of maximum heart rate, which is equivalent to about 40–60% of heart rate reserve (HRR) or about 30–60% of VO_2 max.

The most common form of exercise reported was walking or stationary cycling, with studies reporting benefits of resistance training or arm cycle ergometry in decreasing insulin requirements or improving fasting and postprandial glucose excursions.[27,34,37] We demonstrated that pregnant women can exercise more efficiently during nonweight-bearing exercises.[35] Nonweight-bearing exercise, such as swimming or stationary cycling, is also better tolerated by physically detrained or sedentary individuals. Jovanovic-Peterson and colleagues published a study which tested the use of arm ergometry as a method for improving glucose tolerance in women with GDM.[27] Nineteen women with GDM were assigned to either diet or to an arm ergometry exercise program for 6 weeks. Although the subjects assigned to either the mild exercise or diet program achieved a decrease in blood glucose levels, this began to occur after 6 weeks from enrollment into the study. The reason for the modest glucose tolerance response was due to the type and intensity of exercise (i.e., arm ergometry at low intensity for 20 min).

Table 17.1 Exercise programs for GDM treatment

Study	Subjects	Objective	Methods	Exercise program	Outcome variable	Conclusions
Davenport et al[47]	$n = 20$	To determine the effectiveness of a low-intensity walking program on glycemic control and insulin requirements	Case–control study, matched by age, BMI, and insulin, with two controls for every intervention subject in the walking program	Exercise consisted of low-intensity walking (30% heart rate (HR) reserve) 3–4×/week starting at 25 min/sessions, increasing to 40 min/sessions	Exercise subjects experienced a greater average decrease in post exercise blood glucose (BG) of 2.0 mmol/L and required less insulin (0.16 vs. 0.5 units/kg)	A structured low-intensity walking program lowers fasting and postprandial glucose, decreased amounts of insulin, and leads to fewer insulin injections
Artal et al[48]	$n = 96$	To determine if weight gain restriction impacts pregnancy outcome in obese women with GDM	Sequential enrollment: subjects were provided a eucaloric diet (15–20 kcal/kg/day) and/or supervised exercise and home-based exercise prescription	60% VO_{2max} walk or stationary bike; supervised (lab) or home exercise 30 min/day 5–6 day/week (or more)	Less weight gain/week in diet only subjects compared to exercise+diet (0.1 vs. 0.3 kg/week; $p<0.05$)	Caloric restriction and exercise resulted in lower weight gain with no adverse pregnancy outcomes
Brankston et al[34]	$n = 38$	To examine the effects of circuit-type resistance training on insulin requirements in GDM	Subjects were randomized to diet or diet + resistant exercise. Diet consisted of 24–30 kcal/kg/day	Circuit-type resistance exercise of 8 exercises, 15–20 reps, 2–4 sets; increasing weekly for 4 weeks until delivery (average 2.0 sessions/week)	The diet + resistance exercise subjects were prescribed less insulin (0.2 vs. 0.5 units/kg; ($p<0.05$) and started insulin later in gestation (1.1 vs. 3.7 weeks; $p<0.05$)	Resistance exercise may decrease the need for insulin in GDM pregnancies

Garcia-Patterson, et al[49]	$n = 20$	To examine the effects of postprandial exercise on blood glucose after one bout of exercise	Controlled crossover trial on two separate days (3–7 days apart). BG was assessed after one bout of exercise on study day two	Walking on a flat surface, self-paced, for 1-h and seated during the second hour (one bout of exercise)	Significant differences in (control vs. study day) 1-h postprandial BG excursion (1.8 vs. 1.1 mmol/L; $p<0.001$)	Light postprandial exercise decreases postprandial BG excursion and may prevent the need for insulin
Avery and Walker[38]	$n = 13$	To evaluate the effect of exercise after a session at low and moderate intensity	Repeated measure design to analyze glycemic indices at rest, and after light and moderate intensity exercise	Light intensity at 35% VO_2 max; Moderate intensity at 55% VO_2 max; 30 min each session	After a single bout of exercise BG levels declined after low to moderate exercise but disappeared after 45 min ($p=0.01$)	A dose response to exercise decreases acute BG levels
Avery et al[36]	$n = 33$	To determine the effectiveness of a partially home-based, moderate exercise program	Supervised exercise on a cycle ergometer in the lab with a heart rate monitor. Home exercise with perceived exertion scale and self measured heart rate	70% estimated HR max at 30 min. 3–4×/week; 2×/week supervised and 2×/week home based	No differences in fasting or postprandial BG control. Cardiorespiratory fitness increased by 10% in exercise group and 5% in controls ($p=0.005$)	A partially-home based exercise program did not reduce BG levels but improved cardiorespiratory fitness
Lesser et al[28]	$n = 11$	To examine the effect of one bout of moderate intensity exercise on glycemic excursion following a mixed nutrient meal	Randomized crossover trial to compare BG and insulin levels, with and without exercise 14-h earlier, and following a mixed nutrient meal (600 kcal, 50% carbohydrate, 20% protein, 30% fat)	A single bout of stationary cycling 14-h earlier for 30 min at 60% VO_2 max	No differences in glycemic response or plasma insulin levels following a mixed nutrient meal	A single bout of exercise does not improve postprandial glycemic excursion or plasma insulin levels following a mixed nutrient meal

(continued)

Table 17.1 (continued)

Study	Subjects	Objective	Methods	Exercise program	Outcome variable	Conclusions
Bung et al[37]	$n = 51$	To evaluate the beneficial effects of exercise in women with insulin requiring GDM	Subjects with fasting BG between 105 and 130 mg/dL were randomized to exercise + diet or exercise + insulin. Diet consisted of 30 kcal/kg/day.	Recumbent bicycling in lab consisted of 45 min, divided into 3 sessions of 15 min each with 5-min breaks in between at 50% VO_{2max}	No differences in glycemic control in the exercise compared to the insulin group similar outcome date	Exercise and diet can obviate the need for insulin in GDM.
Jovanovic-Peterson et al[27]	$n = 29$	To evaluate the impact of exercise using an arm cycle ergometer on glucose tolerance in GDM	Diet consisted of 24–30 kcal/kg/day for 6 weeks. Diet + exercise subjects also participated in 3 exercise sessions/week over 6 weeks	Arm cycle ergometer for 20 min at 70% HR max 3×/week for 6 weeks	Diet+exercise lowered A1C, FBG, and 1-h post prandial glucose	Arm ergometer results in improved glycemic control (glycosylated hemoglobin, fasting BG, and 1-h plasma glucose) compared to diet alone

Avery et al randomized 33 women with GDM at less than 34 weeks gestation into an exercise-training program and diet vs. diet alone.[36] Those subjects randomized to exercise training were prescribed 30 min sessions of variable exercise, twice weekly both at home and in the laboratory, at 70% of aerobic capacity throughout pregnancy. The exercising subjects completed three bouts of 30 min exercise each week and the control subjects reported 0.7 exercise bouts each week. In contrast to the Jovanovic-Peterson et al study,[27] the Avery et al study did not identify significant metabolic effects from exercise. However, the authors observed that the exercise intensity and frequency may not have been sufficient, since half of the exercise sessions were conducted at home and were not supervised.

In another study, Lesser et al enrolled six subjects with GDM into a randomized cross-over design study whose objectives were to determine the efficacy of a single cycle ergometry test to affect fasting glycemia, insulin concentration, and insulin excursion following a mixed nutrient meal in a diabetic subject.[28] As expected, one single bout of limited exercise (30 min at approximately 60% aerobic capacity) was insufficient to blunt the glycemic response of a mixed nutrient meal; we have observed that it takes an average of 7–10 days for this type of intervention to achieve therapeutic results.

We randomized GDM women to 45 min cycle ergometry exercise at 50% of aerobic capacity, or 5–7.5 times the resting metabolic rate vs. an insulin and diet program.[37] The exercise subjects had a compliance rate of more than 90%. The average gestational age at delivery was 39 ± 2 weeks for the insulin group and 38 ± 2 weeks for the exercise group. At eight weeks, no significant differences in glycemic control between the groups were observed; euglycemia was obtained within 1 week and maintained thereafter until delivery. No episodes of hypoglycemia were recorded. Both study groups had similar outcomes, suggesting that an exercise regimen can be offered as a safe and efficient therapeutic option to patients with GDM that require insulin.[37]

17.3 Physical Activity and GDM Prevention

Table 17.2 summarizes the literature quantifying the amount of exercise necessary to achieve benefit; the majority of these studies focus on GDM prevention and include pre-pregnancy activity levels. Reduced risk of GDM is seen when women exercise the year before pregnancy and during pregnancy. These studies demonstrate that higher exercise intensities are more frequently observed in the year prior to pregnancy with light–moderate activity during pregnancy. The greatest reduction in GDM or in glycemic measures both before and during pregnancy is observed in exercise programs lasting at least several weeks, whereas single bouts of exercise provided the fewest benefits.[28,38]

Dempsey et al examined the relation between recreational physical activity before and during pregnancy and risk of GDM in a prospective cohort study in 900 women using structured questionnaires.[39] Women who exercised ≥4.2 h/week during the year before pregnancy experienced a 74–76% reduction in risk, even after adjusting for various covariates. Energy expenditure was also associated with a reduced risk of developing GDM such that ≥21.1 MET-hours per week resulted in a 74% risk reduction in GDM.[39] Those that

Table 17.2 GDM studies using epidemiological data or questionnaires

Epidemiological studies						
Study	Subjects	Objective	Methods	Exercise program	Outcome variable	Conclusion
Snapp and Donaldson[50]	$n = 75{,}160$	Assessed the association of maternal exercise during GDM and adverse maternal and infant outcomes	National Maternal Infant Health Survey (NMIHS) to categorize subjects to exercise or nonexercise groups	Reported exercise (leisure time) of at least 30 min, 3×/week or more, for 6 or more months of pregnancy	Exercise subjects were less likely than the nonexercisers to deliver a large for gestational age (LGA) infant	Moderate leisure time physical activity may reduce risk of LGA in women with GDM
Zhang et al[40]	$n = 21{,}765$	Assessed the amount, type, and intensity of pregravid physical activity and association with GDM risk	Nurses' Health Study II data. Physical activity and sedentary behavior was assessed with a questionnaire	Reported physical activity and sedentary behaviors (such as watching TV)	Total amount of physical activity in MET-hours per week; amount of vigorous physical activity (>6 METS) in MET-hours per week	The amount and intensity of pregravid physical activity was associated with GDM risk. ≥40 MET-hours per week of total physical activity with ≥22.1 MET-hours of vigorous physical activity was associated with the lowest relative risk of GDM (30% less risk)
Dye et al[42]	$n = 12{,}776$	To examine if exercise has a preventative role in decreasing the rate of GDM and if associated with BMI	Data from the Central New York Regional Perinatal Data System (population cohort registry)	Categorized as an exerciser if exercised ≥1 ×/week for 30 min or more	Lower rates of GDM in those who exercise but only in women with BMI > 33 kg/m^2 (OR = 1.9)	Exercise during pregnancy may play a role in reducing the incidence of GDM in obese women

Questionnaires						
Oken, et al[51]	$n = 1,896$	To determine the association of television viewing and physical activity before and during pregnancy on risk of GDM	Questionnaires to classify activity before and during pregnancy as sedentary, walking, light–moderate, or vigorous and amount of television viewing	Walking (for fun, not at work);Light–moderate (e.g., bowling, yoga, stretching); Vigorous (e.g., jogging, swimming, cycling, aerobics)	Decreased GDM risk: Vigorous before and none during pregnancy 17%; Vigorous before and light–moderate or vigorous during 51%; no difference in television viewing	Vigorous physical activity before pregnancy and light–moderate physical activity during pregnancy may decrease abnormal glucose tolerance and GDM
Rudra et al[41]	$n = 897$	To examine the relationship of perceived exertion 1 year before pregnancy on risk of GDM	Questionnaires – Seven-Day Physical Activity Recall Minnesota Leisure-Time Physical Activity	Perceived exertion scale (1–10); Energy expenditure calculated as MET-hours per week: 0.1–14.9, 15.0–29.9, ≥30	Maximal perceived exertion decreased risk of GDM by 81% compared to 43% for minimalexertion	The risk of GDM is inversely related to exercise with maximal perceived exertion providing greater benefits than minimal 1-year prior to pregnancy
Dempsey et al[39]	$n = 909$	To examine the relations between recreational physical activity before and during pregnancy on risk of GDM	Interviews to categorize women as inactive or active during pregnancy (using past 7 days) or activity recall 1-year before pregnancy	Energy expenditure was calculated as MET-hours per week from vigorous (e.g., running or aerobics)	Median 21.1 MET-hours per week in the year before pregnancy (56% lower GDM risk) and 28.0 MET-hours per week during pregnancy (74% lower GDM risk)	Women participating in vigorous physical activity before pregnancy and at least light–moderate physical activity during pregnancy were less likely to develop GDM

spent <21.1 MET-hours per week resulted in a GDM risk reduction of 43%.[39] MET-hours per week were calculated by dividing the total number of hours spent on each activity per week by the number of weeks during which the activity was performed, multiplying the result by the activity intensity score reported in METS, and summing all reported activities. Pregnant women who exercise ≥28 MET-hours per week had a 30% reduction in the relative risk of GDM. The study also determined that women who exercise before and during pregnancy have as much as a 70% risk reduction in GDM.

Zhang et al[40] conducted a prospective cohort study to assess whether the amount, type, and intensity of pregravid physical activity were associated with GDM risk. The analysis included 22,000 women who reported at least one prior singleton pregnancy. Physical activity was assessed with a physical activity questionnaire. Both total and vigorous activity scores were significantly and inversely associated with GDM risk. The relative risks of GDM decreased with total pregravid weekly physical activity such that 16 MET-hours per week showed a 17% reduction in GDM risk and 63 MET-hours per week showed a 30% reduction in GDM risk, compared with those that did not exercise. If the amount of pregravid weekly vigorous physical activity increased (vigorous exercise intensity ≥6 METS or ≥21 mL/kg/min) the relative risk for GDM also decreased, by 20 and 30%, respectively, if 6 and 15 MET-hours per week of vigorous physical activity performed. The inverse associations remained statistically significant after controlling for body mass index (BMI) and other covariates.

Rudra et al showed that those who exercised strenuously up to maximal exertion using the Borg scale of perceived exertion in the year before pregnancy had a 43% decreased in the risk for GDM.[41] Women who performed ≥30 MET-hours per week of energy expenditure from physical activity in the year before pregnancy had a 50% decrease in the risk of GDM compared with only a 34% decrease in GDM if the exercise expenditure was less than 14.9 MET-hours per week.[41] These findings suggest a potential benefit for the adoption and continuation of an active lifestyle for women of reproductive age that is of vigorous intensity prior to pregnancy.

In 1997, a study we published utilized a population-based birth registry in Central New York State between October 1995 and July 1996.[42] Approximately 12,800 women were included in the analysis. When stratified by pre-pregnancy BMI, physical activity was associated with reduced rates of GDM among women with a BMI greater than 33 (odds ratio = 1.9, 95% confidence interval 1.2–3.1) The results of this study suggest that for some obese pregnant women, exercise plays a role in reducing the risk for developing GDM during pregnancy.

17.4 Recommendations for GDM and Activity

Experts agree that pregnancy and postpartum are opportune times for modifying life style[43] and risk factors through physical activity and diet.[44] Historically, pregnant women and particularly diabetic pregnant women were precluded from engaging in physical activities out of concern for deleterious effects on the fetus. This changed at the Second International

Workshop Conference on GDM in 1985. Artal et al and a panel of experts recommended exercise as a therapeutic adjunct in mothers with GDM.[45]

Currently, exercise is accepted as an adjunct intervention in the management of diabetes in nonpregnant women. The opinion of ACOG is that pregnant patients should continue to exercise in the absence of either other medical or obstetric complications. The ACOG guidelines recommend 30 min or more of moderate exercise/day on most, if not all, days of the week.[1] The Society of Obstetricians and Gynecologists of Canada (SOGC) suggest that all women should be encouraged to participate in aerobic and strength conditioning exercise as part of a healthy lifestyle during pregnancy.[20]

Our recommendations for the management and prevention of GDM are as presented in Table 17.3. Given that moderate exercise intensity is 3–6 METS,[46] the maximum number

Table 17.3 Artal et al exercise prescription for sedentary, overweight, or obese women with GDM who are unaccustomed to exercise

Previously sedentary, and/or overweight/obese pregnant women	% HRR	% VO_2R	RPE	Target exercise energy expenditure (MET-hours per week)
Weeks 1–3 of training (26 weeks gestational age)	35–39	40–45	12–14	≥16
Weeks 3–6 of training (gestational age 29 weeks)	45–55	50–60	13–15	28
Weeks 6–9 of training (gestational age 32 weeks)	60	65	15–16	28
Weeks 9–12 of training (gestational age 35 weeks)	60	65	15–16	28

% HRR = %VO_2R unless overweight, sedentary and pregnant. In overweight, sedentary, pregnant women %VO_2R is slightly higher by about 5% compared to %HRR until 70% VO_2R, after which %VO_2R and %HRR are about equal.[52] The RPE is rating of perceived exertion from 6 (no exertion) to 20 (maximal exertion)[53]

%HRR accounts for the measured resting heart rate and the measured maximum heart rate which is based on Karvonen's method.[54] For example, let's consider an exercise heart rate for a sedentary overweight pregnant woman with GDM: in the beginning of the program, the %HRR should be about 35–39% HRR. If her resting heart rate is 90 beats/min (after sitting upright in a chair for 5 min) and measured maximum heart rate measured from a graded exercise test to volitional exhaustion (VO_2 max test) is 185 beats/min, then 39% HRR = 0.39·(185–90) + 85 = 122 beats/min. Heart rate at maximum exercise should be measured and *not* estimated as 220 – age because of the large standard deviation of ± beats/min in age predicted maximum heart rate[55] and because of the blunted maximum heart rate of 10–15 beats/min that sometime occurs during pregnancy[52,56,57]

To adhere to the exercise prescription, the pregnant woman should wear a heart rate monitor. If no heart rate monitor is provided, the RPE scale should be followed. Some of the suggested program shown in this table for exercise intensity is based on the ACSM[58] and elsewhere.[52] The target goal for the amount of physical activity per week expended during pregnancy is based on Dempsey et al (2004)[39] which shows a 33% risk reduction in GDM in women who exercise ≥28 MET-hours per week during pregnancy. So for example, one can exercise three METS × 1.6 h/day × 6 days per week = 28.8 MET-hours per week; or one can exercise for less time at a higher intensity to achieve the same expenditure i.e., 5 METS × 0.95 h/day × 6 days per week = 28.5 MET-hours per week. Perceived exertion intensity is a more practical approach.

of MET-hours per week expended is 12 MET-hours. Most subjects can engage safely in additional physical activities.

We recommend that overweight, sedentary pregnant women who have a risk for GDM or have GDM should perform at a minimum level of 16 MET-hours of physical activity, preferably building up to ≥28 MET-hours of physical activity per week. The beginning exercise intensity would be 35–39% of HRR which builds to 60% of HRR at near-term. Any intensity less than 30% HRR and any energy expenditure that is less than 16 MET-hours per week would not be sufficient to bolster fitness benefits or reduce the risk of GDM. Perceived exertion intensity is a more practical approach (of Borg scale 12-14 (out of 20)). In prescribing physical activity to sedentary subjects, it may be more acceptable to discuss a "walking program" than an "exercise program."

Individualizing an exercise program for women who have GDM involves assessing health and physical fitness, developing a program specific to the patient's situation, recommending fluid and food intake, and informing the patient about limitations, contraindications, warning signs, and specific concerns. For the purpose of diabetes management and glycemic control, a walking program performed for at least 30 min/day should suffice.

References

1. ACOG Committee opinion. Number 267, January 2002: exercise during pregnancy and the postpartum period. *Obstet Gynecol*. 2002;99(1):171-173.
2. American Diabetes Association. Gestational diabetes mellitus. *Diabetes Care*. 2003;26 (suppl 1):S103-S105.
3. Metzger BE, Freinkel N. Effects of diabetes mellitus on endocrinologic and metabolic adaptations of gestation. *Semin Perinatol*. 1978;2(4):309-318.
4. Langer O, Berkus M, Brustman L, Anyaegbunam A, Mazze R. Rationale for insulin management in gestational diabetes mellitus. *Diabetes*. 1991;40(Suppl 2):186-190.
5. Dela F, Larsen JJ, Mikines KJ, Ploug T, Petersen LN, Galbo H. Insulin-stimulated muscle glucose clearance in patients with NIDDM. Effects of one-legged physical training. *Diabetes*. 1995;44(9):1010-1020.
6. Holloszy JO. Exercise-induced increase in muscle insulin sensitivity. *J Appl Physiol*. 2005;99(1): 338-343.
7. Mikines KJ, Sonne B, Farrell PA, Tronier B, Galbo H. Effect of physical exercise on sensitivity and responsiveness to insulin in humans. *Am J Physiol*. 1988;254(3 pt 1):E248-E259.
8. Bogardus C, Thuillez P, Ravussin E, Vasquez B, Narimiga M, Azhar S. Effect of muscle glycogen depletion on in vivo insulin action in man. *J Clin Invest*. 1983;72(5):1605-1610.
9. Perseghin G, Price TB, Petersen KF, et al. Increased glucose transport-phosphorylation and muscle glycogen synthesis after exercise training in insulin-resistant subjects. *N Engl J Med*. 1996;335(18):1357-1362.
10. Annuzzi G, Riccardi G, Capaldo B, Kaijser L. Increased insulin-stimulated glucose uptake by exercised human muscles one day after prolonged physical exercise. *Eur J Clin Invest*. 1991;21(1):6-12.
11. Magkos F, Tsekouras Y, Kavouras SA, Mittendorfer B, Sidossis LS. Improved insulin sensitivity after a single bout of exercise is curvilinearly related to exercise energy expenditure. *Clin Sci (Lond)*. 2008;114(1):59-64.
12. Devlin JT, Horton ES. Effects of prior high-intensity exercise on glucose metabolism in normal and insulin-resistant men. *Diabetes*. 1985;34(10):973-979.

13. Devlin JT, Hirshman M, Horton ED, Horton ES. Enhanced peripheral and splanchnic insulin sensitivity in NIDDM men after single bout of exercise. *Diabetes*. 1987;36(4):434-439.
14. Borghouts LB, Keizer HA. Exercise and insulin sensitivity: a review. *Int J Sports Med*. 2000;21(1):1-12.
15. Henriksson J. Influence of exercise on insulin sensitivity. *J Cardiovasc Risk*. 1995;2(4):303-309.
16. van Baak MA, Borghouts LB. Relationships with physical activity. *Nutr Rev*. 2000;58 (3 Pt 2):S16-S18.
17. Henriksen EJ. Invited review: effects of acute exercise and exercise training on insulin resistance. *J Appl Physiol*. 2002;93(2):788-796.
18. Heath GW, Gavin JR III, Hinderliter JM, Hagberg JM, Bloomfield SA, Holloszy JO. Effects of exercise and lack of exercise on glucose tolerance and insulin sensitivity. *J Appl Physiol*. 1983;55(2):512-517.
19. Bassuk SS, Manson JE. Epidemiological evidence for the role of physical activity in reducing risk of type 2 diabetes and cardiovascular disease. *J Appl Physiol*. 2005;99(3):1193-1204.
20. Davies GA, Wolfe LA, Mottola MF, MacKinnon C. Joint SOGC/CSEP clinical practice guideline: exercise in pregnancy and the postpartum period. *Can J Appl Physiol*. 2003;28(3): 330-341.
21. Kristiansen S, Hargreaves M, Richter EA. Exercise-induced increase in glucose transport, GLUT-4, and VAMP-2 in plasma membrane from human muscle. *Am J Physiol*. 1996;270 (1 pt 1):E197-E201.
22. Hansen PA, Nolte LA, Chen MM, Holloszy JO. Increased GLUT-4 translocation mediates enhanced insulin sensitivity of muscle glucose transport after exercise. *J Appl Physiol*. 1998;85(4):1218-1222.
23. Richter EA, Kiens B, Saltin B, Christensen NJ, Savard G. Skeletal muscle glucose uptake during dynamic exercise in humans: role of muscle mass. *Am J Physiol*. 1988;254 (5 pt 1):E555-E561.
24. Wahren J, Felig P, Hagenfeldt L. Physical exercise and fuel homeostasis in diabetes mellitus. *Diabetologia*. 1978;14(4):213-222.
25. Hargreaves M, Meredith I, Jennings GL. Muscle glycogen and glucose uptake during exercise in humans. *Exp Physiol*. 1992;77(4):641-644.
26. Wahren J, Felig P, Ahlborg G, Jorfeldt L. Glucose metabolism during leg exercise in man. *J Clin Invest*. 1971;50(12):2715-2725.
27. Jovanovic-Peterson L, Durak EP, Peterson CM. Randomized trial of diet versus diet plus cardiovascular conditioning on glucose levels in gestational diabetes. *Am J Obstet Gynecol*. 1989;161(2):415-419.
28. Lesser KB, Gruppuso PA, Terry RB, Carpenter MW. Exercise fails to improve postprandial glycemic excursion in women with gestational diabetes. *J Matern Fetal Med*. 1996;5(4):211-217.
29. Battaglia FC, Meschia G. Principal substrates of fetal metabolism. *Physiol Rev*. 1978;58(2): 499-527.
30. Girard J. Gluconeogenesis in late fetal and early neonatal life. *Biol Neonate*. 1986;50(5): 237-258.
31. Artal R, Wiswell R, Romem Y. Hormonal responses to exercise in diabetic and nondiabetic pregnant patients. *Diabetes*. 1985;34(suppl 2):78-80.
32. Soultanakis HN, Artal R, Wiswell RA. Prolonged exercise in pregnancy: glucose homeostasis, ventilatory and cardiovascular responses. *Semin Perinatol*. 1996;20(4):315-327.
33. Artal R, Platt LD, Sperling M, Kammula RK, Jilek J, Nakamura RI. Maternal cardiovascular and metabolic responses in normal pregnancy. *Am J Obstet Gynecol*. 1981;140(2): 123-127.
34. Brankston GN, Mitchell BF, Ryan EA, Okun NB. Resistance exercise decreases the need for insulin in overweight women with gestational diabetes mellitus. *Am J Obstet Gynecol*. 2004;190(1):188-193.

35. Artal R, Masaki DI, Khodiguian N, Romem Y, Rutherford SE, Wiswell RA. Exercise prescription in pregnancy: weight-bearing versus non-weight-bearing exercise. *Am J Obstet Gynecol.* 1989;161(6 Pt 1):1464-1469.
36. Avery MD, Leon AS, Kopher RA. Effects of a partially home-based exercise program for women with gestational diabetes. *Obstet Gynecol.* 1997;89(1):10-15.
37. Bung P, Artal R, Khodiguian N, Kjos S. Exercise in gestational diabetes. An optional therapeutic approach? *Diabetes.* 1991;40(suppl 2):182-185.
38. Avery MD, Walker AJ. Acute effect of exercise on blood glucose and insulin levels in women with gestational diabetes. *J Matern Fetal Med.* 2001;10(1):52-58.
39. Dempsey JC, Sorensen TK, Williams MA, et al. Prospective study of gestational diabetes mellitus risk in relation to maternal recreational physical activity before and during pregnancy. *Am J Epidemiol.* 2004;159(7):663-670.
40. Zhang C, Solomon CG, Manson JE, Hu FB. A prospective study of pregravid physical activity and sedentary behaviors in relation to the risk for gestational diabetes mellitus. *Arch Intern Med.* 2006;166(5):543-548.
41. Rudra CB, Williams MA, Lee IM, Miller RS, Sorensen TK. Perceived exertion in physical activity and risk of gestational diabetes mellitus. *Epidemiology.* 2006;17(1):31-37.
42. Dye TD, Knox KL, Artal R, Aubry RH, Wojtowycz MA. Physical activity, obesity, and diabetes in pregnancy. *Am J Epidemiol.* 1997;146(11):961-965.
43. Kjos SL. Postpartum care of the woman with diabetes. *Clin Obstet Gynecol.* 2000;43(1): 75-86.
44. Dornhorst A, Rossi M. Risk and prevention of type 2 diabetes in women with gestational diabetes. *Diabetes Care.* 1998;21(Suppl 2):B43-B49.
45. Anon. Proceedings of the Second International Workshop-Conference on Gestational Diabetes Mellitus. October 25–27, 1984, Chicago, Illinois. *Diabetes.* 1985;34(suppl 2):1-130.
46. Haskell WL, Lee IM, Pate RR, et al. Physical activity and public health: updated recommendation for adults from the American College of Sports Medicine and the American Heart Association. *Med Sci Sports Exerc.* 2007;39(8):1423-1434.
47. Davenport MH, Mottola MF, McManus R, Gratton R. A walking intervention improves capillary glucose control in women with gestational diabetes mellitus: a pilot study. *Appl Physiol Nutr Metab.* 2008;33(3):511-517.
48. Artal R, Catanzaro RB, Gavard JA, Mostello DJ, Friganza JC. A lifestyle intervention of weight-gain restriction: diet and exercise in obese women with gestational diabetes mellitus. *Appl Physiol Nutr Metab.* 2007;32(3):596-601.
49. Garcia-Patterson A, Martin E, Ubeda J, Maria MA, de Leiva A, Corcoy R. Evaluation of light exercise in the treatment of gestational diabetes. *Diabetes Care.* 2001;24(11): 2006-2007.
50. Snapp CA, Donaldson SK. Gestational diabetes mellitus: physical exercise and health outcomes. *Biol Res Nurs.* 2008;10(2):145-155.
51. Oken E, Ning Y, Rifas-Shiman SL, Radesky JS, Rich-Edwards JW, Gillman MW. Associations of physical activity and inactivity before and during pregnancy with glucose tolerance. *Obstet Gynecol.* 2006;108(5):1200-1207.
52. Davenport MH, Charlesworth S, Vanderspank D, Sopper MM, Mottola MF. Development and validation of exercise target heart rate zones for overweight and obese pregnant women. *Appl Physiol Nutr Metab.* 2008;33(5):984-989.
53. Borg GA. Psychophysical bases of perceived exertion. *Med Sci Sports Exerc.* 1982;14(5): 377-381.
54. Karvonen MJ, Kentala E, Mustala O. The effects of training on heart rate; a longitudinal study. *Ann Med Exp Biol Fenn.* 1957;35(3):307-315.
55. Londeree BR, Moeschberger ML. Effect of age and other factors on maximal heart rate. *Res Q Exerc Sport.* 1982;53:297-303.

56. Mottola MF, Davenport MH, Brun CR, Inglis SD, Charlesworth S, Sopper MM. VO2peak prediction and exercise prescription for pregnant women. *Med Sci Sports Exerc.* 2006;38(8):1389-1395.
57. Heenan AP, Wolfe LA, Davies GA. Maximal exercise testing in late gestation: maternal responses. *Obstet Gynecol.* 2001;97(1):127-134.
58. ACSM. *ACSM's Guidelines for Exercise Testing and Prescription.* 7th ed. Baltimore: Lippincott Williams & Wilkins; 2006.

Nutrition and Weight Recommendations for Treating Gestational Diabetes Mellitus 18

Janet C. King and David A. Sacks

18.1 Introduction

The importance of nutrition in the treatment and management of gestational diabetes mellitus (GDM) is well established. Maternal and fetal needs for a healthy pregnancy outcome need to be met in the context of aberrant regulation of glucose metabolism, the primary fuel for the fetus. Nutrition of women with GDM poses a unique challenge. The primary objective of dietary advice for women with GDM is to maintain maternal normoglycemia while reducing accelerated fetal growth.[1] Since excessive gestational weight gain, particularly fat gain, may exacerbate maternal insulin resistance,[2] dietary recommendations for women with GDM should promote appropriate maternal weight gain. The overall objective of this chapter is to review past and current dietary recommendations for women with GDM and to integrate those recommendations with guidelines for healthy weight gains; complications of obesity during pregnancy are discussed in depth in another chapter in this book. It is important to recognize that the dietary principles promoted for women with GDM will have a lifelong positive impact on maternal health and decrease the risk for developing type 2 diabetes mellitus in the future.

18.2 Historical Evolution of Nutrition Recommendations for Treating GDM

Since the early days of treating women with diabetes during pregnancy, medical nutrition therapy (MNT) has been a cornerstone of management. The first reports of diet therapy for pregnant diabetic women come from Germany in the early twentieth century[3] where diets

J.C. King (✉)
Children's Hospital Oakland Research Institute,
Oakland, CA, USA
e-mail: jking@chori.org

C. Kim and A. Ferrara (eds.), *Gestational Diabetes During and After Pregnancy*,
DOI: 10.1007/978-1-84882-120-0_18,

high in protein and fat (85% of total energy) and, therefore, low in carbohydrate were applied. In severe cases, starvation diets were used. Subsequently, diabetic women at the Joslin Clinic in Boston were treated with a diet providing modest restrictions in energy, i.e., 30 kcal/kg body weight, 1 g protein/kg, and *liberal* amounts of carbohydrate (180–250 g).[4] In 1951, Duncan modified the plan.[5] Because many women were obese or had edema, he based energy and protein intakes on a proportion of the ideal body weight rather than actual body weight. At about the same time, Moss and Mulholland recommended using much higher protein intakes, 2 g protein/kg current body weight.[6] However, they were the first to limit total weight gain to no more than 20 lb or 9.1 kg. In 1952, Reis introduced calorie restriction to keep hyperglycemia and glycosuria under control.[7] Women doing light work were allowed 25 kcal/kg; those doing moderate work were allowed 30 kcal/kg. Based on the erroneous assumption that minimization of weight gain would reduce the incidence of edema, the latter being part of the definition of pre-eclampsia at that time, restrictions in energy intake and weight gain continued through the 1960s.

In 1970, the National Research Council of the National Academy of Sciences (NAS) published a landmark report demonstrating that fetal growth and development were adversely affected by maternal weight gain restriction.[8] This report recommended easing the weight gain restriction for pregnancy from 22 to 30 lb (10–13.6 kg). However, weight gain continued to be restricted for diabetic women to ≤15 lb (6.8 kg) until 1979. At that time, the American Diabetes Association in collaboration with the American Dietetic Association recommended that the NAS weight gain standards for non-diabetic pregnant women should also be applied to diabetic women.[9] They recommended consuming moderate amounts of complex carbohydrates, no refined sugars, and to limit cholesterol and saturated fat intakes.[9]

Thus, since the early 1900s, MNT for pregnant women with diabetes has evolved from energy restricted diets, to moderate energy intakes with high amounts of protein with limited weight gain, to diets restricted in refined carbohydrates and limited amounts of fat. The research basis for these recommendations stems primarily from practical experiences and observations; the efficacy of these dietary regimens on maternal glycemic control and pregnancy outcome has not been studied systematically. Since 2000, individualized dietary prescriptions and exercise goals have been promoted to improve glycemic control, and gestational weight gain recommendations for normal pregnancy were also used for women with GDM.[10, 11] A review of the current recommendations and their evidence base follows.

18.3 Medical Nutrition Therapy for Gestational Diabetes Mellitus

18.3.1 Current Nutrition Recommendations for Women with GDM

The goals of MNT are to achieve and maintain normoglycemia, provide sufficient calories to promote appropriate weight gain, as recommended by the Institute of Medicine (IOM), to avoid maternal ketosis, and to provide adequate nutrients for maternal and fetal health.[12] Upon diagnosis of GDM, the first course of action is to refer the patient to a dietitian for nutritional counseling and development of an individualized meal plan. Thus, MNT is the foundation for the management of GDM. Insulin therapy may be used concurrently with MNT if normoglycemia is not maintained consistently with diet alone. Although there are no universal specific guidelines for managing GDM, the American Diabetes Association, the American College of Obstetricians and Gynecologists, and the American Dietetic Association all recommend individualized counseling for developing a culturally-appropriate food plans emphasizing healthy food choices, portion control, and good cooking practices.[12–14] A modest energy restriction (30% of estimated energy needs) may be recommended for obese women with GDM to reduce blood glucose levels without elevating plasma free fatty acids or inducing ketonuria.[15] However, there are no randomized controlled trials demonstrating which dietary compositions and patterns best promote normoglycemia and optimal maternal and fetal outcomes. Until those data are available, more specific recommendations cannot be made. A review of current information on the maternal diet and management of GDM or pregnancy outcome follows.

18.3.2 Energy Restriction for GDM

A common nutritional goal for all pregnant women is to provide adequate nourishment for the mother and fetus while limiting unnecessary maternal weight and fat gain. Thus, it is not surprising that the energy levels of diet patterns for women with GDM have received a lot of attention. Since 1985, seven studies have reported the effect of energy restricted diets on the outcomes of pregnancy in women who have GDM[16–22] (Table 18.1). Four of the studies were short-term,[18, 20, 21, 23] either 7 days or 4 weeks, making it impossible to determine the effect of maternal energy restriction on birth weight or other indicators of pregnancy outcome. Two short-term studies showed that a severe, 50%, energy restriction from 2,400 to 1,200 kcal/day for 7 days caused ketonemia and ketonuria to develop.[20, 23] However, 24-h mean glucose concentrations and fasting insulin levels declined. A more moderate energy restriction, 1,600–1,800 kcal/day, prevented ketonemia while improving glycemia.[23]

Three studies evaluated the effects of moderate energy restriction ranging from about 1,600–1,800 kcal/day from the time of diagnosis for GDM to term, or about 10–15 weeks.[16, 17, 22] The studies were small and did not have sufficient power to determine the effects of energy restriction on birth weight. Nevertheless, none showed that a modest calorie reduction inhibited fetal growth. Furthermore, ketosis did not develop in any of the studies. One group assessed the impact of energy restriction on the need for insulin therapy in obese women with GDM.[22] In both the energy restricted and control groups, about 17% of the women required insulin therapy, but there was a tendency in the restricted group toward initiating insulin therapy later in gestation and needing a lower maximum daily dosage. A larger trial with more subjects is needed to confirm this finding.

In sum, these studies of moderate energy restriction in GDM women show an improvement in glycemic control measured either by 24-h mean glucose levels, fasting insulin levels, or the amount of exogenous insulin required. The diets tended to reduce weight gain during the treatment period in the third trimester, the gestational age when fetal growth rate reaches a maximum. However, that reduction in maternal weight gain was not associated with a decrease

Table 18.1 Randomized controlled trials of energy restriction and pregnancy outcomes in women with gestational diabetes mellitus[a]

Year [reference] First Author	Study design	Study duration	Population and number [n]	Energy intake, kcal/day	Carbohydrate intake, g/day (as % of kcal)	Gestational weight gain, kg Mean ± SD	Effect on pregnancy outcome
Short-term studies							
Maresh et al[21]	Randomized, cross-over of recently diagnosed GDM women at 28 weeks gestation	4 weeks	Diet Restr[10] Diet Restr +Insulin[10]	1,500–1,800 1,800–2,100	120–150 (33) 150–180 (33)	0.7 kg/week 1.5 kg/week	Diet restriction + insulin reduced serum glucose to that of controls. Diet restriction with or without insulin caused ketonemia
Gillmer et al[18]	Randomized study of recently diagnosed GDM women	4 weeks	Diet Restr[7] Diet Restr + Insulin[8]	1,500–1,800 2,100	120–150 g (~33) 180 g (~33)	−1.7 ± 2.6 +0.9 ± 2.4	Diet restriction with or without insulin caused ketonemia
Magee[20]	Randomized study of obese GDM women	1 week	Kcal Restr[7] Control[5]	1,200 2,400	150 (50) 300 (50)	Not reported	Kcal restriction lower fasting insulin and 24-h mean glucose, but did not change OGTT results. Ketonemia and ketonuria occurred with kcal restriction
Knopp[19]	Randomized study of obese GDM women	1 week	Kcal Restr[7] Control[5]	1,200 2,400	150 (50) 300 (50)	Not reported	Kcal restriction improved fasting and 24 h mean glucose by 22 and 10%. Ketonemia doubled in kcal/restricted group with 33% kcal/restr (1,800 vs. 2,400), no marked ketonuria occurred

Longer-term studies								
Algert[16]	Nonrandomized, observational	Diagnosis to delivery, 10–15 weeks	Obese GDM[22] Lean GDM[31]	1,700–1,800 2,000–3,000	212–225 (50–60) 250–370	10.6 ± 7.7 13.3 ± 4.1		Moderate kcal restriction in obese GDM women reduced weight gain without causing ketonemia. Birth weight slightly higher – 3,922 vs. 3,544 g
Dornhorst[17]	Nonrandomized, observational	Diagnosis to delivery	GDM[35] Non GDM [2337]	1,200–1,800 Not controlled	150–225 (50) Not controlled	4.6 ± 4.9 9.7 ± 5.3		No difference in birth weights or incidence of macrosomia in comparison to a general prenatal non-GDM population
Rae, A.[22]	Stratified Randomized Controlled Trial	Diagnosis to delivery	GDM-kcal restr[66] GDM-control[58]	1,590–1,776 2,010–2,220	210–244 (51) 240–274 (46)	11.6 ± 1.3 9.7 ± 1.5		Kcal restriction did not alter frequency of insulin therapy (17.5% vs. 16.9%), but it lowered the dose (23 vs. 60U). No difference in ketonemia, ketonuria, blood glucose, pregnancy complications, or birth weight

[a]Adapted from Gunderson[92]

in birth weight or an increase in the prevalence of macrosomic infants. Ketosis occurred only with a severe energy restriction to about 1,200 kcal/day; higher intakes ranging from 1,600 to 1,800 kcal/day did not produce ketosis. Since maternal body weight is a primary determinant of energy requirements, it is important to express moderate energy restriction in terms of kcal/kg rather than kcal/day. Algert et al[16] showed that obese women with GDM do not develop ketosis or fetal growth retardation when consuming at least 25 kcal/kg/day. This led the fourth International Workshop-Conference on Gestational Diabetes Mellitus to support moderate caloric restriction for overweight women with GDM with prescriptions as low as "25 kcal/kg actual pregnant body weight."[24] Calorie recommendations for energy intake have not been established for normal weight women with GDM.

18.3.3 Sources and Amount of Dietary Carbohydrate

Glucose transfer occurs in a concentration-dependent manner across the placenta.[1] Thus, maximal transfer across the maternal-fetal gradient occurs following meals when the maternal-fetal glucose gradient is greatest. It is thought, therefore, that accelerated fetal growth among progeny of diabetic women reflects accelerated glucose transfer due to their postprandial blood glucose levels being greater than that observed in non-diabetic women. A clear objective of dietary management for GDM women should therefore be to reduce postprandial glycemia. This can be achieved by either decreasing dietary carbohydrate at the expense of dietary fat, by increasing the proportion of carbohydrate from fiber or low glycemic sources, or both. Since fasting insulin resistance also occurs during pregnancy in normal women and women with GDM, higher fasting glucose levels may contribute to fetal overgrowth along with elevated levels postprandially. Elevated glucose concentrations in the fasting state are a particular problem among obese women.

To date, studies of the effect of the *amount* of dietary carbohydrate on pregnancy outcome in GDM women have been done only in women who were also consuming energy-restricted diets.[25,26] As expected, the studies show that carbohydrate intake as percent of energy is positively correlated with the 1-h postprandial glucose response to a mixed meal.[25,26] Likely because of the normal early morning increase in plasma cortisol ("dawn phenomenon") the response following breakfast tended to be greater than that following lunch or dinner. This suggests the benefit of lower carbohydrate consumption at breakfast than at lunch and dinner. Major et al also demonstrated,[25] that carbohydrate restriction along with a low calorie diet improves infant outcomes. In comparison with 21 women consuming between 45 and 50% of their energy as carbohydrate, women with less than 42% as carbohydrate had fewer large for gestational age (LGA) infants and less cesarean deliveries. This preliminary evidence is not sufficient to conclude that a low carbohydrate/low energy diet should be recommended for all GDM women. It suggests, however, that the benefits of an energy-restricted diet may be enhanced by a concurrent reduction in carbohydrate.

In contrast, Romon et al[27] unexpectedly found that a high carbohydrate diet was associated with a *decreased* incidence of macrosomia in women with GDM. None of the women consuming more than 210 g carbohydrate/day gave birth to a LGA baby. This outcome is difficult to explain. It may reflect a decrease in lipolysis and circulating free fatty acids with higher amounts of dietary carbohydrate. Lower levels of free fatty acids may be associated with an improvement in insulin-stimulated glucose uptake.[28] Thus, a higher intake of carbohydrate may reduce the rise in serum FFA and insulin resistance that in turn lowers the postprandial glycemic response and fetal overgrowth.

The postprandial blood glucose response is primarily determined by the rate of intestinal carbohydrate absorption, with the most rapidly absorbed refined sugars causing the highest response and the more complex, slowly absorbed carbohydrates causing the lowest response. Thus, shifting the *source* of carbohydrates to a higher proportion of complex, low glycemic foods may enable GDM women to maintain normoglycemia with higher carbohydrate intakes. Studies by both Fraser et al and Clapp et al showed that high fiber/low glycemic diets allowed non-diabetic pregnant women to sustain their pre-pregnancy postprandial glycemic response throughout gestation, whereas women consuming a lower fiber/high glycemic diet experienced a 190% increase in their postprandial response by late gestation.[29,30] These findings suggest that the usual maternal insulin resistance and hyperglycemia observed in late pregnancy may reflect the intake of a Westernized, low fiber, high glycemic diet rather than being a normal metabolic response to pregnancy. A prospective, epidemiological cohort study confirmed that the source of dietary carbohydrate influences the risk of GDM. Among 13,110 women in the Nurses' Health Study, high dietary fiber was strongly associated with a reduced GDM risk. Each 10 g/day increment in total fiber intake was associated with a 26% reduction in the risk for GDM. Conversely, a low cereal fiber/high glycemic load diet was associated with a 2.15-fold increased risk for GDM compared to the reciprocal diet.[31] In 2008, a Cochrane review assessed the efficacy of either a high fiber or a low glycemic index diet for preventing GDM.[32] Three trials (107 women) were included in the review,[30,33,34] but the data were insufficient to determine if a diet rich in complex carbohydrates reduced the risk of GDM.

Recently, Moses et al evaluated the effect of a low glycemic diet on the need for insulin therapy in women with GDM. Sixty-three women with GDM were randomly assigned to a low glycemic index (GI) diet or a conventional high fiber, higher GI diet. The need for insulin therapy was significantly reduced in the low GI group, 29% vs. 59% ($p = 0.023$). Furthermore, 9 of the 19 women in the higher GI group were able to avoid the use of insulin by changing to the low GI diet. No differences in fetal growth or other pregnancy complications were observed between the two groups.

Currently, the American Diabetes Association recommends that dietary carbohydrate be limited to about 40–45% of the energy intake for women with GDM with a smaller proportion at breakfast than at lunch or dinner.[3] In contrast, Felig and Naylor recommend greater than 45% of the total energy in the form of low glycemic carbohydrates.[1] Based on the work of Fraser,[30] it has also been suggested that carbohydrate intakes may be as high as 60% if they come primarily from complex sources. An adequately powered, randomized, controlled trial is needed to disentangle the relationship between pregnancy outcomes in GDM women with the amount of fiber and the amount and sources of carbohydrate they consume.

18.3.4
Sources or Types of Dietary Fat

To reduce the risk of dyslipidemia, non-pregnant, diabetic patients are advised to consume diets with less than 10% of the energy intake from saturated fats and less than 300 mg cholesterol/day.[15] However, similar recommendations have not been made for women with

GDM[15] due to the lack of data showing a beneficial effect of dietary fat modifications on the metabolic adjustments of pregnancy in women with GDM. In a small study of women with GDM, Ilic et al[35] found that the addition of fat to a test meal significantly lowered the glycemic and insulin response, presumably due to fat-induced slower gastric emptying and glucose absorption in the presence of more dietary fat. However, it is not prudent to recommend high fat intakes during gestation in order to improve glycemic control in a population at risk for future metabolic disorders, including cardiovascular disease.

To date, the effects of the degree of saturation of fatty acids on glucose tolerance during pregnancy has not been studied in a randomized controlled trial. However, evidence from several case control studies suggests that polyunsaturated fatty acids (PUFAs) may be protective against impaired glucose tolerance (IGT) or GDM whereas high intake of saturated fatty acids is detrimental.[36, 37] Bo et al[36] found that a high intake of saturated fat, as a % of total fat, increased the risk of IGT/GDM twofold whereas the intake of PUFAs reduced the risk by 15% among 504 Italian women. Neither the total amount of dietary fat nor the amount of monounsaturated fatty acids was associated with risk for IGT/GDM. This finding was supported by a subsequent study of 1,698 pregnant women in North Carolina.[38] When the diets of these women were modeled so that their intake of dietary fat was increased by 100 kcal while carbohydrate was reduced by 100 kcal, the risk of IGT and GDM increased by 12% and 9%, respectively. The types of dietary fat were not reported. However, since saturated fat intakes tend to be high in this region of the US, the increased risk of IGT/GDM with more dietary fat may reflect a higher intake of saturated fat and lower PUFAs, as observed in the study of Italian women.[36] A study of 171 Chinese women[37] also found that an increased intake of PUFAs (10.2 vs. 8.5% of total energy), and an associated reduction in saturated fat, lowered the incidence of GDM during pregnancy. It is not known which of the various PUFAs have the strongest impact on GDM risk. Among 1,733 first-trimester gravidas, Radesky and associates[39] found that the intake of omega-3 fatty acids was associated with a small *increased* risk for GDM (11%), but not with IGT risk. Beneficial effects of omega-3 fatty acids on glucose tolerance have been reported in animal models, but there is no evidence that omega-3 fatty acids improve insulin action in humans.[40]

In addition to these nutrient-specific studies, a prospective cohort study of 13,110 women in the Nurses' Health Study[41] reported that a Western-type dietary pattern (i.e., high in red meat, refined sugars, and fried or snack foods) predicted a higher incidence of GDM compared to a prudent diet characterized by a high intake of fruit, green leafy vegetables, poultry and fish. Taken together, all of these data imply that pregnant women at risk for GDM may benefit from diets low in saturated fats and higher in PUFAs, but the findings are insufficient to determine the optimal dietary fatty acid composition for reducing IGT/GDM.

18.3.5 Micronutrient Intakes

An adequate intake of vitamins and minerals for maternal-fetal health is one of the GDM MNT goals.[3] Since there is no evidence that the vitamin/mineral requirements of women with GDM differ from that of healthy pregnant women, the IOM Dietary Reference Intakes (DRIs) are appropriate for planning diets for women with GDM[42] (Table 18.2). The

Table 18.2 Dietary reference intakes (DRIs) for pregnancy that may be used for women with GDM[42]

Nutrient	DRI	Increase %	Rationale for increase	Comment
Energy (kcal/day)	2,855	19%	Maternal and fetal deposition	a
Carbohydrate (g/day)	*175*	35%	Fetal brain glucose utilization	
Total fiber (g/day)	28	12%	Extrapolation based on increased energy intake	b
Protein (g/day)	*71*	54%	Maternal and fetal deposition	
n-6 PUFA (g/day)	13	8%	Median linoleic acid intake from CSFII	c
n-3 PUFA (g/day)	1.4	27%	Median α-linolenic acid intake from CSFII	
Calcium (mg/day)	1100	0%	Adequate adjustments in maternal homeostasis in pregnancy	d
Fluoride (mg/day)	3	0%	Limited data available to suggest increased need in pregnancy	d
Phosphorus (mg/day)	*700*	0%	Adequate adjustments in maternal homeostasis in pregnancy	
Chloride (g/day)	2.3	0%	Limited data available to suggest increased need in pregnancy	d
Potassium (g/day)	4.7	0%	Daily accretion in pregnancy is small	b
Sodium (g/day)	1.5	0%	Daily accretion in pregnancy is small	d
Molybdenum (μg/day)	*50*	11%	Extrapolation based on average maternal weight gain	d
Selenium (μg/day)	*60*	9%	Fetal deposition	
Zinc (mg/day)	*11*	38%	Maternal and fetal deposition	b
Choline (mg/day)	450	6%	Median intake from CSFII	d
Folate (μg/day)	*600*	50%	Maintain normal folate status	e
Niacin (mg/day)	*18*	29%	Maternal and fetal deposition plus increased energy utilization	
Pantothenic acid (mg/day)	6	20%	Maternal and fetal deposition	
Riboflavin (mg/day)	*1.4*	27%	Maternal and fetal deposition plus increased energy utilization	d
Thiamin (mg/day)	*1.4*	27%	Maternal and fetal deposition plus increased energy utilization	d
Vitamin A (μg/day)	*770*	10%	Fetal liver Vitamin A deposition	b

(*continued*)

Table 18.2 (continued)

Nutrient	DRI	Increase %	Rationale for increase	Comment
Vitamin B_{12} (μg/day)	*2.6*	8%	Fetal deposition and changes in maternal absorption	
Vitamin B_6 (mg/day)	*1.9*	46%	Maternal and fetal deposition	[d]
Vitamin C (mg/day)	*85*	13%	Amount needed to prevent scurvy in infant and estimated fetal transfer	[d]
Biotin (μg/day)	30	0%	Limited data available to suggest increased need in pregnancy	[d]
Vitamin D (μg/day)	5	0%	Daily accretion in pregnancy is small	
Vitamin E (mg/day)	*15*	0%	Circulating concentrations normally increase in pregnancy; lack of clinical deficiency	
Vitamin K (μg/day)	90	0%	Comparable concentrations in pregnancy; lack of clinical deficiency	

[a]For healthy moderately active individuals, third trimester; requirements for first trimester are not increased above non-pregnancy and requirements for second trimester are 2,708 kcal/d. Subtract 7 kcal/day for females for each year of age above 19 years.

[b]Percent increase for pregnant women 14–18 is slightly *lower* than for age 19–30 year.

[c]Percent increase for pregnant women 31–50 year is slightly *higher* than for age 19–30 year.

[d]Percent increase for pregnant women 14–18 year is slightly *higher* than for age 19–30 year.

[e]Low maternal folate status in very early pregnancy (before women typically know they have conceived) has been associated with the birth of offspring with a neural tube defect (NTD). Therefore, the non-pregnant DRI for women in their child-bearing years was formulated for preventing NTDs. In view of evidence linking the use of supplements containing folic acid before conception and during early pregnancy with reduced risk of NTDs in the fetus, it is recommended that all women capable of becoming pregnant take a supplement containing 400μg of folic acid every day, in addition to the amount of folate consumed in a healthy diet.

[f]Adapted from Ritchie and King.[43]

MyPyramid (www.MyPyramid.gov) translates the DRIs into a food intake pattern. Using this pattern for pregnant women will assure that the recommended intakes of all micronutrients except iron and vitamin E will be adequate for pregnancy.[43] The shortfall in iron and vitamin E can be provided easily by a vitamin-mineral supplement with at least 10 mg iron and 9 mg vitamin E.

Although there is no evidence that the dietary need for micronutrients differs between GDM and healthy women, there is evidence of an abnormal metabolism of some micronutrients in non-pregnant patients with type 2 diabetes.[44] Urinary zinc excretion tends to be elevated in diabetic patients, possibly because zinc becomes chelated with glycosylated amino acids or peptides and excreted with those compounds. But, elevated urinary zinc is not always associated with reduced serum zinc concentrations in diabetic patients. Studies of diabetic pregnant rats suggest that zinc transport to the fetus is reduced, but there is no evidence that this occurs in humans. A study of 504 Italian pregnant women[45] found that women with lower intakes and serum levels of zinc were more likely to be hyperglycemic. A similar inverse relationship was seen for selenium. There was no evidence, however, that the low intakes of zinc and selenium *caused* gestational hyperglycemia or that increased intakes of these trace elements lowers blood glucose levels.

Lower serum and urinary magnesium levels have been observed among women with type 1 diabetes or GDM.[44] However, evidence that poor magnesium status increases the risk of hyperglycemia in non-pregnant or pregnant individuals is lacking. It is proposed that lower serum magnesium levels among diabetic patients reflect a positive effect of exogenous insulin on cellular magnesium uptake, leading to a decline in serum magnesium. No maternal or fetal health outcomes have been linked to low serum magnesium levels in women with GDM who are receiving exogenous insulin.

Since chromium is thought to be required for normal insulin function,[41] the effects of supplemental chromium on glycemic control have been studied in healthy and GDM pregnant women. Jovanovic-Peterson and Peterson[46] found that chromium picolinate supplements (4 μg/kg/day) reduced hemoglobin A1c, glucose, and insulin levels compared with the patients' baseline levels and improved glucose tolerance. However, other studies of chromium supplementation during pregnancy do not support those findings. In a prospective study of 425 women (396 healthy and 29 with GDM), serum chromium levels did not differ between the two groups of women when they enrolled for prenatal care or when they were screened for GDM in the second trimester.[47] Gunton et al also reported that serum chromium concentrations were not related to glucose intolerance in late pregnancy.[48] In addition, a meta-analysis of 15 RCTs concluded that the effects of supplemental chromium on glucose, insulin, or glycated hemoglobin in type 2 diabetic subjects were inclusive.[49] Thus, there is no expectation that chromium supplementation would benefit women with GDM. Nor is there any evidence that poor chromium status increases the risk of GDM.

There is some evidence for an association between GDM and circulating maternal 25-hydroxy vitamin D (25(OH)D), a form of vitamin D. Zhang et al found plasma 25(OH) D at 16 weeks gestation to be significantly lower in women who subsequently developed GDM than in controls matched by season of conception, with the relation remaining significant after adjustment for maternal age, race, family history of diabetes, and pre-pregnancy BMI. There was a 1.29-fold increase in risk of GDM for every 12.5 nmol/L decrease in plasma 25(OH)D in non-Hispanic white subjects.[50] Another study found a borderline significant inverse association between fasting plasma glucose and serum 25(OH)D at mid-gestation after adjusting for ethnicity, age, and BMI, but the odds ratio for GDM did not have any significance.[51] This relationship between vitamin D status and GDM may be linked to maternal obesity since the incidence of both GDM and poor vitamin D status are associated with obesity.

In sum, at this time there is no evidence supporting an enhanced requirement for any micronutrient among GDM women.

18.4 Guidelines for Weight Gain During Pregnancy

The IOM recently published revised guidelines for weight gain during pregnancy for all pregnant women.[2] Progressive decrements in total pregnancy weight gain were proposed for each of four categories of prepregnancy body mass index (BMI, in kg/m^2) (Table 18.3). These guidelines were based on analyses of data demonstrating the amount of weight gain for women in each prepregnancy body mass index BMI category associated with delivery of a term baby weighing between 6.6 and 8.8 pounds. The only difference between these recommendations and those released in 1990[11] is that an upper level was established for obese women with BMIs greater than 30 kg/m^2. In 1998, the National Heart, Lung and Blood Institute (NHLBI) published a similarly hierarchical set of criteria categorizing prepregnancy BMI.[52] In addition to the four classes, the NHLBI created three subclasses of the heaviest (obese) group (Table 18.4). The NHLBI criteria were endorsed by the World

Table 18.3 Institute of Medicine categories of prepregnancy BMI and weight gain recommendations for pregnancy for these categories[3]

Category	BMI (kg/m^2)	Total weight gain		Rate of weight gain second and third trimester	
		In kg	In lbs	In kg/week	In lbs/week
Underweight	<18.5	12.5–18	28–40	0.44–0.58	1.0–1.3
Normal	18.5–24.9	11.5–16	25–35	0.35–0.50	0.8–1.0
Overweight	25–29.9	7.0–11.5	15–25	0.23–0.33	0.5–0.7
Obese	≥30	5.0–9.0	11–20	0.17–0.27	0.4–0.6

Table 18.4 1998 National Heart, Lung, and Blood Institute and World Health Organization categories of pre-pregnancy BMI[52,53] and 2002 National Institutes of Health weight gain recommendations for pregnancy for these categories[54]

Category	BMI (kg/m^2)	Total weight gain	
		In kg	In lbs
Underweight	<18.5	12.2–18.1	27–40
Normal	18.5–24.9	11.3–15.9	25–35
Overweight	25–29.9	6.8–11.3	15–25
Obese	≥30	≤6.8	≤15
Class 1	30–34.9		
Class 2	35–39.9		
Class 3	≥40 or ≥35 with comorbidities		

Health Organization,[53] and in 2002, the National Institutes of Health[54] published guidelines for weight gain for each of the NHLBI categories of pre-pregnancy BMI.

It is of great concern that over the past few decades there has been a marked increase in obesity. One third of all women in the US are obese. With the increase in obesity, there has been a concomitant decrease in small-for-dates neonates, and an increase in large-for-dates neonates.[55] Furthermore, an increase in the proportion of pregnant women who gain more weight than is recommended for their pre-pregnancy BMI has been reported.[56]

Some medical societies concerned with women's health are non-specific in their recommendations for weight gain by diabetic women during pregnancy, while others endorse the IOM, NHLBI, and NIH guidelines (Tables 18.3 and 18.4). The American Diabetes Association recommends that all diabetic women follow a diet during pregnancy that provides adequate energy intake to maintain normoglycemia, appropriate weight gain, and avoidance of ketonemia. Weight reduction is discouraged, although a caloric reduction of 30% of daily energy needs for obese women who have GDM is permissible.[57] The American Association of Clinical Endocrinologists advises only that weight gain should be monitored during pregnancy without commenting on caloric content.[58] The American Dietetic Association recommends following the IOM guidelines for weight gain for women who have pregestational or GDM.[59] While offering no guidelines for weight gain for women who have pregestational diabetes, the American College of Obstetricians and Gynecologists suggests adequate nutrients for appropriate weight gain, avoidance of ketosis, and a cautious caloric restriction of no more than 33% for obese women who have GDM.[60] They recommend following the IOM guidelines for all obese pregnant women.[61]

Since studies of nonpregnant individuals have shown that even small reductions in body weight improve glycemic control,[62] Artal et al[63] initiated an intervention program to restrict weight gain in obese women with GDM. A total of 96 women were studied with 39 women in a kcal restricted diet plus exercise group and 57 women in a kcal restricted diet only group. The addition of exercise to a kcal restricted diet lowered weekly weight gain from 0.3 to 0.1 kg ($p<0.05$). The incidence of LGA tended to be higher among the women who gained weight versus those who lost weight or had no weight change (10 vs. 1 macrosomic baby), but the difference did not reach statistical significance ($p=0.12$). No adverse pregnancy outcomes were observed with weight maintenance or loss. It is unfortunate that the effect of weight loss or maintenance versus gain on glycemic control was not reported. However, the study suggests that prevention of excessive weight gain or, possibly, weight maintenance among high-risk, obese pregnant women may reduce the risk of fetal over-growth.

18.4.1 Rationale for Individualized Weight Gain Recommendations

That there is an association between maternal obesity during pregnancy and adverse maternal, fetal, neonatal, and childhood outcomes is of little dispute. Much of the research pertaining to the independent relationship between maternal weight gain and adverse outcomes has focused on weight gain in obese pregnant women. A number of studies of large patient populations have focused primarily on the relationships between weight gain during pregnancy and either pre-eclampsia, birth weight, or both. In studies of unselected populations of singleton births, controlling for such confounders as maternal age, ethnicity, and parity, an independent relationship has been reported between adverse outcomes and maternal weight gain exceeding 16 kg for all prepregnancy BMI groups,[64] and maternal weight gain of 5–10 kg for women whose prepregnancy BMI is ≥30 kg/m^2.[65] Similar findings have been reported for women whose pregnancy weight gain exceeded that recommended for BMI category by the IOM.[66,67,68] Some have,[68] and some have not[69] found the effects of pre-pregnancy BMI and pregnancy weight gain to be additive. Two population-based studies calculated the weight gain that was associated with the lowest incidence of a variety of adverse maternal and perinatal outcomes. One study found the optimal weight gain for obese women to be less than 13 pounds.[70] The other study found the optimal weight change to be a gain of 10–25 pounds for class I and 0–9 pounds for class II, and a weight loss of 0–9 pounds for women with class III obesity.[71]

A study of an unselected population of pregnant women found that the average weekly weight gain before 16 weeks and between 28 and 32 weeks was significantly less than that of the respective succeeding 4 week periods.[72] It appears that not only absolute weight gain but also the distribution of weight gain per trimester may be associated with the incidence of pregnancy complications. A study designed to look at the independent relationship of weight gain during each trimester and clinical outcomes analyzed data of patients who did not have diabetes or hypertension as well as those who were not obese.[73] The mean weight gain was greatest in second trimester (7.7 kg) while that in first and third were respectively 2.1 kg and 6.6 kg. In multivariable analysis, weight gain in second trimester, either alone or in combination with weight gain in first and third trimester, was most strongly associated with birth weight.

After adjustment for confounders (e.g., maternal age, parity, prepregnancy BMI), studies of both gestational and pregestational diabetic women have shown independent positive relationships between maternal weight gain and adverse maternal and fetal outcomes. In women who have GDM, weight gains in excess of those recommended by the IOM were associated with an increased risk of LGA neonates and the need for augmenting diet therapy with insulin therapy to maintain acceptable levels of maternal glycemia.[74] In another report,[75] women who were screened for GDM with the 50-g glucose screening test and whose glucose results were <140 mg/dL and who gained ≤40 pounds during pregnancy had a significantly lower risk of having a macrosomic neonate within each of five incremental categories of the test results than did women who gained >40 pounds. Within the group found to have GDM, those who gained ≤40 pounds had a lower risk of a macrosomic neonate compared with women whose weight gain was >40 pounds (respectively 13.5% vs. 29.3%; $p=0.018$). It appears that weight gain may be more influential than maternal glucose concentrations for developing fetal macrosomia since the risk of macrosomia was greater when a normal GST occurred with a weight gain of more than 40 pounds compared with that of women with one abnormal glucose tolerance test result and a weight gain of less than 40 pounds.[74] Another study that combined the data of pregestational and gestational diabetic women reported positive independent relationships between LGA neonates and both prepregnancy BMI ≥30 and gestational weight gain.[76] In contrast, among women with type 1 diabetes there was no relationship between gestational weight gain and the incidence of LGA neonates,[77] but there was an independent relationship between LGA neonates and hemoglobin A1c concentrations during the second half of pregnancy. Finally, in another study that defined weight gain by subtracting the sum of maternal prepregnancy, neonatal, and placental weights from the maternal weight at term, there was no difference between weight gain and the incidence of

LGA among women with either type 1, gestational, or no diabetes.[78] The data from this study suggest that factors other than maternal weight gain, such as selective maternal-fetal transfer of energy, may influence fetal over-growth.

In summary, in the face of the burgeoning population of overweight and obese reproductive age women, analysis of contemporary data to establish ideal weight gain parameters for women who do and who do not have diabetes is indicated. In both diabetic and non-diabetic women, weight gains during pregnancy as well as maternal hyperglycemia appear to each have an independent relationship with adverse maternal and perinatal outcomes. The relative influence of each of these factors requires further exploration, however.

18.5 Effect of Cultural Beliefs and Practices on Dietary Practices

Many immigrants from developing economy nations are sustained by their indigenous cultural beliefs. Some also arrive bearing little formal education, poor language skills, little experience with and knowledge of the necessities of health care, and how to obtain them. Among immigrants from Mexico (and likely among those from other cultures) information about diet comes most often from family and friends. Thus, incorporating the spouses and members of these women's social networks is an important component of education regarding a healthy diet during pregnancy.[79]

The so-called "Hispanic paradox" refers to the observation, primarily among Mexican immigrants, that despite having a number of demographic characteristics generally associated with adverse pregnancy outcomes (e.g., poverty, limited education, limited access to medical care) Mexican-American women have a lower incidence of low birth weight and prematurity than do Caucasians, Asians, and other people of color living in the USA.[80, 81] That these findings are more prevalent among first generation Mexican immigrant women than among those born in the U.S. may be more easily explained by elements of cultural background than by genetics.[54] In one study,[74] Mexico-born immigrant women were found to consume diets that contained significantly more calories, fiber, folate, vitamins A, C, and E, and zinc than did those of second generation women. When members of both groups who took diet supplements during pregnancy were compared, these differences remained significant except for the amounts of vitamin C consumed. Among the women born in Mexico, the longer they had lived in the USA, the lower their dietary content of calories, fiber, folate, vitamins A, C, and E, iron, and zinc.[82]

Some dietary beliefs and practices are shared by different Asian cultures. In Chinese, Korean, Vietnamese, and Asian subcontinent societies, a balance between the yin, or cool, female, soft, breath forces, and the yang, or hot, male, strong, blood forces, is thought to be necessary to achieve health and well-being for oneself and one's baby. Pregnancy is a "hot" state. Thus, only cold foods are to be consumed. In contrast, the post-partum period is a "cold" period, and only hot foods such as hot water and tea, ginger, vinegar, pigs' feet, and high protein meats are to be consumed. Red meats are an exception and are to be avoided because it is thought that they are slow healing. Brown seaweed soup is consumed during pregnancy and in the first 20 days following delivery. It is thought that brown seaweed soup benefits women postpartum because it cleanses the blood and increases milk production.[83,84] It is interesting that acculturation of Asian women may alter some less healthy dietary customs as well as healthy habits. For example, among Punjabi women living in Canada for 5 years or less, some requested a change from traditional high fat foods to foods with a lower fat content.[85]

In general, there has been little research into the effects of traditional Asian pregnancy diets and birth outcomes. One Australian study reported that there were no significant group differences in total energy intake, maternal weight gain, and birth weight between pregnant immigrants following a traditional Vietnamese diet and those consuming a non-traditional diet.[86] Clearly, more research is needed on acculturation, nutrient intakes, and pregnancy outcomes. A list of beliefs and practices pertaining to pregnancy from several cultures is found in Table 18.5. Understanding these beliefs should help the health care provider to guide the pregnant immigrant to incorporate other healthy dietary practices into their traditional diets.

Table 18.5 Traditional cultural beliefs regarding diet during pregnancy and the puerperium

Mexico Drinking milk during pregnancy causes large babies and difficult births *Ruda con chocolate* (garden rue, an herb, with chocolate) speeds up labor, while chamomile tea is good for labor. *Epizote* (a Mexican herb) cleanses the stomach after delivery. Because birth marks are the result of unsatisfied cravings (*antojos*), it is best to give in to these cravings.
China See text re: "hot" and "cold" foods Avoid shellfish because it may cause a rash on the baby (*www.hawcc.hawaii.edu/nursing/RNChinese02*) Pineapple may cause miscarriages (*www.hawcc.hawaii.edu/nursing/RNChinese02*) Squid and crab may cause the uterus to become sticky (*www.hawcc.hawaii.edu/nursing/RNChinese02*) Coconut milk causes the baby to have good skin quality (*www.hawcc.hawaii.edu/nursing/RNChinese02*) Soup of papaya, fish with papaya, and salty foods increase milk production (*www.hawcc.hawaii.edu/nursing/RNChinese02*)
Vietnam See text re: "hot" and "cold" foods
Korea See text re: "hot" and "cold" foods See text re: brown seaweed soup (*Park*) Food prohibitions including sources of protein: e.g., chicken, squid, pork, fish (*Pritham*)
Punjabi Increased milk intake prevents chloasmae. (*Grewal*) *Soonf* (fennel seeds) roasted in brown sugar induces labor (*Grewal*)

18.6 Lactation in Mothers Who Had GDM

There is no evidence that having had GDM interferes with initiating lactation. However, maternal obesity is a risk factor for lactation failure and, therefore, the prevalence of breast-feeding may be lower among obese women who had GDM. The reported associations between breastfeeding and a reduced risk of childhood obesity are compelling reasons to help obese mothers overcome lactation difficulties.[87] Because lactogenesis is promoted by maternal-fetal contact, one of the simplest ways to promote lactation among obese women is to limit maternal-newborn separation, and to assist the mother in finding comfortable ways to help the infant latch onto the breast. Obese women with larger breasts often have excess periareolar adipose tissue that flattens the areola and nipple making it more difficult for the infant to grasp the nipple.[88]

The energy and nutrient demands for lactating women exceed those of pregnancy.[89] Given the elevated nutrient requirements of lactation, women need dietary counseling on how to plan meals that are nutrient-dense without exceeding their energy requirements. The MyPyramid food pattern developed for lactating women can assist the women in making wise food choices, http://www.mypyramid.gov/mypyramidmoms/index.html.

The postpartum period is also a good time to help obese women who had GDM lose weight and, therefore, reduce their risk for GDM in a subsequent pregnancy. A randomized intervention trial of breastfeeding overweight mothers found that those who reduced energy intake (−500 kcal/day) or who participated in aerobic exercise (45 min/4 days each week) had babies that grew similarly to those of women who were not on an energy-restricted diet or who did not exercise regularly.[90] There is some evidence that energy restriction alone causes a greater loss of lean body mass compared to exercise in combination with energy restriction.[91]

18.7 Conclusions and Research Needed

GDM modifies the metabolism of carbohydrate and fat during pregnancy. Thus, medical nutritional therapy is the cornerstone for treating the disorder. Currently, the American Diabetic Association and the American Dietetic Association recommend developing individualized food plans for each patient that will achieve and maintain normal glycemia, provide sufficient energy to support an appropriate weight gain and avoid maternal ketosis, and supply adequate nutrients for maternal and fetal health. Specific dietary guidelines have not been established for accomplishing these goals. The limited studies of diet therapies for GDM women are observational case reports of a small number of women. Although varying degrees of energy restriction have been used for nearly 100 years to manage GDM, no large-scale, randomized, controlled trials have examined the appropriate energy need per kg body weight for improving glycemic control without ketosis and fetal growth restriction. There is some evidence that the efficacy of an energy-restricted diet is mediated by the amount and type of dietary carbohydrate.

Further studies of this interaction between dietary energy and carbohydrate are needed in women who have GDM. Also, the efficacy of the amount and type of dietary carbohydrate and how it is distributed in the diet throughout the day on improving maternal glycemic control, the need for insulin therapy, and reducing fetal over-growth has not been determined independent of the amount of dietary energy. An assessment of the amount and type of dietary fat for healthy pregnancy outcomes in GDM women is also needed.

Since there is no evidence that the amount of weight gained by GDM women to support optimal fetal growth differs from that of healthy women, the American Diabetes Association recommends that the IOM guidelines for gestational weight gain in healthy women be used for women with GDM. Examination of the effect of restricting weight gain on maternal glycemic control pregnancy outcome is needed to determine if different standards should be established for overweight or obese women with GDM.

Finally, it is important to remember that GDM is a risk factor for future type 2 diabetes and cardiovascular disease. Thus, the dietary counseling provided to GDM women should be based on principles of good life-long dietary habits, and the recommended food patterns should consider the woman's cultural background. This will enhance the likelihood of continuing the recommended food pattern into the postpartum period and, eventually, reducing the risk of GDM and associated morbidities in the mother and her child.

References

1. Dornhorst A, Frost G. The principles of dietary management of gestational diabetes: reflection on current evidence. *J Hum Nutr Diet*. 2002;15:145-156; quiz 157-149.
2. Rasmussen K, Yaktine A. *Weight Gain During Pregnancy: Reexamining the Guidelines*. Washington DC: National Academies Press; 2009.
3. Thomas AM, Gutierrez YM. *Gestational Diabetes Mellitus*. Chicago, IL: American Dietetic Association; 2005.
4. White P. Diabetes complicating pregnancy. *Am J Obstet Gynecol*. 1937;33:380-385.
5. Duncan G. *Diabetes Mellitus: Principles & Treatment*. Philadelphia, PA: WB Saunders; 1951.
6. Moss J, Mulholland H. Diabetes and pregnancy: with special reference to the prediabetic state. *Ann Intern Med*. 1951;34:678-691.
7. Reis R, DeCosta E, Allweiss M. *Diabetes and Pregnancy*. Springfield, IL: Charles C Thomas; 1952.
8. Committee on Maternal Nutrition, Food and Nutrition Board. *Maternal Nutrition and the Course of Pregnancy*. Washington, DC: National Academy of Sciences; 1960.
9. Association AD, Association AD. Principles of nutrition and dietary recommendations for patients with diabetes mellitus. *Diabetes Care*. 1979;2:520-523.
10. American Diabetes Association. Evidence-based nutrition principles and recommendations for the treatment and prevention of diabetes and related complications. *Diabetes Care*. 2002;25:202-212.
11. Institute of Medicine. Food and Nutrition Board. Nutrition during Pregnancy. Part I. Weight Gain. Part II. Nutrient Supplements. National Academy Press, Washington, D.C; 1990.
12. American Dietetic Association. *Medical nutrition Therapy Evidence-Based Guides for Practice: Nutrition Practice Guidelines Type 1 and Type 2 Diabetes Mellitus (CD-ROM)*. Chicago, Ill: American Dietetic Association; 2001.

13. American College of Obstetricians and Gynecologists. Pregestational diabetes mellitus. Practice bulletin no. 60. *Obstet Gynecol*. 2005;105:675-685.
14. Metzger B, Buchanan T, Coustan D, et al. Summary and recommendations of the fifth international workshop-conference on gestational diabetes mellitus. *Diabetes Care*. 2007;30:S251-S260.
15. American Diabetes Association. Nutrition principles and recommendations in diabetes. *Diabetes Care*. 2004;27:S36-S46.
16. Algert S, Shragg P, Hollingsworth DR. Moderate caloric restriction in obese women with gestational diabetes. *Obstet Gynecol*. 1985;65:487-491.
17. Dornhorst A, Nicholls JS, Probst F, et al. Calorie restriction for treatment of gestational diabetes. *Diabetes*. 1991;40(suppl 2):161-164.
18. Gillmer MD, Maresh M, Beard RW, Elkeles RS, Alderson C, Bloxham B. Low energy diets in the treatment of gestational diabetes. *Acta Endocrinol Suppl (Copenh)*. 1986;277:44-49.
19. Knopp RH, Magee MS, Raisys V, Benedetti T, Bonet B. Hypocaloric diets and ketogenesis in the management of obese gestational diabetic women. *J Am Coll Nutr*. 1991;10:649-667.
20. Magee MS, Knopp RH, Benedetti TJ. Metabolic effects of 1200-kcal diet in obese pregnant women with gestational diabetes. *Diabetes*. 1990;39:234-240.
21. Maresh M, Gillmer MD, Beard RW, Alderson CS, Bloxham BA, Elkeles RS. The effect of diet and insulin on metabolic profiles of women with gestational diabetes mellitus. *Diabetes*. 1985;34(suppl 2):88-93.
22. Rae A, Bond D, Evans S, North F, Roberman B, Walters B. A randomised controlled trial of dietary energy restriction in the management of obese women with gestational diabetes. *Aust N Z J Obstet Gynaecol*. 2000;40:416-422.
23. Kopp W. Role of high-insulinogenic nutrition in the etiology of gestational diabetes mellitus. *Med Hypotheses*. 2005;64:101-103.
24. Metzger B, Coustan D. Summary and recommendations of the Fourth International Workshop-Conference on Gestational Diabetes Mellitus. The Organizing Committee. *Diabetes Care*. 1998;21:B161-B167.
25. Major CA, Henry MJ, De Veciana M, Morgan MA. The effects of carbohydrate restriction in patients with diet-controlled gestational diabetes. *Obstet Gynecol*. 1998;91:600-604.
26. Peterson CM, Jovanovic-Peterson L. Percentage of carbohydrate and glycemic response to breakfast, lunch, and dinner in women with gestational diabetes. *Diabetes*. 1991;40:172-174.
27. Romon M, Nuttens MC, Vambergue A, et al. Higher carbohydrate intake is associated with decreased incidence of newborn macrosomia in women with gestational diabetes. *J Am Diet Assoc*. 2001;101:897-902.
28. Sivan E, Homko CJ, Whittaker PG, Reece EA, Chen X, Boden G. Free fatty acids and insulin resistance during pregnancy. *J Clin Endocrinol Metab*. 1998;83:2338-2342.
29. Clapp JF III. Effect of dietary carbohydrate on the glucose and insulin response to mixed caloric intake and exercise in both nonpregnant and pregnant women. *Diabetes Care*. 1998;21:B107-B112.
30. Fraser RB, Ford FA, Milner RD. A controlled trial of a high dietary fibre intake in pregnancy–effects on plasma glucose and insulin levels. *Diabetologia*. 1983;25:238-241.
31. Zhang C, Liu S, Solomon CG, Hu FB. Dietary fiber intake, dietary glycemic load, and the risk for gestational diabetes mellitus. *Diabetes Care*. 2006;29:2223-2230.
32. Tieu J, Crowther CA, Middleton P. Dietary advice in pregnancy for preventing gestational diabetes mellitus. *Cochrane Database Syst Rev*. 2008:CD006674.
33. Clapp JF III. Maternal carbohydrate intake and pregnancy outcome. *Proc Nutr Soc*. 2002;61:45-50.
34. Moses RG, Luebcke M, Davis WS, et al. Effect of a low-glycemic-index diet during pregnancy on obstetric outcomes. *Am J Clin Nutr*. 2006;84:807-812.
35. Ilic S, Jovanovic L, Pettitt DJ. Comparison of the effect of saturated and monounsaturated fat on postprandial plasma glucose and insulin concentration in women with gestational diabetes mellitus. *Am J Perinatol*. 1999;16:489-495.

36. Bo S, Menato G, Lezo A, et al. Dietary fat and gestational hyperglycaemia. *Diabetologia*. 2001;44:972-978.
37. Wang Y, Storlien LH, Jenkins AB, et al. Dietary variables and glucose tolerance in pregnancy. *Diabetes Care*. 2000;23:460-464.
38. Saldana TM, Siega-Riz AM, Adair LS. Effect of macronutrient intake on the development of glucose intolerance during pregnancy. *Am J Cin Nutr*. 2004;79:479-486.
39. Radesky JS, Oken E, Rifas-Shiman SL, Kleinman KP, Rich-Edwards JW, Gillman MW. Diet during early pregnancy and development of gestational diabetes. *Paediatr Perinat Epidemiol*. 2008;22:47-59.
40. Riserus U. Fatty acids and insulin sensitivity. *Curr Opin Clin Nutr Metab Care*. 2008;11:100-105.
41. Zhang C, Schulze M, Solomon C, Hu FB. A prospective study of dietary patterns, meat intake and the risk of gestational diabetes mellitus. *Diabetologia*. 2006;49:2604-2613.
42. Otten J, Hellwig J, Meyers L. *Dietary Reference Intakes: the essential guide to nutrient requirements*. Washington, D.C: National Academies Press; 2006.
43. Ritchie L, King JC. Nutrient recommendations and dietary guidelines for pregnant women. In: Lammi-Keefe C, Couch S, Philipson E, eds. *Handbook of Nutrition and Pregnancy*. Totowa, NJ: Humana Press; 2008:3-25.
44. Catalano PM, Kirwan JP, Haugel-de Mouzon S, King J. Gestational diabetes and insulin resistance: role in short- and long-term implications for mother and fetus. *J Nutr*. 2003;133:1674S-1683S.
45. Bo S, Lezo A, Menato G, et al. Gestational hyperglycemia, zinc, selenium, and antioxidant vitamins. *Nutrition*. 2005;21:186-191.
46. Jovanovic-Peterson L, Peterson CM. Vitamin and mineral deficiencies which may predispose to glucose intolerance of pregnancy. *J Am Coll Nutr*. 1996;15:14-20.
47. Woods S, Ghodsi V, Engel A, Miller J, James S. Serum chromium and gestational diabetes. *J Am Board Fam Med*. 2008;21:153-157.
48. Gunton J, Hams G, Hitchman R, McElduff A. Serum chromium does not predict glucose tolerance in late pregnancy. *Am J Cin Nutr*. 2001;73:99-104.
49. Althuis MD, Jordan NE, Ludington EA, Wittes JT. Glucose and insulin responses to dietary chromium supplements: a meta-analysis. *Am J Clin Nutr*. 2002;76:148-155.
50. Zhang C, Qiu C, Hu FB, et al. Maternal plasma 25-hydroxyvitamin D concentrations and the risk for gestational diabetes mellitus. *PLoS One*. 2008;3:e3753.
51. Clifton-Bligh RJ, McElduff P, McElduff A. Maternal vitamin D deficiency, ethnicity and gestational diabetes. *Diabet Med*. 2008;25:678-684.
52. National Institutes of Health. Department of Health and Human Services. National Hearth, Lung, and Blood Institute. Clinical guidelines on the identification, evaluation, and treatment of overweight and obesity in adults.1998.
53. World Health Organizaton. *Obesity: Preventing and Managing the Global Epidemic*. Report of a WHO consultation presented the World Health Organization: 3-5 June 1997; Geneva, Switzerland; 1998.
54. US Department of Health and Human Services National Institutes of Health NIH Publication No. 06–5130. Healthy eating and physical activity across your life-span: fit for two: tips for pregnancy. NIDDK weight-control information network. 2002.
55. Committee on the Impact of Pregnancy Weight on Maternal and Child Health. National Research Council. Influence of Pregnancy Weight on Maternal and Child Health: Workshop Report: 1-49; 2007
56. Helms E, Coulson CC, Galvin SL. Trends in weight gain during pregnancy: a population study across 16 years in North Carolina. *Am J Obstet Gynecol*. 2006;194:e32-e34.
57. American Diabetes Association. Nutrition Recommendations and Interventions for Diabetes: a position statement of the American Diabetes Association. *Diabetes Care*. 2008;31(suppl 1): S61-S78.

58. Rodbard HW, Blonde L, Braithwaite SS, et al; AACE Diabetes Mellitus Clinical Practice Guidelines Task Force. American Association of Clinical Endocrinologists medical guidelines for clinical practice for the management of diabetes mellitus. *Endocr Pract.* 2007;13 (suppl 1):1-68.
59. American Dietetic Association. Position of the American Dietetic Association. Nutrition and lifestyle for a healthy pregnancy outcome. *J Am Diet Assoc.* 2008;108:553-561.
60. ACOG Practice Bulletin. Clinical Management Guidelines for Obstetrician-Gynecologists Number 64, July 2005 (Replaces Committee American Association of Clinical Endocrinologists medical guidelines for clinical practice for the management of diabetes mellitus). *Endocr Pract.* 2007;13(suppl 1):1-68.
61. Opinion Number 238. Hemoglobinpathies in pregnancy. *Obstet Gynecol.* 2000;106:203-210.
62. ACOG Committee Opinion number 315. Obesity in pregnancy. *Obstet Gynecol.* 2005;106: 671-675.
63. Klein S, Sheard NF, Pi-Sunyer X, et al. Weight management through lifestyle modification for the prevention and management of type 2 diabetes: rationale and strategies. A statement of the American Diabetes Association, the North American Association for the Study of Obesity, and the American Society for Clinical Nutrition. *Am J Clin Nutr.* 2004;80:257-263.
64. Artal R, Catanzaro RB, Gavard JA, Mostello DJ, Friganza JC. A lifestyle intervention of weight-gain restriction: diet and exercise in obese women with gestational diabetes mellitus. *Appl Physiol Nutr Metab.* 2007;32:596-601.
65. Cedergren M. Effects of gestational weight gain and body mass index on obstetric outcome in Sweden. *Int J Gynaecol Obstet.* 2006;93:269-274.
66. Jensen DM, Ovesen P, Beck-Nielsen H, et al. Gestational weight gain and pregnancy outcomes in 481 obese glucose-tolerant women. *Diabetes Care.* 2005;28:2118-2122.
67. Hedderson MM, Weiss NS, Sacks DA, et al. Pregnancy weight gain and risk of neonatal complications: macrosomia, hypoglycemia, and hyperbilirubinemia. *Obstet Gynecol.* 2006;108: 1153-1161.
68. Stotland NE, Cheng YW, Hopkins LM, Caughey AB. Gestational weight gain and adverse neonatal outcome among term infants. *Obstet Gynecol.* 2006;108:635-643.
69. Kabali C, Werler MM. Pre-pregnant body mass index, weight gain and the risk of delivering large babies among non-diabetic mothers. *Int J Gynaecol Obstet.* 2007;97:100-104.
70. Jain NJ, Denk CE, Kruse LK, Dandolu V. Maternal obesity: can pregnancy weight gain modify risk of selected adverse pregnancy outcomes? *Am J Perinatol.* 2007;24:291-298.
71. Cedergren MI. Optimal gestational weight gain for body mass index categories. *Obstet Gynecol.* 2007;110:759-764.
72. Kiel DW, Dodson EA, Artal R, Boehmer TK, Leet TL. Gestational weight gain and pregnancy outcomes in obese women: how much is enough? *Obstet Gynecol.* 2007;110:752-758.
73. Dawes MG, Grudzinskas JG. Patterns of maternal weight gain in pregnancy. *Br J Obstet Gynaecol.* 1991;98:195-201.
74. Abrams B, Selvin S. Maternal weight gain pattern and birth weight. *Obstet Gynecol.* 1995; 86:163-169.
75. Cheng YW, Chung JH, Kurbisch-Block I, Inturrisi M, Shafer S, Caughey AB. Gestational weight gain and gestational diabetes mellitus: perinatal outcomes. *Obstet Gynecol.* 2008; 112:1015-1022.
76. Hillier TA, Pedula KL, Vesco KK, et al. Excess gestational weight gain: modifying fetal macrosomia risk associated with maternal glucose. *Obstet Gynecol.* 2008;112:1007-1014.
77. Ray JG, Vermeulen MJ, Shapiro JL, Kenshole AB. Maternal and neonatal outcomes in pregestational and gestational diabetes mellitus, and the influence of maternal obesity and weight gain: the DEPOSIT study. Diabetes Endocrine Pregnancy Outcome Study in Toronto. *QJM.* 2001;94:347-356.

78. Nielsen GL, Dethlefsen C, Moller M, Sorensen HT. Maternal glycated haemoglobin, pregestational weight, pregnancy weight gain and risk of large-for-gestational-age babies: a Danish cohort study of 209 singleton Type 1 diabetic pregnancies. *Diabet Med.* 2007;24:384-387.
79. Lepercq J, Hauguel-De Mouzon S, Timsit J, Catalano PM. Fetal macrosomia and maternal weight gain during pregnancy. *Diabetes Metab.* 2002;28:323-328.
80. Thornton PL, Kieffer EC, Salabarria-Pena Y, et al. Weight, diet, and physical activity-related beliefs and practices among pregnant and postpartum Latino women: the role of social support. *Matern Child Health J.* 2006;10:95-104.
81. Report of final natality statistics AND National Center for health statistics. *Monthly Vit Statist Rep.* 1997;45:6-8.
82. Gutierrez YM. Cultural factors affecting diet and pregnancy outcome of Mexican American adolescents. *J Adolesc Health.* 1999;25:227-237.
83. Harley K, Eskenazi B, Block G. The association of time in the US and diet during pregnancy in low-income women of Mexican descent. *Paediatr Perinat Epidemiol.* 2005;19:125-134.
84. Park KJ, Peterson LM. Beliefs, practices, and experiences of Korean women in relation to childbirth. *Health Care Women Int.* 1991;12:261-269.
85. Pritham UA, Sammons LN. Korean women's attitudes toward pregnancy and prenatal care. *Health Care Women Int.* 1993;14:145-153.
86. Grewal SK, Bhagat R, Balneaves LG. Perinatal beliefs and practices of immigrant Punjabi women living in Canada. *J Obstet Gynecol Neonatal Nurs.* 2008;37:290-300.
87. Mitchell J, Mackerras D. The traditional humoral food habits of pregnant Vietnamese-Australian women and their effect on birth weight. *Aust J Public Health.* 1995;19:629-633.
88. Owen CG, Martin RM, Whincup PH, Davey-Smith G, Gillman MW, Cook DG. The effect of breastfeeding on mean body mass index throughout life: a quantitative review of published and unpublished observational evidence. *Am J Clin Nutr.* 2005;82:1298-1307.
89. Jevitt C, Hernandez I, Groer M. Lactation complicated by overweight and obesity: supporting the mother and newborn. *J Midwifery Womens Health.* 2007;52:606-613.
90. O'Connor D, Houghton L, Sherwood K. Nutrition issues during lactation. In: Lammi-Keefe C, Couch S, Philipson E, eds. *Handbook of Nutrition and Pregnancy.* Totowa, NJ: Humana Press; 2008.
91. Lovelady C, Garner K, Moreno K, Williams J. The effect of weight loss in overweight, lactating women on the growth of their infants. *N Engl J Med.* 2000;342:449-453.
92. Gunderson EP. Gestational diabetes and nutritional recommendations. *Curr Diab Rep.* 2004;4:377-386.

Pharmacological Treatment Options for Gestational Diabetes

19

Oded Langer

19.1 Introduction

Gestational diabetes mellitus, or GDM, is defined as carbohydrate intolerance first diagnosed during pregnancy.[1] In the United States, approximately 135–200,000 women annually develop GDM; this is in addition to those pregnant women already afflicted with either type 1 or type 2 diabetes.[2] There has been a significant increase (approaching 33%) in the incidence of type 2 diabetes with its recognized parallel risk for obesity[3] as well as the insidious rise of adolescent obesity in the offspring of diabetic women.[4]

Maternal hyperglycemia and the resultant fetal hyperinsulinemia are central to the pathophysiology of diabetic complications of pregnancy. These complications include congenital malformations, an increase in neonatal intensive care unit admission, and birth trauma. In addition, there is an increased rate of accelerated fetal growth, neonatal metabolic complications, and risk of stillbirth.[5,6]

The definition of GDM is problematic, since several million type 2 diabetic women are not diagnosed until pregnancy.[1] These women are usually classified as having GDM; thus, GDM actually represents a mixture of women with abnormal carbohydrate tolerance test results in pregnancy and those with previously undiagnosed type 2 diabetes. The prevalence of GDM varies in direct proportion to the prevalence of type 2 diabetes in a given population, ethnic group, or geographic area. As a result, studies report varying rates of population prevalence and complications. In the US, reported prevalence rates range from 1 to 14%.[7] The similarities between type 2 diabetes and GDM as to risk factors, metabolic abnormalities, and endocrine abnormalities provide the rationale for proposing that GDM is an "early" type 2 diabetes and thus represents the same disease with a different name.

Type 2 diabetes and GDM are heterogeneous disorders whose pathophysiology is characterized by peripheral insulin resistance, impaired regulation of hepatic glucose production, and declining β-cell function. The primary events in both are deficits in insulin secretion, followed by peripheral insulin resistance. Glucose intolerance follows β-cell

O. Langer
Department of Obstetrics and Gynecology, St Luke's-Roosevelt Hospital Center, University Hospital of Columbia University, New York, NY, USA
e-mail: odlanger@chpnet.org

C. Kim and A. Ferrara (eds.), *Gestational Diabetes During and After Pregnancy*, DOI: 10.1007/978-1-84882-120-0_19, © Springer-Verlag London Limited 2010

dysfunction (impairment in the first phase of insulin secretion). In the second phase, the release of newly synthesized insulin is impaired. When tight glycemic control is achieved, there may follow a reversal of the effects of glucose toxicity that produce the intrapancreatic (desensitization of β-cells) or extra-pancreatic effect.[8–11]

It has become self-evident that the treatment goal for pregnant and nonpregnant diabetic patients is to optimize the glycemic profile. This is customarily performed in the pregnant diabetic woman with the trial of diet therapy and the addition of pharmacological therapy (insulin or oral antidiabetic drugs such as glyburide) when glycemic control cannot be achieved by diet alone. Therefore, investigators have chosen blood glucose control as the primary outcome variable when comparing drugs designed to reduce levels of glycemia.[12–15]

In this chapter, I briefly discuss the pathophysiology of GDM and diabetes and how these relate to the therapies for GDM. I briefly review medical nutrition therapy and physical activity, followed by a more detailed review of pharmacologic therapies. Particular attention is paid to the sulfonylureas or oral agents, specifically regarding safety during and after pregnancy for mothers and offspring, effectiveness for glycemic control, and cost.

19.2 Pathophysiology

Autoimmunity is a major component of the pathophysiology of insulin-dependent diabetes mellitus (type 1) characterized by β-cell destruction. The autoimmune systems responsible for β-cell demise are actively functioning prior to the appearance of clinical diabetes. Markers for this deterioration are islet-cell and insulin autoantibodies, antibodies to glutamic acid decarboxylase, and other β-cell antigens. Viruses, dietary factors, and exposure to chemicals have also been implicated in the development of type 1 diabetes.

The pathophysiology of type 2 diabetes is characterized by increased hepatic glucose production, abnormal insulin secretion, and increased insulin resistance, all contributors to hyperglycemia. The increase in hepatic glucose production is a secondary phenomenon related mainly to the decrease in insulin action and increased glucagon secretion. During normal pregnancy, the marked reduction of insulin sensitivity could be compensated by a reciprocal increase in β-cell secretion. Therefore, pregnancy may be characterized as a state of hyperinsulinemia and insulin resistance as a response to the diabetogenic effects on normal carbohydrate metabolism.

Women who develop GDM have a higher insulin resistance prior to conception, often in association with obesity. Insulin resistance results in decreased glucose uptake in skeletal muscles, white adipose tissue, and the liver, as well as suppression of hepatic glucose production. The β-cell adaptation to insulin resistance is impaired in GDM women and may be a universal response to the insulin resistance, since it is found in many ethnic groups. Women with a history of GDM have an increased risk of developing type 2 diabetes later in life. The reported risk ranges from 6.8 to 92% when the results of an impaired glucose tolerance (IGT) test are combined with overt diabetes, and is 3–50% for overt diabetes alone.[16] Furthermore, there is a 2–4 fold (27–38%) increased rate of metabolic syndrome in women with previous GDM. This rate is even higher in previous obese GDM (tenfold) and GDM-treated with diet (sevenfold).[17–21]

19.3 The Rationale and Fundamental Structure of Intensified Therapy

Intensified therapy is an approach to achieving established levels of glycemic control. It incorporates memory-based self-monitoring blood glucose, multiple injections of insulin or its equivalent, diet, and an interdisciplinary team effort. These integrally related components often make the difference between success and failure in diabetes management. We demonstrated in a large prospective study that intensified therapy, in comparison to the conventional approach, resulted not only in improved perinatal outcome, regardless of ethnic origin, with similar compliance for diet and insulin therapies.[21–23]

Diabetes-related complications can be decreased for both pregnant and nonpregnant patients with intensified therapy that results in improved glycemic control.[15–24] However, there is a paucity of data addressing the glucose profile in nondiabetic pregnancies. Recently, two studies of nondiabetic pregnant women addressed the characteristics of normoglycemia in day-to-day settings during the third trimester. One study using self-monitoring blood glucose[25] reported a gradual increase in mean blood glucose in the third trimester. Our study[25] used a system that measured continuous blood glucose in obese and nonobese nondiabetic women. These studies imply that currently recommended clinical thresholds may be associated with improved pregnancy outcome, but they are not the equivalent of the biological norm in the nondiabetic pregnant state. For example, a threshold of <140 mg/dL postprandial and/or 120 mg/dL preprandial was reported to be associated with a decreased rate of anomalies, while a mean blood glucose of <100–110 mg/dL was linked to decreased rates of large-for-gestational-age infants (LGA) or macrosomia.[26–28] Therefore, different thresholds of glycemia are required to minimize specific complications in the pregnant diabetic patient.

Regardless of the treatment modality used, the goal is always to achieve the established level of glycemic control that will diminish the rate of hypoglycemia and ketosis and maximize perinatal outcome. Although there is ample evidence that there is an association between diabetes control and the occurrence of maternal/fetal complications, this association does not prove cause and effect. It does, however, provide the rationale to attempt to control the glucose levels.

19.4 Diet and Exercise: Ancillary Modalities for Glucose Control

For all types of diabetes, the underlying foundation of treatment is diet. The essential principle of nutritional therapy is to achieve and maintain the maternal blood glucose profile comparable to that of the nondiabetic woman. Two current approaches are recommended: (1) decrease the proportion of carbohydrates to 40–50% in a daily regimen of 3 meals and

3–4 snacks and, (2) use of lower glycemic index carbohydrates for approximately 60% of daily intake. The assignment of daily caloric intake is similar for gestational and pregestational diabetes and is calculated based on pre-pregnancy body mass index (BMI).[29]

The second component of a diabetes treatment protocol is exercise. In isolation, it is not a cure for diabetes, however, exercise acts to improve insulin sensitivity and glucose tolerance. I believe that a tempered exercise program, when pregnant diabetic women are not only willing but also able (socio-economic limitations, obesity, multi-parity) to participate may improve postprandial blood glucose levels and insulin sensitivity.[30,31] Hypoglycemic reactions during and after exercise may be positive markers of improved insulin sensitivity. Low blood glucose necessitates adjustment of the insulin dose and carbohydrate intake. Extra monitoring is warranted after evening exercise, as glucose uptake increases for several hours after exercise and can cause nocturnal hypoglycemia.

19.5 Alternative Routes in Pharmacological Therapy

When diet therapy fails to achieve established levels of glycemic control, insulin and oral hypoglycemic and antihyperglycemic agents are the validated alternatives to treatment. When pharmacological therapy is a consideration for management, several questions need to be addressed. Who should receive it? How long should a patient remain on diet therapy before the introduction of pharmacological treatment? What is the required dose in order to achieve the established level of glycemic control?

19.6 Insulin Therapy

In GDM, opinions of authoritative bodies differ regarding the threshold of fasting plasma glucose for the initiation of pharmacological therapy (glyburide, metformin or insulin). Furthermore, the amount of insulin required to achieve targeted levels of glycemic control is still debated. This debate is, in part, due to study subjects' differing ethnicities, as well as their rates of obesity (Table 19.1). Regardless of these confounding factors, the ultimate measure should always be the rate of study participants who achieved the targeted level of glycemia.

We evaluated 57 GDM women with normal OGTT postpartum and found a biphasic increase in insulin requirements. The first phase was characterized by a significant weekly increase up to the 30th week of gestation; from 31 to 39 weeks the insulin dose remained unchanged. Insulin requirements for obese patients were 0.9 units/kg and for nonobese subjects 0.8 units/kg. There was a significant difference in variability as measured by the coefficient of variation (45 vs. 25%, $p<0.01$), respectively. These findings suggest that GDM women need weekly visits during the 20th–30th weeks of gestation for insulin adjustment. Moreover, the total insulin dose required to reach the established level of glycemic control for the majority of patients ranges from 40 to 90 units (body-weight dependent).[32]

Table 19.1 Studies reporting the use of oral hypoglycemic and antihyperglycemic agents in pregnancy; success of therapy

	Design	Number of patients					Achievement of good control
		Type of patients	Glyburide	Reg. insulin	Metformin	Other	
Langer et al[14]	RCT	GDM	201	203			82 and 88%
Conway et al[62] 100	Prospective observational	GDM	75				84%
Kremer and Duff[52]	Prospective observational	GDM	73				81%
Chmait et al[65]	Prospective observational	GDM	69				82%
Gilson and Murphy[66]	Prospective observational	GDM	22	22			82%
Fines et al[67]	Retrospective case–control	GDM	40	44			NA
Glueck et al (2002)[74]	Prospective observational	PCOS			42		
	Prospective and retrospective observational	PCOS		39	33	39 without metformin	
Hellmuth et al (2001)[63]	Prospective observational	GDM		42	50	68 sulfonylurea	
Notelovitz[64]	RCT	GDM and Type-2 diabetes		52		tolbutamide, chlorpropramide	80% using oral hypoglycemic and 36% using insulin
Yogev et al[77]	Prospective	GDM	25	30		27 diet-treated	Mean blood glucose similar in all groups

Another question frequently confronted by clinicians is which form of insulin should be recommended for the pregnant diabetic patient. Human insulin became widely available in the 1980s when the preferred method of production was recombinant DNA technology. This led to the availability of mutant insulin (insulin analogs) during the mid-1990s that were designed primarily to have improved pharmacokinetic features for subcutaneous administration. In pregnancy, however, human insulin is recommended since the use of insulin analogs has not been adequately tested in GDM.

There is little or no difference between insulin lispro, insulin aspart, and human insulin in receptor binding, metabolic, and mitogenic potency with a slight increased binding of insulin lispro to the receptor for IGF-1.[33–36] Mounting evidence of the beneficial effects of insulin lispro in type 1 and type 2 nonpregnant diabetic subjects include decreased frequency of severe hypoglycemic episodes, limited postprandial glucose excursions, and a possible decrease in glycosylated hemoglobin when the drug is administered by continuous subcutaneous infusion. In addition, insulin lispro provides greater convenience in the timing of administration (analogs administered up to 15 min after start of a meal compared to soluble insulin taken 30 min before the meal).[33–36]

In pregnancy, data on insulin lispro are limited and abstracted from studies with relatively small sample sizes. Most of these reports demonstrated an improvement in glycemic control, an increase in patient satisfaction, a decrease in hypoglycemic episodes, but no data on maternal and neonatal outcome. This omission limits the ability to draw any firm conclusions about the efficacy of insulin lispro in comparison to human insulin in pregnancy.

19.7 Oral Antidiabetic Drugs in GDM Treatment

Oral hypoglycemic and antihyperglycemic agents are successfully used in the treatment of nonpregnant type 2 diabetes. Each may be used alone or in combination with other oral agents or insulin. Oral antidiabetic agents are convenient to use, less invasive than insulin, and relatively less expensive. Therefore, they can become the drug of choice when dietary modifications fail to reduce hyperglycemia. Oral antidiabetic agents are used in the United States especially to provide type 2 diabetes patients with support in maintaining the tight glucose control that lowers their risk for microvascular complications. Both the United Kingdom Prospective Diabetes Study (UKPDS) and the Diabetes Control and Complications Trial (DCCT) studies[23,37] strongly support the use of intensive therapy in patients with type 1 and type 2 diabetes to achieve and maintain near-normal HbA1c levels and to prevent diabetic complications.

Recently, opinions have shifted towards the use of these drugs during pregnancy. In fact, the use of glyburide has replaced insulin as first-line drug treatment of GDM in many obstetric practices.[35,38] In addition, many experts and authoritative bodies in the United States have recommended the use of glyburide (sulfonylurea) as an alternative pharmacological therapy to insulin in pregnancy.[36,39–42] Others, however, have recommend further evaluation.[43–45]

The rationale is significantly lower in glyburide vs. insulin-treated by three main factors:

1. GDM and patients with IGT have a milder hyperglycemia in comparison to type 2 diabetic individuals. Since oral antidiabetic agents can decrease the glycemic profile in type 2 diabetes, it is reasonable to hypothesize that they will be even more effective in the treatment of GDM.
2. There is a similarity in the pathogenesis of type 2 diabetes and GDM. In addition to the insulin secretion and resistance abnormalities found in both conditions, there is a loss of the first-phase insulin secretion with a striking lag time between the post-prandial rise in glucose and the presence of significant insulin at the peripheral sites. This will result in an early increase in postprandial glucose values. Since second-generation sulfonylurea agents are rapid in onset and have short duration of action, it makes them ideal agents to treat very early stages of type 2 and possibly GDM patients.
3. The UKPDS, a randomized trial of type 2 diabetes, supported the efficacy of these drugs and in particular the use of glyburide.[23]

The UKPDS,[23] the largest prospective study evaluating the impact of oral antidiabetic agents on the outcome of type 2 diabetes, demonstrated that in 70% of patients a desirable level of glucose control was achieved with the use of sulfonylurea-glyburide. The most favorable effect was obtained within the first 5 years of the disease (70% of the patients treated with glyburide achieved the desired goal). In years 3, 6, and 9, the desired goals were achieved by fewer than 55, 40, and 30% of patients, respectively, using a single agent (insulin, sulfonylurea, or metformin). With greater deterioration in β-cell function, multiple therapies will eventually be needed in the majority of patients to achieve glycemic target levels.

The study also demonstrated a 25% reduction of risk, primarily attributed to microvascular complications, and a trend toward fewer macrovascular complications after intensive therapy vs. conventional therapy. Improved glycemic control rather than a specific therapy was the primary factor responsible for the reduced risk of complications because all treatments (e.g., insulin, sulfonyurea, metformin) had similar risk reduction. The objective of the study's glucose threshold (HbA1c<7) was to decrease microvascular complications, however, this threshold is insufficient to decrease pregnancy-related complications. In comparison to the UKPDS success rate in achieving glycemic control in type 2 diabetes with the use of glyburide, women with GDM who characteristically have a milder glycemic profile should have an equal or greater success in achieving glycemic control with the use of antidiabetic agents.[46,47]

As with type 1 and type 2 diabetes, the use of oral agents is a pragmatic alternative to insulin therapy in pregnancy because of ease of administration and patient satisfaction with a noninvasive treatment. However, these reasons alone, although valid, are not adequate to introduce a new drug if improvement in pregnancy outcome as well as cost effectiveness is not associated with its use. Therefore, several relevant outcomes will be addressed.

19.8 Does Glyburide Cross the Placenta?

In order for a drug to be potentially functional and safe in pregnancy, it should not cross the placenta and/or not be detrimental to the fetus at clinically significant concentrations. We demonstrated that glyburide (glibenclamide) does not cross the human placenta from the maternal to fetal circulation in significant amounts. Since the placenta of the diabetic mother is characterized by dilation of capillaries, relatively immature villous structure and chronic disturbances in intervillous circulation, we studied the placentas of both nondiabetic and diabetic mothers. There was virtually no transport of the drug even with maternal concentrations 3–4 times higher than peak therapeutic levels. We also demonstrated that first generation sulfonylureas diffused across the placenta most freely.[48–51] Furthermore, in mothers treated with therapeutic plasma concentrations of glyburide, the drug was undetectable in the cord blood (using high-performance liquid chromatography) of their neonates.[14] Our findings were confirmed by multiple studies, all reassuring that neither glyburide nor its metabolite cross the placenta. Several studies shed additional light on the reason why glyburide does not cross the placenta, confirming its safety in pregnancy.[42,52–54]

19.9 Are Patients Who Use Oral Agents at a Higher Risk for Developing Congenital Malformations than those on Insulin?

The concern over congenital anomalies and the effect on the fetus, mainly hypoglycemia and growth stimulation, were reported as case studies using first generation sulfonylureas in small-sample retrospective studies.[55–57] For example, the results of a study of increased rate of congenital malformations involved 20 type 2 patients with hyperglycemia before conception (HbA1c>8). Thus, it is impossible to define if the rate of anomalies was due to the use of the drug or the existing hyperglycemia.[58] In contrast, several studies demonstrated that the cause of anomalies in oral hypoglycemic agent users is associated with altered maternal glucose metabolism, and not the drug. Towner et al, in a study of 332 type 2 patients, demonstrated that mode of therapy (oral agents or insulin) was not associated with anomalies, however level of glycemia and maternal age were significant contributors to their development.[59] Moreover, a recent meta-analysis failed to demonstrate an increased risk of fetal anomalies with sulfonylurea drugs.[60,61]

19.10 Is Glyburide as Effective as Insulin in Controlling Blood Glucose?

Several retrospective and randomized studies evaluated the efficacy of oral agents during pregnancy with an 80–85% reported success rate. The majority of studies demonstrated that these agents were comparable to insulin in their ability to achieve established levels of glycemic control and pregnancy outcome[52,62–72] (Table 19.2).

Table 19.2 Studies reporting the use of oral hypoglycemic and antihyperglycemic agents in pregnancy; neonatal outcome

		Number of patients				
	Design	Glyburide	Insulin	Metformin	Complications	LGA
Langer et al[14]	RCT	201	203		No difference in metabolic complications, congenital anomalies and perinatal mortality	12 and 13%
Conway et al[62]	Prospective observational	75			NA	NA
Kremer and Duff[52]	Prospective observational	73				19% Macrosomia
Chmait et al[65]	Prospective observational	69			Cesarean section 36%	7% Macrosomia
Gilson and Murphy[70]	Prospective observational	22	22		No significant difference in the rate between insulin and glyburide treated groups	No significant difference between insulin and glyburide groups
Fines et al[67]	Retrospective case–control	40	44		No difference in ponderal index between the groups	Less macrosomia in the glyburide group (5/40 vs. 11/44)
Glueck et al[74]	Prospective observational			42	GDM developed in 7.1% of patients	
	Prospective and retrospec-tive observational			33	GDM developed in 3% of patients treated with metformin vs. 27% without treatment	

(continued)

Table 19.2 (continued)

	Design	Number of patients			Complications	LGA
		Glyburide	Insulin	Metformin		
Hellmuth et al[63]	Prospective observational		42	50	No significant difference in neonatal morbidity. Higher rate of preeclampsia (32 vs. 10%) and perinatal mortality (11.6 vs. 1.3%) in metformin group	
Notelovitz[64]	RCT		52		No significant difference in perinatal mortality, metabolic complications and congenital anomalies	
Yogev at al[25,77]	Prospective	25	30		Significant lower rate of maternal hypoglycemia In glyburide group	

Although showing similar rates of success to those in our study, many studies showed significantly higher rates of adverse outcomes. In a randomized controlled trial, we compared glyburide with the traditional insulin therapy in 404 GDM women. The primary outcome was the ability to achieve established levels of glycemic control; insulin and glyburide had comparable results. Moreover, adequate glycemic control was obtained with significantly fewer hypoglycemic episodes in the glyburide group vs. the insulin group. Importantly, complications that have been anecdotally attributed to the drug due to transplacental passage were not observed. The insulin and glyburide-treated patients showed comparable results in cord-serum insulin concentrations, incidence of macrosomia, increased ponderal index, LGA infants, neonatal metabolic complications (hypoglycemia, polycythemia, and hyperbilirubinemia), respiratory complications, and cesarean delivery.[14] Finally, although not measured in our study, the acceptability of the pill over an injection is an additional advantage of the drug.

Recently, the results of a large randomized study compared the use of metformin and insulin in pregnancy.[73] This trial of 751 women demonstrated that the infants of mothers taking metformin showed comparable results to those in the insulin group. Although glyburide and metformin have not been compared in clinical trails, in the current study, 46% of subjects in the metformin group required supplemental insulin while in our study[14] only 4% of women treated with glyburide needed insulin in order to achieve targeted levels of glycemic control. These differences may be the result of varying study criteria as well as different populations and differing target levels for glucose control achieved in each study. In fact, the rate of macrosomia and LGA in the metformin study was twofold higher than that in the glyburide study. Similar findings regarding the effect of metformin use in pregnancy in retrospective studies suggested a decreased rate of abortion and GDM in polycystic ovarian syndrome patients.[74, 75]

19.11 Is Glyburide as Effective as Insulin at all GDM Severity Levels?

We analyzed the association among glyburide dose, severity of GDM, and selected maternal and neonatal factors. Glyburide and insulin are equally efficacious for GDM treatment at all severity levels of diabetes when fasting plasma glucose results on the oral glucose tolerance test were between 95 and 139 mg/dL. Over 80% of GDM patients requiring pharmacological intervention achieved the established levels of glycemic control with either glyburide or insulin. The majority of patients (71%) will require, on average, a 10 mg daily dose of glyburide to achieve glycemic control. Furthermore, in all disease severity levels, glyburide-treated and insulin-treated subjects had comparable success rates in achieving the targeted levels with similar pregnancy outcome.[76] Again, achieving the established level of glycemic control, not the mode of pharmacological therapy, is the key to improving pregnancy outcome in GDM.

The varying reported rates of outcomes of interest in the glyburide studies (glycemic control and perinatal outcomes) may be explained by a number of factors. When comparing different studies' success rates in achieving glycemic control, different criteria for targeted levels of glycemic control influence the results. Furthermore, different populations (ethnic and geographic groups) and sample size, as well as quality and method of glucose testing (self-monitoring, postprandial, preprandial, or mean blood glucose) will also influence the definition of success in a given study. Finally, the physician factor with respect to patient-care, provider communication, and drug administration (dose and algorithms) were shown to significantly affect the failure rate to achieve targeted levels of control. Therefore, it is not surprising that studies reported similar success rates in achieving desired levels of glycemic control for insulin or glyburide-treated patients but with unacceptable perinatal outcome in both groups, i.e., LGA and/or macrosomic rates of approximately 30–45%.

19.12 Does the Rate of Maternal Hypoglycemia Increase During Glyburide Therapy?

Hypoglycemia is the main side effect of glyburide treatment in nonpregnant women. However, the majority of type 2 diabetic persons who used this drug in the nonpregnant state are older than the average gravida. Thus, the severity of the hypoglycemia may be less pronounced in the younger age group of GDM women. In our study[77] we used a continuous glucose monitoring system that recorded data every 5 min for 72 continuous hours, capturing 288 measurements/day. We found that asymptomatic hypoglycemic events, defined as more than 30 consecutive minutes of glucose values below 50 mg/dL, were found in 63% of the insulin-treated GDM compared with 28% in the glyburide-treated women. Thus, although some laboratory hypoglycemic episodes (using self-monitoring blood glucose or laboratory plasma values) may be identified during pharmacological therapy, the rate of these episodes will be significantly lower in glyburide vs. insulin-treated women (Table 19.3).

19.13 Is Glyburide Therapy Less Costly than Insulin Therapy in Diabetic Treatment?

Care providers must consider costs with the selection of therapy. This becomes an even more important factor when medications that are similar in their effectiveness and safety are available. Goetzel and Wilkins performed a cost analysis of insulin vs. glyburide in the treatment of GDM. They found that glyburide is considerably less costly than insulin, even when the cost of educating the new insulin user is minimized (15 min/patient). The strongest determinant was the medication cost, with an average savings/patient of $166–$200 based on year 2000 rates.[78]

19.14 Should Lactating Mothers Use Oral Agents?

In general, women are encouraged to breastfeed their newborn infants. A common concern is whether the drugs taken by the mother will affect the wellbeing of the child. As a rule of thumb, a concentration of drug ≥10% in the breast milk is of potential concern. When

Table 19.3 Selected pregnancy outcome variables in metformin, glyburide, and insulin treatment when compared with nondiabetic women[15,73]

	Metformin vs. insulin		Glyburide vs. insulin		Nondiabetic
LGA (%)	19.3	18.6	12.0	13.0	11.9
Macrosomia (%)	22.9	21.4	7.2	4.7	8.1
Ponderal index >2.85	–	–	9.0	12.0	22.0
Overall cesarean section (%)	22.9	23.2	23.0	24.0	13.7
Congenital malformation (%)	4.1	3.2	2	2	–
Preeclampsia (%)	8.3	6.8	6.0	6.0	7.6
Chronic HTN (%)	8.5	7.3	6.0	9.1	6.2
5 Min Apgar score <7 (%)	0.8	0.3	3.1	4.2	2.5
Neonatal ICU admission (%)	12.7	12.2	6.0	7.0	4.7
Hypoglycemia (%) <40 mg/dL	15.2	18.6	9.0	6.0	2.5
Polycythemia (%) >60%	–	–	2.0	3.0	1.4
Hyperbilirubinemia (%) >11 mg/dL	8	8.4	6.0	4.0	6.4
Hypocalcemia (%) <8 mg/dL	–	–	1.0	1.0	NA
Respiratory complications (%)	3.3	4.3	2.0	3.0	2.1
Shoulder dystocia	–	–	1.5	1.6	0.5

LGA large-for-gestational age infants (>90th percentile); *HTN* hypertension; *ICU* intensive care unit

Macrosomia = ≥4,000 g

metformin was evaluated, infant blood level was 0.28% of weight, normalized to maternal dose.[79] There was no trace of glyburide identified in breast milk of these infants.[80]

19.15 Summary

Although not universally accepted, the introduction of insulin analogs (mainly lispro), oral hypoglycemic agents (mainly glyburide) and intensified therapy has profoundly altered the management approach to treatment of diabetes in pregnancy, with outcomes comparable to the general population. The benefit of insulin analog is the reduction of nocturnal hypoglycemic episodes and postprandial levels, as well as the ease of patient use. With the establishment of efficacy of glyburide and possibly metformin, there is an equally effective alternative to insulin therapy. Glyburide is a cost-effective, patient friendly and, therefore, potentially compliance-enhancing therapy that produces perinatal outcome in GDM pregnancies comparable to the traditional insulin therapy. For GDM patients who require pharmacological therapy, glyburide is the drug of choice; thereafter, patients who fail to achieve glycemic control should begin insulin therapy.

The major obstacles to the creation of evidence-based criteria to guide benefit/risk in pharmacological therapy in obstetrics is the fear of the potential adverse drug effects on the fetus and, therefore, a resultant paucity of research. The history of the U.S. Food and Drug Administration regulations for prescription drug labeling in pregnancy adds an additional layer of difficulty. The ethical, legal, and medical rhetoric surrounding this dilemma may have exaggerated the potential for fetal harm. There may be greater risk to the fetus in withholding certain medications than in prescribing them. The current evidence-based data for both insulin lispro and glyburide support their use in pregnancy.[81,82]

References

1. American College of Obstetricians and Gynecologists Committee on Practice Bulletin – Obstetrics. ACOG Practice Bulletin. Clinical management guidelines for obstetrician-gynecologists. Number 30, September 2001. Gestational diabetes. *Obstet Gynecol*. 2001;98(3): 525-538.
2. American Diabetes Association. Diagnosis and Classification of Diabetes Mellitus. *Diabetes Care*. 2006;29(suppl 1):S43-S48.
3. Mokdad AH, Serdula MK, Dietz WH, et al. The spread of the obesity epidemic in the United States, 1991-1998. *JAMA*. 1999;282(16):1519-1522.
4. Silverman BL, Rizzo TA, Cho NH, et al. Long-term effects of the intrauterine environment. *Diabetes*. 1996;21(suppl 2):142-149.
5. Suhonen L, Hiilesmaa V, Teramo K. Glycemic control during early pregnancy and fetal malformations in women with type 1 diabetes mellitus. *Diabetologia*. 2000;43:79-82.
6. Lauenborg J, Mathiesen E, Ovesen P, et al. Audit on stillbirths in women with pregestational type 1 diabetes. *Diabetes Care*. 2003;26(5):1385-1388.
7. US Preventive Services Task Force. Agency for Healthcare Research and Quality. Department of Health and Human Services; 1996.
8. Reaven GM. The role of insulin resistance in human disease. *Diabetes*. 1998;37:1595-1607.
9. Olefsky JM. Pathogenesis of non-insulin dependent diabetes (type 2). In: DeGroot LJ, Nesser GM, Cahill JC, eds. *Endocrinology*. 2nd ed. Philadelphia: WB Saunders; 1989:1369-1388.
10. Buchanan TA, Xiang AH, Peters RK. Response of pancreatic B-cells to improved insulin sensitivity in women at high risk for type 2 diabetes. *Diabetes*. 2000;49:782-788.
11. Catalano PM, Kirwan JP, Haugel-de Mouzon S, et al. Gestational diabetes and insulin resistance: Role in short- and long-term implications for mother and fetus. *J Nutr*. 2003;133: 1674S-1683S.
12. Langer O. Maternal glycemic criteria for insulin therapy in gestational diabetes mellitus. *Diabetes Care*. 1998;21(suppl 2):B91-B98.
13. Schade DS, Jovanovic L, Schneider J. A placebo-controlled randomized study of glimepiride in patients with type 2 diabetes mellitus for whom diet therapy is unsuccessful. *J Clin Pharm*. 1998;38:636-641.
14. Langer O, Conway DL, Berkus MD, Xenakis EMJ, Gonzales O. A comparison glyburide and insulin in women with gestational diabetes mellitus. *N Engl J Med*. 2000;343(16):1134-1138.
15. Langer O, Rodriguez DA, Xenakis EMJ, et al. Intensified vs. conventional management of gestational diabetes. *Am J Obstet Gynecol*. 1994;170:1036-1047.

16. Kim C, Herman WH, Vijan S. Efficacy and cost of postpartum screening strategies for diabetes among women with histories of gestational diabetes mellitus. *Diabetes Care*. 2007;30(5): 1102-1106.
17. Bo S, Menato G, Lezo A, et al. Dietary fat and gestational hyperglycaemia. *Diabetologia*. 2001;44:972-978.
18. Lauenborg J, Mathiesen E, Hansen T, et al. The prevalence of the metabolic syndrome in a Danish population of women with previous gestational diabetes mellitus is three-fold higher than in the general population. *J Clin Endocrin Met*. 2005;90(7):4004-4010.
19. Hofman PL, Regan F, Jackson WE, et al. Premature birth and later insulin resistance. *NEJM*. 2004;351(21):2179-2187.
20. Weiss R, Dziura J, Burgert TS, et al. Obesity and the metabolic syndrome in children and adolescents. *NEJM*. 2004;350(23):2362-2374.
21. Langer N. Is cultural diversity a factor in self-monitoring blood glucose in gestational diabetes? *J Assoc Minor Phys*. 1995;6(2):73-77.
22. Langer N, Langer O. Emotional adjustment to diagnosis and intensified treatment of gestational diabetes. *Obstet Gynecol*. 1994;84(3):329-334.
23. UK Prospective Diabetes Study Group 33. Intensive blood glucose control with sulphonylureas or insulin compared with conventional treatment and risk of complications in patients with type 2 diabetes. *Lancet*. 1998;352:837-853.
24. Parretti E, Mecacci F, Papini M, et al. Third-trimester maternal glucose levels from diurnal profiles in non-diabetic pregnancies: Correlation with sonographic parameters of fetal growth. *Diabetes Care*. 2001;24:1319-1323.
25. Yogev Y, Ben-Haroush A, Chen R, et al. Diurnal glycemic profile in obese and normal weight non-diabetic pregnant women. *Am J Obstet Gynecol*. 2004;191(5):1655-1660.
26. Langer O, Conway DL. Level of glycemia and perinatal outcome in pregestational diabetes. *J Matern Fetal Med*. 2001;9(1):35-41.
27. Langer O. A spectrum of glucose thresholds may effectively prevent complications in the pregnant diabetic patient. *Semin Perinatol*. 2002;26(3):196-205.
28. Langer O. Is normoglycemia the correct threshold to prevent complications in the pregnant diabetic? *Diabet Rev*. 1996;4(1):2-10.
29. Mazze R, Langer O. Medical nutrition therapy. In: Langer O, ed. *The Diabetes in Pregnancy Dilemma*. Maryland: University Press of America; 2006:251-263.
30. Artal R. Exercise: The alternative therapeutic intervention for gestational diabetes. *Clin Obstet Gynecol*. 2003;46(2):479-487.
31. Artal R. Exercise: the logical intervention for diabetes in pregnancy. In: Langer O, ed. *The Diabetes in Pregnancy Dilemma*. Maryland: University Press of America; 2006:285-295.
32. Langer O, Anyaegbunam A, Brustman L, et al. Gestational diabetes: insulin requirements in pregnancy. *Am J Obstet Gynecol*. 1987;157(3):669-675.
33. Jovanovic L, Ilic S, Pettitt, et al. Metabolic and immunologic effects of insulin lispro in gestational diabetes. *Diabetes Care*. 1999;22:1422-1427.
34. Hirsch IB. Insulin analogues. *N Engl J Med*. 2005;352:174-183.
35. Gabbe SG, Graves CR. Management of diabetes mellitus complicating pregnancy. *Obstet Gynecol*. 2003;102:857-868.
36. Saade G. Gestational diabetes mellitus: a pill or a shot? *Obstet Gynecol*. 2005;105:456-457.
37. The Diabetes Control and Complications Trial Research Group. The effect of intensified treatment of diabetes on the development and progression of long-term complications in insulin-dependent diabetes mellitus. *N Engl J Med*. 1993;329:977-986.
38. Ecker JL, Greene MD. Gestational diabetes – setting limits, exploring treatments. *N Engl J Med*. 2008;358(19):2061-2063.
39. Greene MF. Oral hypoglycemic drugs for gestational diabetes. *N Eng J Med*. 2000;343: 1178-1179 [editorial].

40. Cefalo RC. A comparison of glyburide and insulin in women with gestational diabetes mellitus. *Obstet Gynecol Surv*. 2001;56:126-127.
41. Kirschbaum TH. Medical complications of pregnancy. In: *Yearbook of Obstetrics, Gynecology, and Women's Health*. Mosby: St. Louis; 2002:103-106.
42. Koren G. The use of glyburide in gestational diabetes: an ideal example of "bench to bedside. *Pediatr Res*. 2001;49:734.
43. American Diabetes Association. Position statement on gestational diabetes mellitus. *Diabetes Care*. 2004;27(suppl 1):S88-S90.
44. Coustan DR. Oral hypoglycemic agents for the Ob/Gyn. Contemp Ob/Gyn. 2001;April:45-63.
45. Jovanovic L. The use of oral agents during pregnancy to treat gestational diabetes. *Curr Diab Rep*. 2001;1:69-70.
46. American Diabetes Association. Implications of the United Kingdom Prospective Diabetes Study. *Diabetes Care*. 2000;23(suppl 2):S27-S31.
47. Anon. The effects of intensive treatment of diabetes on the development and progression of long-term complications in insulin-dependent diabetes mellitus. *N Engl J Med*. 1993;329:977-986.
48. Elliot B, Langer O, Schenker S, et al. Insignificant transfer of glyburide occurs across the human placenta. *Am J Obstet Gynecol*. 1991;165:807-812.
49. Elliot B, Schenker S, Langer O, et al. Comparative placental transport of oral hypoglycemic agents: a model of human placental drug transfer. *Am J Obstet Gynecol*. 1994;171:653-660.
50. Elliot B, Langer O, Schussling F. A model of human placental drug transfer. *Am J Obstet Gynecol*. 1997;176:527-530.
51. Ng WW, Miller RK. Transport of nutrients in the early human placenta: amino acid, creatinine, vitamin B12. *Trophoblastic Res*. 1983;1:121-133.
52. Kremer CJ, Duff P. Glyburide for the treatment of gestational diabetes. *Am J Obstet Gynecol*. 2004;190(5):1438-1439.
53. Nanovskaya TN, Nekhayeva I, Hankins G, Ahmed M. Effect of human serum albumin on transplacental transfer of glyburide. *Biochem Pharmacol*. 2006;72:632-639.
54. Nanovskaya TN, Nekhayeva IA, Patrikeeva SL, et al. Transfer of metformin across the dually perfused human placental lobule. *Am J Obstet Gynecol*. 2006;195:1081-1085.
55. Kovo N, Haroutiunian S, Feldman N, et al. Determination of metformin transfer across the human placenta using dually perfused ex-vivo placental cotyledon model [abstract]. *Am J Obstet Gynecol*. 2005;193(6):S85.
56. Kemball ML, McIvert C, Milner RDG, et al. Neonatal hypoglycemia in infants of diabetic mothers given sulfonylurea drugs in pregnancy. *Arch Dis Child*. 1970;45:696-701.
57. Zucker P, Simon G. Prolonged symptomatic neonatal hypoglycemia associated with maternal chloropropamide therapy. *Pediatrics*. 1968;42:824-825.
58. Piacquadio K, Hollingsworth DR, Murphy H. Effects of in-utero exposure to oral hypoglycemic drugs. *Lancet*. 1991;338:866-869.
59. Towner D, Kjos SL, Leung B, et al. Congenital malformations in pregnancies complicated by NIDDM. *Diabetes Care*. 1995;18(11):1446-1451.
60. Gutzin S, Kozer E, Magee L, et al. The safety of oral hypoglycemic agents in the first trimester of pregnancy: a meta-analysis. *Can J Clin Pharmacol*. 2003;10(4):179-183.
61. Gilbert C, Valois M, Koren G. Pregnancy outcome after first-trimester exposure to metformin: a meta-analysis. *Fertil Steril*. 2006;86(3):658-663.
62. Conway DL, Gonzales O, Skiver D. Use of glyburide for the treatment of gestational diabetes: the San Antonio experience. *J Matern Fetal Neonatal Med*. 2004;15(1):51-55.
63. Hellmuth E, Damm P, Molsted-Pedersen L. Oral hypoglycaemic agents in 118 diabetic pregnancies. *Diabet Med*. 2001;17(7):507-511.
64. Notelovitz M. Sulphonylurea therapy in the treatment of the pregnant diabetic. *S Afr Med J*. 1971;45(9):226-229.

65. Chmait R, Dinise T, Moore T. Prospective observational study to establish predictors of glyburide success in women with gestational diabetes mellitus. *J Perinatol.* 2004;24 (10): 617-622.
66. Gilson G, Murphy N. Comparison of oral glyburide with insulin for the management of gestational diabetes mellitus in Alaska native women. *Am J Obstet Gynecol.* 2002;187:6(S), S152 [A #336].
67. Fines V, Moore T, Castle S. A comparison of glyburide and insulin treatment in gestational diabetes mellitus on infant birthweight and adiposity. *Am J Obstet Gynecol.* 2003;189:6(S), S108 [A #161].
68. Velazquez MD, Bolnick J, Cloakey D, et al. The use of glyburide in the management of gestational diabetes. *Obstet Gynecol.* 2003;101(suppl):88S.
69. Pendsey SP, Sharma RR, Chalkhore SS. Repaglinde: a feasible alternative to insulin in management of gestational diabetes mellitus. *Diabetes Res Clin Pract.* 2002;56(suppl 1):S46 [OR103].
70. Jacobson GF, Ramos GA, Ching JY, Kirby RS, Ferrara A, Field DR. Comparison of glyburide and insulin for the management of gestational diabetes in a large managed care organization. *Am J Obstet Gynecol.* 2005;193:118-124.
71. Langer O, Most O, Monga S. Glyburide: predictors of treatment failure in gestational diabetes (Abstract). *Am J Obstet Gynecol.* 2006;195(6):S136.
72. Moretti ME, Rezvani M, Koren G. Safety of glyburide for gestational diabetes: a meta-analysis of pregnancy outcomes. *Ann Pharmacother.* 2008;42:483-490.
73. Rowan JA, Hague WM, Gao W, Battin MR, Moore MP. Metformin versus insulin for the treatment of gestational diabetes. *N Engl J Med.* 2008;358:2003-2015.
74. Glueck CJ, Wang P, Kobayashi S, Phillips H, Sieve-Smith L. Metformin therapy throughout pregnancy reduces the development of gestational diabetes in women with polycystic ovary syndrome. *Fertil Steril.* 2002;77(3):520-525.
75. Moore LE, Briery CM, Clokey D, et al. Metformin and insulin in the management of gestational diabetes mellitus: preliminary results of a comparison. *J Reprod Med.* 2007;52(11):1011-1015.
76. Langer O, Yogev Y, Xenakis EM, Rosenn B. Insulin and glyburide therapy: dosage, severity level of gestational diabetes and pregnancy outcome. *Am J Obstet Gynecol.* 2005;192:134-139.
77. Yogev Y, Ben-Haroush A, Chen R, et al. Undiagnosed asymptomatic hypoglycemia: diet, insulin, and glyburide for gestational diabetic pregnancy. *Obstet Gynecol.* 2004;104:88-93.
78. Goetzel L, Wilkins I. Glyburide compared to insulin for the treatment of gestational diabetes mellitus: a cost analysis. *J Perinatol.* 2002;22:403-406.
79. Hale TW, Kristensen JH, Hacket LP, et al. Transfer of metformin into human milk. *Diabetologia.* 2002;45:1509-1514.
80. Feig DS, Briggs GG, Kmenser JM. Transfer of glyburide and glipzide into breast milk. *Diabetes Care.* 2005;28:1851-1855.
81. Ryan EA. Glyburide was as safe and effective as insulin in gestational diabetes. *EBM.* 2001;6:79.
82. Landon M, Durnwald C. Glyburide: the new alternative for treating gestational diabetes? *Am J Obstetrics Gynecol.* 2005;193:1-2.

Section VII

Postpartum Implications for GDM in Women

Risk for Maternal Postpartum Diabetes 20

Catherine Kim

20.1 Introduction

Gestational diabetes mellitus (GDM) confers a sevenfold risk for future diabetes, independent of other significant risk factors such as weight, visceral adiposity, and physical activity.[1,2] Up to a third of women with diabetes may have been affected by prior GDM.[3] This chapter reviews the factors affecting postpartum diabetes risk in women with a GDM history. Methodological issues include varying diagnostic criteria for GDM and postpartum diabetes. The discussion of risk factors begins with traditional risk factors for glucose tolerance as they apply to women with a GDM history, and further describes several risk factors for postpartum maternal diabetes unique to GDM women. These latter factors arise from the index diagnosis of GDM, and include glucose levels obtained from prenatal diagnostic testing, earlier onset of glucose intolerance during pregnancy, elevated glucose levels during pregnancy, and the need for hypoglycemic medication during pregnancy. The chapter concludes with studies that examine GDM women's future cardiovascular disease risk.

20.2 Factors Affecting Estimates of Postpartum Diabetes Risk: Diagnostic Criteria

In a 1991 review, John B. O'Sullivan observed: "Although the variability in diabetes incidence rates is wide, there is broad general agreement on the predictive nature of gestational blood glucose levels,"[4] a statement that still holds. His report, including his own landmark studies of Boston City Hospital women with GDM, noted postpartum diabetes cumulative incidences ranging from 5 to 87%.[4] He further noted that differing criteria for the index GDM diagnosis and postpartum diabetes diagnosis contributed unnecessary variation in

C. Kim
Department of Obstetrics and Gynecology,
University of Michigan, Ann Arbor, MI, USA
e-mail: cathkim@med.umich.edu

C. Kim and A. Ferrara (eds.), *Gestational Diabetes During and After Pregnancy*,
DOI: 10.1007/978-1-84882-120-0_20, © Springer-Verlag London Limited 2010

risk estimates. In other words, apart from diabetes risk factors themselves, methodological issues affect estimates of postpartum diabetes risk. Diagnostic criteria for the index diagnosis of GDM define the population and therefore the denominator of postpartum diabetes risk estimates. Background screening rates also affect postpartum diabetes risk estimates by reducing the number of high-risk women with GDM who had undetected glucose tolerance preceding pregnancy. Diagnostic criteria for postpartum diabetes define the outcome. Finally, cohort retention, particularly if the cohort loses high-risk women, also influences postpartum diabetes risk estimates. The following section reviews each of these issues.

20.2.1 Diagnostic Criteria for GDM

As discussed in chapter 3, the criteria for the index diagnosis of GDM vary significantly across medical organizations and centers. In general, the lower the glucose cut-offs, the broader the range of risk in the population subsequently diagnosed with GDM. Identification of a greater proportion of pregnant women with GDM necessarily leads to a greater denominator, and a decreased proportion subsequently identified with postpartum glucose intolerance. Conversely, more specific, but less sensitive GDM criteria lead to fewer women identified with GDM. However, a greater proportion of these women are subsequently identified as having postpartum glucose intolerance.

Ferrara et al demonstrated this in their study, in which two sets of GDM diagnostic criteria were applied to women who underwent glucose tolerance testing during pregnancy.[5] Of these women, 3.2% had GDM by National Diabetes Data Group criteria. Of the same women, 4.8% had GDM by Carpenter and Coustan criteria, which uses lower glucose cut-offs. With the lower cut-offs, the prevalence of GDM increased by approximately 50%. However, the additional populations identified tended to be low risk; relative increments were greatest in low-risk age and ethnic groups, specifically women aged <25 years (70%) and in whites (58%). Thus, although the denominator, women with GDM, increased, the additional women identified were at similar or lower risk when compared with the original National Diabetes Data Group cohort.

20.2.2 Background Screening for Diabetes

Diabetes screening is not routine in non-pregnant women of reproductive age. The American Diabetes Association (ADA) recommends screening for diabetes beginning at age 45 years in the absence of risk factors,[6] and other medical organizations such as the United States Preventive Services Task Force (USPSTF)[7] and the World Health Organization (WHO)[8] do not categorically recommend screening unless other risk factors for diabetes or cardiovascular disease are present.

No studies examine how background detection rates might affect postpartum diabetes risk estimates. More frequent background diabetes screening in non-pregnant women prior to conception might lead to greater identification of women with preconception diabetes, and decrease the number of women identified with GDM.[9] However, since background screening rates occur in the setting of changing risk factors rates, such as obesity and multiparity, it is difficult to isolate the impact of background screening.

20.2.3 Diagnostic Criteria for Postpartum Glucose Intolerance

Criteria for postpartum glucose intolerance vary between medical organizations. The primary debate is whether screening should consist of performance of a postpartum fasting glucose alone vs. a 75-g oral glucose tolerance test (OGTT). The 2007 Fifth International Workshop-Conference on GDM recommends that a 75-g OGTT be performed ≥6 weeks postpartum to screen for maternal glucose intolerance.[10] The Australasian Diabetes in Pregnancy Society also endorses the 75-g OGTT. The 2003 Canadian Diabetes Association guidelines prefer the 75-g OGTT, but state that the fasting glucose is acceptable.[11] As of 2007, the United Kingdom-based National Institute for Health and Clinical Excellence (NICE) recommends a postpartum fasting glucose only, specifically without the OGTT.[12] In 2009, the American College of Obstetricians and Gynecologists stated that screening should be performed and notes that the OGTT demonstrates greater sensitivity than the fasting glucose, but that fasting glucose is acceptable,[13] a contrast with its previous agnostic recommendations regarding screening.

The diabetes screening guidelines of other medical organizations adopt the guidelines for general at-risk populations. The 1999/2006 WHO guidelines recommend a 75-g OGTT.[8,14] The 1997/2003 ADA guidelines recommend a fasting glucose in general practice, although the guidelines recognize the OGTT as a valid diagnostic method.[6,15] The USPSTF does not make specific recommendations for postpartum screening among women with GDM, perhaps reflecting its lack of support for GDM screening during pregnancy.[16]

While organizations differ as to whether or not to obtain the 2-h glucose, the cut-offs for diabetes are similar across groups: fasting glucose of 7.0 mmol/L or 126 mg/dL and, if obtained, a 2-h glucose of 11.1 mmol/L or 200 mg/dL after a 75-g challenge. The fasting glucose value of 126 mg/dL was chosen due to its threshold association with retinopathy.[17] The 2-h criterion of 200 mg/dL corresponded with both all-cause and cardiovascular disease mortality, as well as providing roughly the same risk as a fasting glucose of 126 mg/dL.[17]

The glucose test results may also be used to determine the presence of impaired glucose regulation (IGR).[14] IGR consists of impaired fasting glucose (IFG) and/or impaired glucose tolerance (IGT). The ADA defines IFG as a fasting glucose level ≥100 mg/dL or 5.6 mmol/L[15] and the WHO defines IFG as a fasting glucose level ≥110 mg/dL or 6.1 mmol/L.[8] The ADA defines IGT as a 2-h glucose 140–199 mg/dL or 7.8–11.0 mmol/L, as does the WHO. The IFG cut-off was chosen based on review of receiver operator curves (ROCs) for diabetes prediction and the disagreement between ADA and WHO was based on whether ROCs should be the basis for cut-offs.[8,15] The IGT cut-off was initially chosen more arbitrarily, although the 2-h glucose does correspond with cardiovascular mortality and future diabetes.[8,15] In addition, Diabetes Prevention Program participants were required to have IGT and did respond to diabetes prevention interventions.[17,18]

More sensitive criteria result in greater estimates of postpartum diabetes risk. The OGTT is more sensitive than the fasting glucose alone because the fasting glucose and 2-h glucose capture overlapping, but not identical populations. Fasting glucose may reflect hepatic insulin resistance and early-phase insulin secretion, whereas glucose levels obtained after a glucose challenge may reflect peripheral insulin resistance and later-phase insulin secretion.[19] Women may have defects in either.[19] In the National Health and Examination Survey III, 44% of adults ≥40 years with IGR met both the 2-h and fasting criteria.[20] Fourteen percent met the fasting criteria but not the 2-h criteria, and 41% met the 2-h criteria alone.[20] In the European DECODE study, only 28% of IGR participants met both criteria, and 31% met the 2-h criteria only.[21]

The greater sensitivity of the OGTT is complicated by the greater variability in the 2-h glucose level compared with the fasting glucose.[22] The day-to-day intraindividual coefficients of variation range from 6.4 to 11.4% for fasting glucose and 14.3 to 16.7% for the 2-h glucose.[22,23] In addition, the OGTT has greater initial cost and inconvenience, drawbacks cited by the ADA and NICE.[6,12,15] Finally, there is a lack of consensus regarding utility of intervening for prediabetes states,[7] for cardiovascular disease prevention,[17] and for mortality prevention.[17]

The debate over which diabetes screening test is optimal extends to postpartum women with a GDM history. Among these women, as in the general population, the fasting glucose and 2-h glucose identify distinct groups. In several postpartum GDM cohorts, approximately 5–10% of women have IFG only, about 10–15% have IGT only, and 10–15% have both.[24–27] Other studies have also found limited sensitivity of fasting glucose for IGR and DM in postpartum GDM women,[28,29] particularly for IGR.[29] To our knowledge, no studies examine the diagnostic properties of the HbA1c in the postpartum population. Therefore, despite the convenience of the HbA1c assay, its value for diagnosis is still unknown for postpartum GDM women.

Several issues unique to women with recent GDM could potentially influence choice of screening test in this population. First, women with recent GDM might benefit from more sensitive screening strategies, since diabetes poses risk to future pregnancies. Specifically, this risk includes congenital anomalies of cardiac malformations, neural tube defects, and limb dysgenesis. All are strongly associated with HbA1c before conception.[30] Second, women with GDM are, on average, approximately 10–20 years younger than other populations diagnosed with IGR and diabetes.[9,31] Women with GDM who develop diabetes face relatively prolonged dysglycemia, which could potentially place them at higher risk for diabetes complications than the general population. Earlier identification could lead to reduction of complications. In the Diabetes Control and Complications Trial and its follow-up, intensive treatment reduced microvascular complications, with effects persisting after discontinuation of the trial.[32] In statistical models, the postpartum OGTT is generally more advantageous among women with recent GDM if diabetes identification is the endpoint.[33] Finally, earlier identification of IGR could lead to preventive efforts.

20.2.4 Ascertainment Bias: Performance of Postpartum Screening and Cohort Retention

Regardless of the screening criteria used, multiple reports demonstrate that performance of postpartum screening for those with a GDM history has been the exception, rather than the rule.[24,26,27,34–36] While performance of screening has improved over the past decade, almost half of the women with a GDM history do not undergo screening of any kind or undergo screening with tests such as glycosylated hemoglobins.[27,37] Before 2010, the latter tests have not been recommended as screening tests due to relatively decreased sensitivity and specificity.[17]

Reasons why women forego screening are speculative, but include women's low perception of diabetes risk,[38] lack of healthcare provider perception of risk,[39,40] and lack of other steps necessary for screening such as lab slip distribution or test-ordering.[39,41] The reasons why women forego screening may also differ between study populations. Russell et al found that screened and unscreened women had similar glucose levels during pregnancy,[35] but screened women were more likely to attend the postpartum visit, suggesting that barriers to the postpartum visit also presented barriers to screening. In contrast, Smirnakis et al found that greater than 90% attended a postpartum visit, suggesting that attendance of the postpartum visit was not the major barrier.[34]

Quality improvement studies on this topic are few. In Texas, Hunt and Conway noted that screening performance improved with nurse case-management,[26] including mailed reminders, telephone calls, and home visits. In a Canadian study, where postpartum OGTT costs are not billed to the patient as in most developed countries aside from the United States, mailed reminders increased screening rate.[42] Ferrara et al also noted that referral to a nurse case-management program for general GDM management during pregnancy increased screening fourfold after pregnancy (personal communication).

Infrequent postpartum screening leads to missed diagnoses of postpartum glucose intolerance. In addition, low performance of postpartum screening could bias estimates of future diabetes risk if screened women were different than unscreened women. In a systematic review of studies examining conversion to type 2 diabetes, Nicholson et al found that 75% of studies included reported a loss to follow-up greater than 20%.[43] In particular, retrospective cohorts including only women who have undergone the postpartum test might misrepresent risk. If women who were not screened were at lower or higher risk than women who were screened, this would overestimate and underestimate diabetes risk estimates, respectively. Indeed, women who are not screened may have greater prevalence of risk factors for diabetes, including elevated glucose levels,[26,34] prior macrosomia,[24] poorer education,[27] obesity,[27] and macrosomia.[27]

20.3 Factors Affecting Estimates of Postpartum Diabetes Risk: Risk Factors for Maternal Postpartum Diabetes

Methodological issues aside, postpartum diabetes risk estimates also reflect the underlying glucose tolerance of the population. While risk factors for diabetes among women with GDM vs. women in the general population overlap, there are several key differences. Women with a GDM history are distinct from the general population in that they have exhibited glucose intolerance when exposed to the greater metabolic demands of pregnancy. Risk factors that predict diabetes in the general population do not always predict diabetes among women with histories of GDM. Also, information on traditional diabetes risk factors, particularly lifestyle behaviors, is more limited among women with a GDM history than other at-risk populations for diabetes due to lack of study.

Several risk factors unique to GDM women predict postpartum glucose intolerance and arise from the index diagnosis of GDM. Glucose levels obtained from prenatal diagnostic testing reflect underlying maternal glucose intolerance and are associated with postpartum diabetes. Earlier onset of glucose intolerance during pregnancy, elevated glucose levels during pregnancy, and levels that require treatment with hypoglycemic medication are also associated with future maternal diabetes risk.

20.3.1 Measures of Glucose Intolerance During the Index GDM Pregnancy

20.3.1.1 Fifty-Gram Screening Test and Diagnostic OGTT

Glucose intolerance during the index GDM pregnancy, reflected by the glucose values on the 50-g glucose challenge screening test as well as the diagnostic prenatal OGTT, are associated with postpartum hyperglycemia and diabetes.[44–49] Due to variation in diagnostic testing procedures for GDM, as well as the continuous relationship between glucose values and future risk, no single glucose value consistently identifies women at risk for future diabetes.[44]

As discussed in the chapters regarding the guidelines for diagnosis of GDM and its prevalence, the 50-g glucose challenge is often, but not always, performed during pregnancy as the baseline screening test for GDM. The glucose value from this screen is independently associated with postpartum hyperglycemia,[44] even after adjustment for women's prenatal OGTT values.[49]

The glucose values on the diagnostic prenatal OGTT, whether measured as area under the curve or as tertiles for individual values, and whether measured as part of a 75- or 100-g OGTT, predict greater maternal postpartum glucose intolerance.[24,45–55] As fasting and post-challenge glucose values detect different populations at risk for glucose intolerance in non-pregnant adults, fasting and post-challenge values on the prenatal OGTT are associated with postpartum hyperglycemia to different degrees and in different groups of pregnant women. Women with a greater number of abnormal tests, i.e., elevated fasting or post-challenge values, are at greater risk for diabetes.[24] The prenatal glucose area under the curve reflects an average of all of the prenatal OGTT values and reflects any abnormality in glucose metabolism, although the area under the curve does not distinguish between specific defects.

Elevations in any of the glucose values from the prenatal OGTT are associated with greater postpartum diabetes risk, but fasting glucose and 1-h glucose may be more strongly associated with postpartum diabetes than 2- and 3-h values.[44–53,56]

While not commonly used in clinical practice, several measures may more precisely capture specific defects in glucose metabolism.[24,44,51,52,55] These measures most commonly involve proxies for insulin secretion and sensitivity rather than direct measures using euglycemic clamp studies.[57] Proxies for insulin secretion include insulin and glucose ratios measured after a glucose load[58] or C-peptide-to-glucose levels.[24] Insulin sensitivity is commonly represented by fasting insulin or by equations incorporating fasting insulin and fasting glucose levels.[59] In pregnant women with GDM, both insulin resistance and insulin secretion are independently associated with postpartum diabetes even after adjustment for prenatal OGTT levels.[24,51,55]

20.3.1.2
Medications During the Index GDM Pregnancy

Treatment required during the index GDM pregnancy may also reflect underlying glucose intolerance. Pregnancies requiring sulfonylureas[27] or insulin[45,46,48–50,60–63] may reflect greater glucose intolerance than pregnancies requiring lifestyle management only. Class A2 GDM is GDM requiring insulin therapy because of fasting levels ≥105 mg/dL; this particular category of GDM is associated with postpartum diabetes even after adjustment for the actual fasting glucose level as well as other prenatal OGTT levels.[49] Women eventually placed on insulin or a sulfonylurea may still be at higher risk for future diabetes after adjustment for A2 class.[27,45,46,60] Treatment status may provide additional predictive value, because treatment may reflect progression of insulin resistance and/or β-cell dysfunction later in the pregnancy, whereas prenatal OGTT levels reflect glucose metabolism at the time of diagnosis. However, treatment may reflect other health-care delivery factors such as greater likelihood of follow-up, compliance with medication, and compliance with a postpartum OGTT.[27]

20.3.1.3
Gestational Age at the Time of GDM Diagnosis

Testing for GDM generally occurs between 24 and 28 weeks of pregnancy. However, testing may occur earlier if the healthcare provider suspects glucose intolerance. Earlier gestational age at time of diagnosis, indicating earlier onset of glucose intolerance, has been associated with greater risk of postpartum diabetes,[47–49,52,61,62,64,65] even after consideration of the degree of elevation in glucose levels.[48–50] This association is driven by pregnancies diagnosed at extremes of gestational age, as this risk was not significantly elevated when women in the middle of the gestational age distribution were included.[47–49,52,66]

20.3.2
Other Risk Factors for Future Diabetes: Adiposity

Anthropometric factors reflect adiposity, a step in the causal pathway of insulin resistance.[67] While adiposity is generally associated with future glucose intolerance, different anthropometric measures reflect different types of adiposity, which in turn are associated with future diabetes to differing degrees. Greater central or visceral adiposity, as reflected by waist circumference and waist-hip ratio, has stronger risk for GDM than subcutaneous adiposity or traditional measures of body mass.[68] Central adiposity has also been associated with defects in both insulin secretion and sensitivity among women with a GDM history.[69]

The association of future diabetes with preconception[24,47,50,52,61,62] and prenatal adiposity measures[45,53,60,61,70] tends to be less robust than postpartum assessments,[46,54,62,63,71–74] which are more proximal to diabetes onset. Obviously, adiposity measurements across the three periods still correlate highly. Preconception and prenatal associations with diabetes did not always remain robust in multivariate analyses including prenatal OGTT glucose levels.[48, 51, 53, 75–77] This suggests that prenatal adiposity effects upon metabolism were reflected by prenatal OGTT glucose.

20.3.3 Other Risk Factors for Future Diabetes: Sociodemographic Factors

The association between traditional sociodemographic risk factors and postpartum maternal diabetes is not as strong in women with a GDM history as in the general population. This may reflect that women with GDM are already at high-risk, and the factors that predispose them to GDM have minimal additional predictive value for postpartum maternal diabetes.[2] With a few exceptions,[62, 63, 74] maternal age at the time of GDM diagnosis has not been associated with future maternal diabetes,[45, 47, 48, 51–53, 60, 61, 65, 66, 71, 75, 78] although older age predicts glucose intolerance in the general population.[79] This may be because maternal age already predicts the onset of GDM itself,[80] as noted in chapter 5. The lack of association may also be due to the narrow range in maternal age in GDM women, since maternal age generally does not exceed 50 years.

Non-white race is associated with greater diabetes risk in the general population of women, even after adjustment for body mass.[81] Among women with GDM, within-study comparisons of race for future diabetes incidence have sometimes found greater diabetes risk among non-white women,[82, 83] but this finding has not been consistent across studies.[66] This may reflect the fact that higher-risk racial-ethnic groups, such as Latinas and Asians, have already developed GDM.[84] Alternatively, it may reflect that these comparisons are relatively uncommon, due to the homogeneity of the populations within most studies. Between-study comparisons suggest a lower incidence of diabetes among non-Hispanic white women[85] compared with women of non-white race/ethnicity,[86] but definitive conclusions are hard to draw due to selection criteria that differ across studies.

Family history of type 2 diabetes[45, 47, 52, 53, 71, 75, 76, 87] has generally not been associated with maternal postpartum diabetes in GDM women, perhaps for the same reasons that age and race have not. While parity[53, 60, 73, 75, 78, 87] has not been associated with postpartum diabetes in GDM women in most studies, grand multiparity,[63] an additional pregnancy after the index pregnancy,[54] and number of GDM pregnancies are associated with postpartum diabetes risk.[46,49]

20.3.4 Other Risk Factors for Future Diabetes: Lifestyle Behaviors

Surprisingly little information exists regarding behaviors and future diabetes risk among women with a GDM history. Chapter 5 presents evidence that physical activity levels[88] and dietary habits[85] are risk factors for the index diagnosis of GDM, but reports do not comment upon these factors for postpartum maternal diabetes. Chapters 21 and 22, respectively, discuss the diabetes risk associated with various hormonal contraceptives and breastfeeding.

20.3.5 Other Risk Factors for Diabetes: Non-Glucose Factors

Among the general population of women, inflammatory and endothelial factors are associated with glucose intolerance.[89,90] Among women with a GDM history, studies are relatively few. The role of inflammatory markers is discussed in more detail in Chapter 10.

Autoantibodies, including antibodies to islet cells, insulin, the tyrosine phosphatases, and glutamic acid decarboxylase, are associated with the development of type 1 diabetes in the general population and among women with a GDM history.[91] Fuchtenbusch et al found that the degree of diabetes risk was associated with the number of antibodies present.[92] In a 2007 report, de Leiva et al reviewed 17 studies examining autoantibody status and development of diabetes.[91] Autoantibodies were generally associated with diabetes development except in four smaller studies. Of note, adjustment for other factors, particularly glucose levels, was not performed in most studies. The prevalence of antibodies was examined in primarily non-Hispanic white populations, which have a relatively decreased prevalence of type 2 diabetes as compared with type 1 diabetes. Therefore, the additional predictive value of autoantibodies is not yet established.

20.4 Cardiovascular Risk

Among the general population of women, blood pressure levels, low high-density lipoprotein cholesterol (HDL), and high triglycerides are associated with type 2 diabetes.[93] Among women with a GDM history, blood pressure levels[24,71,72,82,94] and HDL and triglyceride levels[24,71,72,82,94,95] have also been associated with diabetes and IGR. Levels of blood pressure and lipids were usually within normal range and related to glucose continuously, without a threshold effect, making it difficult to use these factors for diabetes risk stratification. In a cross-sectional analysis, Kim et al found that women with a GDM history who do not have diabetes may not have increased risk of other cardiovascular risk factor abnormalities.[96] As of publication, we are unaware of any prospective studies that have examined the sequence of cardiovascular risk factor evolution, including glucose, blood pressure, lipids, and inflammatory and endothelial markers, among women with a GDM history.

As GDM is associated with elevations in cardiovascular risk factors, it is not surprising that GDM is associated with vascular dysfunction and future cardiovascular disease. Heitritter et al found that women with a GDM history had greater vascular resistance, lower stroke volume, and lower cardiac output than women without a GDM history.[97] Bo et al found that women with a GDM history also had increased intimal medial thickness compared to women without a history.[98] In a cross-sectional study, Carr et al found that women with a GDM history were more likely to have metabolic syndrome and to experience cardiovascular events than women without a GDM history, and moreover, that these cardiovascular events occurred at a younger age.[99] Shah et al found that this increased risk of cardiovascular events, although low, seemed to be primarily attributable to their greater risk of diabetes.[100] They noted that the evolution of cardiovascular risk factor abnormalities and diabetes was not studied, and thus, diabetes did not necessarily precede the diagnosis of other cardiovascular risk factors.[100]

20.5 Conclusions and Research Needed

GDM and its attendant controversies in diagnosis and follow-up highlight the importance of examining pregnancy diseases for their impact on postpartum maternal health. While medical care has traditionally treated prenatal and postpartum care as separate, glucose tolerance does not respect this boundary. Postpartum studies of GDM women are relatively few compared to prenatal and peripartum examinations. Limiting factors include women's low risk perception for future diabetes[38] in conjunction with their provider's low risk perception,[39,40] the socioeconomically disadvantaged profile of GDM women in the United States,[101] and lack of continuity of care between pregnancy healthcare providers and postpartum providers. Greater attention needs to be devoted to improving postpartum screening and consensus on screening guidelines.

Currently, no large prospective cohort studies of GDM and non-GDM women exist. Such studies would establish diabetes conversion rates and incidence of other chronic disease. Such studies would be useful in establishing postpartum screening criteria for GDM women by comparing morbidities associated with fasting value, the 2-hour value, HbA1c, and the variation in each of these tests.

Most importantly, interventions for women with recent GDM need to be developed, in order to improve postpartum screening and maternal chronic disease prevention. The value of intervention for IGR women or diabetic women with a GDM history is assumed to be similar to the general population, but has not been independently established. Such interventions also need to be evaluated for their long-term effects on offspring. Successful interventions would leverage the tight interrelationship between maternal and child health during the unique condition of pregnancy, and in doing so, avert disease in an efficient and cost-effective manner.

References

1. Bellamy L, Casas J, Hingorani A, Williams D. Type 2 diabetes mellitus after gestational diabetes: a systematic review and meta-analysis. *Lancet*. 2009;373:1773-1779.
2. Gunderson E, Lewis C, Tsai A, et al. A 20-year prospective study of childbearing and incidence of diabetes in young women, controlling for glycemia before conception: the Coronary Artery Risk Development in Young Adults (CARDIA) Study. *Diabetes*. 2007;56:2990-2996.
3. Cheung N, Byth K. Population health significance of gestational diabetes. *Diabetes Care*. 2003;26:2005-2009.
4. O'Sullivan J. Diabetes mellitus after GDM. *Diabetes*. 1991;29:131-135.
5. Ferrara A, Hedderson M, Quesenberry C, Selby J. Prevalence of gestational diabetes mellitus detected by the National Diabetes Data Group or the Carpenter and Coustan plasma glucose thresholds. *Diabetes Care*. 2002;25:1625-1630.

6. American Diabetes Association. Diagnosis and classification of diabetes mellitus. *Diabetes Care*. 2008;31:S55-S60.
7. Norris S, Kansagara D, Bougatsos C, Fu R; U.S. Preventive Services Task Force. Screening adults for type 2 diabetes: a review of the evidence for the U.S. Preventive Services Task Force. *Ann Intern Med*. 2008;148:846-854.
8. World Health Organization. *Definition and Diagnosis of Diabetes Mellitus and Intermediate Hyperglycemia: A Report of WHO/IDF Consultation*. Geneva, Switzerland: World Health Organization; 2006.
9. Lawrence J, Contreras R, Sacks D. Trends in the prevalence of pre-existing diabetes and gestational diabetes mellitus among a racially/ethnically diverse population of pregnant women, 1999-2005. *Diabetes Care*. 2008;31:899-904.
10. Metzger B, Buchanan T, Coustan D, et al. Summary and recommendations of the Fifth International Workshop-Conference on Gestational Diabetes Mellitus. *Diabetes Care*. 2007; 30:S251-S260.
11. Meltzer S, Feig D, Ryan E, Thompson D, Snyder J. Gestational diabetes mellitus. Canadian Diabetes Association. Clinical Practice Guidelines Expert Committee. 2003 Practice Guidelines; 2003. Available at: http://www.diabetes.ca/cpg2003/downloads/gdm.pdf. Accessed 01.08.08.
12. National Institute for Health and Clinical Excellence (NICE). *Diabetes in Pregnancy: Management of Diabetes and its Complications from Preconception to the Postnatal Period*. London: National Collaborating Centre for Women's and Children's Health; 2008.
13. ACOG Committee on Obstetric Practice. Postpartum screening for abnormal glucose tolerance in women who had gestational diabetes mellitus. *Obstet Gynecol*. 2009;113:1419-1421.
14. World Health Organization. *Definition, Diagnosis, and Classification of Diabetes Mellitus and its Complications: Report of a WHO Consultation. Part 1. Diagnosis and Classification of Diabetes Mellitus*. Geneva, Switzerland: World Health Organization; 1999.
15. The Expert Committee on the Diagnosis and Classification of Diabetes Mellitus. Follow-up report on the diagnosis of diabetes mellitus. *Diabetes Care*. 2003;26:3160-3167.
16. United States Preventive Services Task Force. Screening for gestational diabetes mellitus: U.S. Preventive Services Task Force recommendation statement. *Ann Intern Med*. 2008; 148:759-765.
17. The Expert Committee on the Diagnosis and Classification of Diabetes Mellitus. Report of the expert committee on the diagnosis and classification of diabetes mellitus. *Diabetes Care*. 1997;20:1183-1197.
18. Knowler W, Barrett-Connor E, Fowler S, et al. Reduction in the incidence of type 2 diabetes with lifestyle intervention or metformin. *N Engl J Med*. 2002;346:393-403.
19. Nathan D, Davidson M, DeFronzo R, et al. Impaired fasting glucose and impaired glucose tolerance: implications for care. *Diabetes Care*. 2007;30:753-759.
20. Harris M, Eastman R, Cowie C, Flegal K, Eberhardt M. Comparison of diabetes diagnostic categories in the U.S. population according to 1997 American Diabetes Association and 1980-1985 World Health Organization diagnostic criteria. *Diabetes Care*. 1997;20:1859-1862.
21. DECODE Study Group. Will new diagnostic criteria for diabetes mellitus change phenotype of patients with diabetes? *BMJ*. 1998;317:371-375.
22. Mooy J, Grootenhuis P, de Vries H, et al. Intra-individual variation of glucose, specific insulin and proinsulin concentrations measured by two oral glucose tolerance tests in a general Caucasian population: the Hoorn Study. *Diabetologia*. 1996;39:298-305.
23. Feskens E, Bowles C, Kromhout D. Intra- and interindividual variability of glucose tolerance in an elderly population. *J Clin Epidemiol*. 1991;44:947-953.
24. Pallardo F, Herranz L, Garcia-Ingelmo T, et al. Early postpartum metabolic assessment in women with prior gestational diabetes. *Diabetes Care*. 1999;22:1053-1058.
25. Kitzmiller J, Dang-Kilduff L, Taslimi M. Gestational diabetes after delivery: short-term management and long-term risks. *Diabetes Care*. 2007;30:S225-S235.

26. Hunt K, Conway D. Who returns for postpartum glucose screening following gestational diabetes mellitus? *Am J Obstet Gynecol*. 2008;198(404):e401-e406.
27. Ferrara A, Peng T, Kim C. Trends in postpartum diabetes screening and subsequent diabetes and impaired glucose regulation among women with histories of gestational diabetes mellitus: a TRIAD Study. *Diabetes Care*. 2009;32(2):269-274.
28. Reinblatt S, Morin L, Meltzer S. The importance of a postpartum 75 gram oral glucose tolerance test in women with gestational diabetes. *J Obstet Gynaecol Can*. 2006;28:690-694.
29. Agarwal M, Punnose J, Dhatt G. Gestational diabetes: implications of variation in post-partum follow-up criteria. *Eur J Obstet Gynecol Reprod Biol*. 2004;113:149-153.
30. Ray J, O'Brien T, Chan W. Preconception care and the risk of congenital anomalies in the offspring of women with diabetes mellitus: a meta-analysis. *Q J Med*. 2001;94:435-444.
31. Harris M, Flegal K, Cowie C, et al. Prevalence of diabetes, impaired fasting glucose, and impaired glucose tolerance in U.S. adults: the Third National Health and Nutrition Examination Survey. *Diabetes Care*. 1998;21:518.
32. Anon. Retinopathy and nephropathy in patients with type 1 diabetes four years after a trial of intensive therapy. The Diabetes Control and Complications Trial/Epidemiology of Diabetes Interventions and Complications Research Group. *N Engl J Med*. 2000;342:381-389.
33. Kim C, Herman W, Vijan S. Efficacy and cost of postpartum screening strategies for diabetes among women with histories of gestational diabetes mellitus. *Diabetes Care*. 2007;30:1102-1106.
34. Smirnakis K, Chasan-Taber L, Wolf M, Markenson G, Ecker J, Thadhani R. Postpartum diabetes screening in women with a history of gestational diabetes. *Obstet Gynecol*. 2005;106:1297-1303.
35. Russell M, Phipps M, Olson C, Welch H, Carpenter M. Rates of postpartum glucose testing after gestational diabetes mellitus. *Obstet Gynecol*. 2006;108:1456-1462.
36. Kim C, Tabaei B, Burke R, et al. Missed opportunities for diabetes screening among women with a history of gestational diabetes. *Am J Public Health*. 2006;96:1-9.
37. Clark H, van Walraven C, Code C, Karovitch A, Keely E. Did publication of a clinical practice guideline recommendation to screen for type 2 diabetes in women with gestational diabetes change practice? *Diabetes Care*. 2003;26:265-268.
38. Kim C, McEwen L, Piette J, Goewey J, Ferrara A, Walker E. Risk perception for diabetes among women with histories of gestational diabetes mellitus. *Diabetes Care*. 2007;30:2281-2286.
39. Gabbe S, Gregory R, Power M, Williams S, Schulkin J. Management of diabetes mellitus by obstetrician-gynecologists. *Obstet Gynecol*. 2004;103:1229-1234.
40. Gabbe S, Hill L, Schmidt L, Schulkin J. Management of diabetes by obstetrician-gynecologists. *Obstet Gynecol*. 1998;91:643-647.
41. Kim C, McEwen L, Kerr E, et al. Preventive counseling among women with histories of gestational diabetes mellitus. *Diabetes Care*. 2007;30:2489-2495.
42. Clark H, Graham I, Karovitch A, Keely E. Do postal reminders increase postpartum screening of diabetes mellitus in women with gestational diabetes mellitus? A randomized controlled trial. *Am J Obstet Gynecol*. 2009;200:e1-e7.
43. Nicholson W, Wilson L, Witkop C, et al. Therapeutic management, delivery, and postpartum risk assessment and screening in gestational diabetes. *Evid Rep Technol Assess (Full Rep)*. 2008;162:1-96.
44. Retnakaran R, Qi Y, Sermer M, Connelly P, Zinman B, Hanley A. Isolated hyperglycemia at 1-hour on oral glucose tolerance test in pregnancy resembles gestational diabetes in predicting postpartum metabolic dysfunction. *Diabetes Care*. 2008;31(7):1275-1281.
45. Cheung N, Helmink D. Gestational diabetes: the significant of persistent fasting hyperglycemia for the subsequent development of diabetes mellitus. *J Diabetes Complicat*. 2006;20:21-25.
46. Steinhart J, Sugarman J, Connell F. Gestational diabetes is a herald of NIDDM in Navajo women. *Diabetes Care*. 1997;20:943-947.
47. Cho N, Lim S, Jang H, Park H, Metzger B. Elevated homocysteine as a risk factor for the development of diabetes in women with a previous history of gestational diabetes mellitus: a 4-year prospective study. *Diabetes Care*. 2005;28:2750-2755.

48. Kjos S, Peters R, Xiang A, Henry O, Montoro M, Buchanan T. Predicting future diabetes in Latino women with gestational diabetes. *Diabetes*. 1995;44:586-591.
49. Schaefer-Graf U, Buchanan T, Xiang A, Peters R, Kjos S. Clinical predictors for a high risk for the development of diabetes mellitus in the early puerperium in women with recent gestational diabetes mellitus. *Am J Obstet Gynecol*. 2002;186:751-756.
50. Catalano P, Vargo K, Bernstein I, Amini S. Incidence and risk factors associated with abnormal postpartum glucose tolerance in women with gestational diabetes. *Am J Obstet Gynecol*. 1991; 165:914-919.
51. Buchanan T, Xiang A, Kjos S, Trigo E, Lee W, Peters R. Antepartum predictors of the development of type 2 diabetes in Latino women 11-26 months after pregnancies complicated by gestational diabetes. *Diabetes*. 1999;48:2430-2436.
52. Jang H, Yim C, Han K, et al. Gestational diabetes mellitus in Korea: prevalence and prediction of glucose intolerance at early postpartum. *Diabetes Res Clin Pract*. 2003;61:117-124.
53. Metzger B, Cho N, Roston S, Radvany R. Prepregnancy weight and antepartum insulin secretion predict glucose tolerance five years after gestational diabetes mellitus. *Diabetes Care*. 1993;16:1598-1605.
54. Peters R, Kjos S, Xiang A, Buchanan T. Long-term diabetogenic effect of a single pregnancy in women with prior gestational diabetes mellitus. *Lancet*. 1996;347:227-230.
55. Buchanan T, Xiang A, Kjos SL, et al. Gestational diabetes: antepartum characteristics that predict postpartum glucose intolerance and type 2 diabetes in Latino women. *Diabetes*. 1998;47:1302-1310.
56. Retnakaran R, Zinman B, Connelly P, Sermer M, Hanley A. Impaired glucose tolerance of pregnancy is a heterogeneous metabolic disorder as defined by the glycemic response to the oral glucose tolerance test. *Diabetes Care*. 2006;29:57-62.
57. Hanson R, Pratley R, Bogardus C, et al. Evaluation of simple indices of insulin sensitivity and insulin secretion for use in epidemiologic studies. *Am J Epidemiol*. 2000;151:190-198.
58. Phillips D, Clark P, Hales C, Osmond C. Understanding oral glucose tolerance: comparison of glucose or insulin measurements during the oral glucose tolerance test with specific measurements of insulin resistance and insulin secretion. *Diabet Med*. 1994;11:286-292.
59. Matthews D, Hosker J, Rudenski A, Naylor B, Treacher D, Turner R. Homeostasis model assessment: insulin resistance and beta-cell function from fasting plasma glucose and insulin concentrations in man. *Diabetologia*. 1985;28:412-419.
60. Lobner K, Knopff A, Baumgarten A, et al. Predictors of postpartum diabetes in women with gestational diabetes mellitus. *Diabetes*. 2006;55:792-797.
61. Greenberg L, Moore T, Murphy H. Gestational diabetes mellitus: antenatal variables as predictors of postpartum glucose intolerance. *Obstet Gynecol*. 1995;86:97-101.
62. Dalfra M, Lapolla A, Masin M. Antepartum and early postpartum predictors of type 2 diabetes development in women with gestational diabetes mellitus. *Diabetes Metab*. 2001;27:675-680.
63. Henry OA, Beischer NA. Long-term implications of gestational diabetes for the mother. Baillieres Clin Obstet Gynaecol. 1991;5(2):461-483.
64. Bartha J, Martinez-del-Fresno P, Comino-Delgado R. Postpartum metabolism and autoantibody markers in women with gestational diabetes mellitus diagnosed in early pregnancy. *Am J Obstet Gynecol*. 2001;184:965-970.
65. Persson B, Hanson U, Hartling S, Binder C. Follow-up of women with previous GDM: insulin, C-peptide, and proinsulin responses to oral glucose load. *Diabetes*. 1991;40:136-141.
66. Dacus J, Meyer N, Muram D, Stilson R, Phipps P, Sibai B. Gestational diabetes: postpartum glucose tolerance testing. *Am J Obstet Gynecol*. 1994;171:927-931.
67. Shuldiner A, Yang R, Gong D. Resistin, obesity, and insulin resistance–the emerging role of the adipocyte as an endocrine organ. *N Engl J Med*. 2001;345:1345-1346.
68. Branchtein L, Schmidt M, Mengue S, Reichelt A, Matos M, Duncan B. Waist circumference and waist-to-hip ratio are related to gestational glucose tolerance. *Diabetes Care*. 1997;20:509-511.

69. Ward W, Johnston C, Beard J, Benedetti T, Porte D Jr. Abnormalities of islet beta-cell function, insulin action, and fat distribution in women with histories of gestational diabetes: relationship to obesity. *J Clin Endocrinol Metab*. 1985;61:1039-1045.
70. Bian X, Gao P, Xiong X, Xu H, Qian M, Liu S. Risk factors for development of diabetes mellitus in women with a history of gestational diabetes mellitus. *Chin Med J (Engl)*. 2000; 113: 759-762.
71. Cho N, Jan J, Park J, Cho Y. Waist circumference is the key risk factor for diabetes in Korean women with history of gestational diabetes. *Diabetes Res Clin Pract*. 2006;71:177-183.
72. Pallardo L, Herranz L, Martin-Vaquero P, Garcia-Ingelmo T, Grande C, Janez M. Impaired fasting glucose and impaired glucose tolerance in women with prior gestational diabetes are associated with a different cardiovascular profile. *Diabetes Care*. 2003;26:2318-2322.
73. Linne Y, Barkeling B, Rossner S. Natural course of gestational diabetes mellitus: long term follow-up of women in the SPAWN study. *BJOG*. 2002;109:1227-1231.
74. Grant P, Oats J, Beischer N. The long-term follow-up of women with gestational diabetes. *Aust N Z J Obstet Gynaecol*. 1986;26:17-22.
75. Lam K, Li D, Lauder I, Lee C, Kung A, Ma J. Prediction of persistent carbohydrate intolerance in patients with gestational diabetes. *Diabetes Res Clin Pract*. 1991;12:181-186.
76. Coustan D, Carpenter M, O'Sullivan P, Carr S. Gestational diabetes: predictors of subsequent disordered glucose metabolism. *Am J Obstet Gynecol*. 1993;168:1139-1145.
77. Kaufmann R, McBride P, Amankwah K, Huffman D. Gestational diabetes diagnostic criteria: long-term maternal follow-up. *Am J Obstet Gynecol*. 1995;172:621-625.
78. Kjos S, Shoupe D, Douyan S, et al. Effect of low-dose oral contraceptives on carbohydrate and lipid metabolism in women with recent gestational diabetes: results of a controlled, randomized, prospective study. *Am J Obstet Gynecol*. 1990;163:1822-1827.
79. Heikes K, Eddy D, Arondekar B, Schlessinger L. Diabetes risk calculator: a simple tool for detecting undiagnosed diabetes and pre-diabetes. *Diabetes Care*. 2008;31:1040-1045.
80. Solomon C, Willett W, Carey V, et al. A prospective study of pregravid determinants of gestational diabetes mellitus. *JAMA*. 1997;278:1078-1083.
81. Shai I, Jiang R, Manson J, et al. Ethnicity, obesity, and risk of type 2 diabetes in women: a 20-year follow-up study. *Diabetes Care*. 2006;29:1585-1590.
82. Kousta E, Efstathiadou Z, Lawrence N, et al. The impact of ethnicity on glucose regulation and the metabolic syndrome following gestational diabetes. *Diabetologia*. 2006;49:36-40.
83. Ali Z, Alexis S. Occurrence of diabetes mellitus after gestational diabetes mellitus in Trinidad. *Diabetes Care*. 1990;13:527-529.
84. Ferrara A, Kahn H, Quesenberry C, Riley C, Hedderson M. An increase in the incidence of gestational diabetes mellitus: Northern California. *Obstet Gynecol*. 2004;103:526-533.
85. Zhang C, Schulze M, Solomon C, Hu F. A prospective study of dietary patterns, meat intake, and the risk of gestational diabetes mellitus. *Diabetologia*. 2006;49:2604-2613.
86. Kim C, Newton K, Knopp R. Gestational diabetes and incidence of type 2 diabetes mellitus: a systematic review. *Diabetes Care*. 2002;25:1862-1868.
87. Damm P, Kuhl C, Bertelsen A, Molsted-Pedersen L. Predictive factors for the development of diabetes in women with previous gestational diabetes mellitus. *Am J Obstet Gynecol*. 1992;167:607-616.
88. Zhang C, Solomon C, Manson J, Hu F. A prospective study of pregravid physical activity and sedentary behaviors in relation to the risk for gestational diabetes mellitus. *Arch Intern Med*. 2006;166:543-548.
89. Meigs J, Hu F, Rifai N, Manson J. Biomarkers of endothelial dysfunction and risk of type 2 diabetes mellitus. *JAMA*. 2004;291:1978-1986.
90. Hu F, Meigs J, Li T, Rifai N, Manson J. Inflammatory markers and risk of developing type 2 diabetes in women. *Diabetes*. 2004;53:693-700.
91. de Leiva A, Mauricio D, Corcoy R. Diabetes-related autoantibodies and gestational diabetes. *Diabetes Care*. 2007;30:S127-S133.

92. Fuchtenbusch M, Ferber K, Standl E, Ziegler A. Prediction of type 1 diabetes postpartum in patients with gestational diabetes mellitus by combined islet cell autoantibody screening: a prospective multicenter study. *Diabetes*. 1997;46:1459-1467.
93. Hu F, Stampfer M, Haffner S, Solomon CG, Willett W, Manson J. Elevated risk of cardiovascular disease prior to clinical diagnosis of type 2 diabetes. *Diabetes Care*. 2002;25:1129-1134.
94. Rivero K, Portal V, Vieria M, Behle I. Prevalence of the impaired glucose metabolism and its association with risk factors for coronary artery disease in women with gestational diabetes. *Diabetes Res Clin Pract*. 2008;79:433-437.
95. Xiang A, Kawakubo M, Kjos S, Buchanan T. Long-acting injectable progestin contraception and risk of type 2 diabetes in Latino women with prior gestational diabetes mellitus. *Diabetes Care*. 2006;29:613-617.
96. Kim C, Cheng Y, Beckles G. Cardiovascular disease risk profiles in women with histories of gestational diabetes without current diabetes. *Obstet Gynecol*. 2008;112:875-883.
97. Heitritter S, Solomon C, Mitchell G, Skali-Ounis N, Seely E. Subclinical inflammation and vascular dysfunction in women with previous gestational diabetes mellitus. *J Clin Endocrinol Metab*. 2005;90:3983-3988.
98. Bo S, Valpreda S, Menato G, et al. Should we consider gestational diabetes a vascular risk factor? *Atherosclerosis*. 2007;194:e72-e79.
99. Carr D, Utzschneider K, Hull R, et al. Gestational diabetes mellitus increases the risk of cardiovascular disease in women with a family history of type 2 diabetes. *Diabetes Care*. 2006;29:2078-2083.
100. Shah B, Retnakaran R, Booth G. Increased risk of cardiovascular disease in young women following gestational diabetes. *Diabetes Care*. 2008;31(8):1668-1669.
101. Kim C, Sinco B, Kieffer E. Racial and ethnic variation in access to healthcare, provision of healthcare services, and rating of health among women with a history of gestational diabetes mellitus. *Diabetes Care*. 2007;30:1459-1465.

Contraception Before and After GDM

21

Monique Hedderson

21.1 Introduction

Gestational diabetes (GDM) is a common pregnancy complication and its prevalence has increased 35–90% during the last decade.[1] Parity is a risk factor for GDM, therefore preventing unwanted pregnancies by encouraging effective contraceptive use with minimal metabolic side effects in reproductive age women is important. Women with prior GDM are at high risk of developing type 2 diabetes mellitus (T2DM), with up to 50% diagnosed with diabetes within 5 years after delivery.[2] Currently , postpartum screening for T2DM among women with a history of GDM is suboptimal[3] and women with prior GDM may have undiagnosed diabetes or impaired glucose tolerance after pregnancy. Pregnancy occurring in women with suboptimal glucose control increases the risk of congenital malformations and the risk has been shown to increase with increasing degree of maternal hyperglycemia.[4] Therefore, contraception use in women with prior GDM is essential to ensure a planned pregnancy occurs when glucose status is normalized. Preventing an additional unwanted pregnancy may also reduce the risk of subsequent diabetes, since one additional pregnancy has been shown to be associated with a threefold increased risk of T2DM in women with previous GDM.[5] Therefore, women with a history of GDM need safe and efficient methods of contraception postpartum that do not enhance their already elevated risk of developing T2DM. This chapter reviews the efficacy and effects on glucose metabolism of the various contraception options available for women with prior GDM including: postpartum lactational amenorrhea, barrier methods, combination oral contraceptives (COCs), progesterone-only contraception, intrafallopian devices, and intrauterine devices (IUDs).

M. Hedderson
Kaiser Permanente Northern California's Division of Research, Oakland, CA, USA
e-mail: Monique.m.hedderson@kp.org

C. Kim and A. Ferrara (eds.), *Gestational Diabetes During and After Pregnancy*,
DOI: 10.1007/978-1-84882-120-0_21,

21.2 Hormonal Contraceptive Use Before Pregnancy and Risk of GDM

GDM is defined as carbohydrate intolerance first recognized during pregnancy and its incidence has increased 35–90% during the last decade.[1] Parity is a risk factor for GDM, therefore preventing unwanted pregnancies by encouraging effective contraceptive use in reproductive age women is important. The increase in incidence of GDM during the last decade coincided with the availability of two new forms of progestin only contraception, Norplant and Depo-Provera (depot medroxyprogesterone acetate [DMPA])[6] in the U.S. The synthetic progestins used in several forms of hormonal contraceptives are structurally related to testosterone and may produce androgenic side effects. The metabolic effects of androgens include reduced glucose tolerance[7] and weight gain.[8] Therefore, women who have taken hormonal contraceptives, especially progestin dominant forms before pregnancy, may be more vulnerable to the metabolic stress induced by placental hormones in late pregnancy,[9] and may be more likely to develop GDM.

To date there has been only one study examining hormonal contraceptive use before pregnancy and risk of GDM. In a nested case–control study, Hedderson et al examined the effects of hormonal contraceptives, including COCs, progestin-only oral contraceptives (POCs) and DMPA use, on subsequent risk of GDM categorized by the androgenicity of the progestin component. There was a suggestion that compared with no hormonal contraceptive use, use of a low-androgen hormonal contraceptive before pregnancy was associated with a slight (16%) reduction in risk of GDM, whereas use of a high-androgen hormonal contraceptive was associated with a modest (43%) increase in GDM risk.[10] These results suggest that some forms of hormonal contraceptives may actually be beneficial and others detrimental in terms of their metabolic effects and the subsequent risk of GDM during pregnancy. It is important to understand whether hormonal contraceptives that are widely used increases the risk of GDM, especially for high risk women, such as women who are overweight or obese. It is also crucial to understand the risks and benefits of the contraceptive choices available for women with a history of GDM who are at high risk of developing GDM in a subsequent pregnancy and of progressing to T2DM.

21.3 Hormonal Contraceptive Use After Pregnancy

21.3.1 Postpartum Lactational Amenorrhea

Lactation amenorrhea method (LAM) is defined as the informed use of breastfeeding as a contraceptive method.[11] LAM is a form of contraception available to women with GDM during the immediate postpartum period while breastfeeding. LAM can delay ovulation and provide 98% efficacy in protection from pregnancy in the first 6 months postpartum[12, 13] when practiced correctly. To practice LAM effectively, women must begin breastfeeding immediately after delivery, avoid supplementation, and breastfeed frequently (i.e., at least every 4 h during the daytime and 6 h during the night). When other contraceptive methods are used in conjunction with exclusive breastfeeding there is an extremely low failure rate. However, LAM is a transitional form of contraception, since the method is less effective when menses returns, 6 months have elapsed postdelivery, or when supplementing infant feeding is used. Therefore, it is crucial that women be educated regarding the factors affecting its efficacy if they are planning to use this as their only form of contraception. Another method of contraception should be initiated if 6 months have elapsed since delivery, menses returns, or the woman begins to supplement feed her infant.

One concern with the use of LAM for birth control in women with a history of GDM is that it is unpredictable when the return of menstruation and ovulation occurs. Breastfeeding in women with a history of GDM may have additional metabolic benefits for both mother and her infant and should be encouraged; breastfeeding is discussed in greater detail in a separate chapter in this book. Therefore, for women with GDM, a strong endorsement of breastfeeding can be coupled with LAM and recommendation of an additional barrier method, such as condoms. This option is especially good for women who are reluctant to use medications such as hormonal contraception while breastfeeding, due to concerns about hormonal effects on the quality and quantity of milk and fear of passing hormones to the infant.

21.3.2 Barrier Methods

Barrier methods include condoms, diaphragm, cervical cap, and spermicides, and can be used by women with a history of GDM since they do not affect glucose tolerance. However, when used alone, condoms have a high typical failure rate of approximately 15%.[14] As mentioned above, when these methods are used in conjunction with LAM it greatly improves their success rate. The success of these methods requires proper use and strong motivation by both the patient and partner. However, when these criteria cannot be met, intrauterine or hormonal contraceptives might be preferable. The use of condoms should be recommended for women who are engaging in sexual activity with multiple partners as a means to protect against sexually transmitted diseases.

21.3.3 Combination Oral Contraceptives

COC pills contain both progestin and estrogen and are used by more than ten million women in the U.S.[15] The type of progestin varies, although in the U.S., the estrogen component is always ethinyl estradiol. It is generally believed that the estrogen component, ethinyl estradiol, has no net effect on glucose tolerance and insulin sensitivity.[16] However, ethinyl estradiol adversely influences hemostatic and renin-angiotensin systems to increase thrombotic risk.[17] Oral estrogens have also been shown to increase high-density lipoprotein (HDL) cholesterol, decrease low-density lipoprotein (LDL) cholesterol, and to increase triglycerides, globulins, and blood pressure.[18] Therefore, low dose estrogen formulas are recommended and women with hypertension or other cardiovascular risk factors are contraindicated from taking COCs.

Alterations in carbohydrate metabolism in women using COCs are thought to be related primarily to the progestin component. The synthetic progestins used in hormonal contraception are structurally related to testosterone and may also produce androgenic side effects. The metabolic effects of androgens include reduced glucose tolerance[7] and weight gain.[8] The degree of androgenicity in COCs is determined by the dose and type of progestin and whether and to what degree it is opposed by estrogen. The progestin components most widely used in today's COCs are either "second-generation" (e.g., levonorgestrel or norgestimate) or "third-generation" (desogestrel or gestoden). The third generation progestins were specifically formulated to decrease the androgenic side effects. There are also "fourth-generation" progestins, such as drospirenone, dienogest and nomegestrol acetate that have aldosterone antagonist properties, and appear to have no androgenic effects and exhibit partial anti-androgenic activity.[19] The overall metabolic effects of any given COC will depend on the net of the type and dose of each hormonal component.

21.4 Effects of COC on Glucose Metabolism Use in Healthy Populations

Early metabolic studies of COCs suggested that formulations with higher doses of the more androgenic forms of progestins (such as norgestrel and levonorgestrel) were associated with greater alterations of glucose metabolism, often resulting in higher levels of fasting insulin.[20–25] Newer formulations of COCs, with lower doses of progestins, have since been formulated to decrease the androgenic side effects. Since then, several studies have examined the effects of low dose formulations on glucose metabolism among women with normal glucose tolerance.

21.5 Randomized Trials

A recent Cochrane review identified all randomized controlled trials examining hormonal contraceptives and carbohydrate metabolism in women without diabetes; they identified 14 trials with enough data to analyze. Glucose values were often better among women using COCs that had desogestrel than other pills, but the insulin results were not consistent.[26] However, the authors noted there have been few studies that compared specific types of contraceptives and many had small numbers of participants and large losses to follow-up. In addition, it was noted that no studies examined whether carbohydrate response to COCs is different in women who are overweight or obese. While there is limited data available on how the new fourth generation COCs (Yaz, Yasmin, etc.) affect glucose metabolism, one small RCT found that Yasmin, a combined low-dose COC with

30 µg of ethinyl estradiol and 3 mg of the novel progestogen drospirenone, as well as the reference Marvelon, containing 30 µg ethinyl estradiol and 150 µg desogestrel, had little impact on carbohydrate metabolism when used for 1 year.[27] In addition, this study found that Yasmin resulted in a beneficial increase in ratio of total HDL and suggests a potential cardioprotective benefit.[28]

21.6 Epidemiologic Studies

Kim et al examined the cross-sectional association between current OC use and fasting glucose, fasting insulin, and diabetes in the CARDIA study, a large study ($n=1940$) of young African-American and white women.[29] After adjusting for extensive covariate data, current use of a COC was associated with lower fasting glucose levels and lower odds of diabetes, but higher insulin levels. They also examined the longitudinal association between COC use and incident diabetes at 10 years of follow-up but found no association, although they had extremely small numbers of participants who developed diabetes. In this study, women primarily used one type of COC and they were unable to examine whether the association varied by the progestin component of the COC. These results suggested that use of COC in healthy young women might actually be beneficial for glucose tolerance and could have important clinical implications, however, they need to be replicated, preferably in a prospective study.

There have been two large population-based prospective cohort studies in the US on COC use and T2DM risk. Both were conducted in the Nurses' Health Study and no significant increase in risk of type 2 diabetes was observed with the older high-dose estrogen–progestin formulations[30] or in the newer low-dose estrogen–progestin COCs.[31] However, both of these studies were limited to predominantly white women and neither was able to examine whether the effects varied by progestin type.

One recent large population-based cohort study in Finland examined COC use and levonorgestrel-releasing IUD use compared with no use of hormonal contraceptives. They found oral contraception users were more insulin resistant, had higher lipid and insulin levels, and lower homeostatic model assessment (HOMA) and insulin sensitivity compared with IUD users[32] and nonusers. They examined second vs. third-generation COC use and actually found users of third-generation COCs had higher levels of C-reactive protein (CRP), total cholesterol, HDL, triglycerides, insulin resistance, and insulin secretion compared with users of second-generation COCs, contrary to what would be expected. This latter study is the only large cohort study to date to find significant metabolic effects of COCs and it needs to be replicated in other studies.

21.7 Effects of COCs in Women with Diabetes

In general, the few studies examining short-term use of low-dose COC use in diabetic women suggest the changes in insulin sensitivity, glucose tolerance, lipid metabolism, and the coagulation/thrombotic system are minimal and similar to findings in healthy women.[33,34]

However, these studies were conducted more than a decade ago and more information examining how the various forms of COCs effect glucose metabolism and diabetic women are needed.

21.8 Effects of COCs Among Women with a History of GDM

There have been a few studies examining the effects of low-dose COCs compared with nonhormonal contraception in women with a history of GDM. Kjos et al conducted a randomized-controlled trial of Hispanic women with a history of GDM and found no difference in glucose tolerance and no adverse effects on lipids with short-term use of two low-dose COCs compared with noncontraceptive users.[35] Skouby found no effects of low-dose triphasic COC (ethinyl estradiol and levonorgestrel) on glucose tolerance in 16 women with previous GDM and in 19 normal women after treatment for 2 and 6 months.[36] In another small study with 6 women with a history of GDM and 6 women without GDM history, Skouby et al found a slight decrease in insulin sensitivity among women with previous GDM after using a low-dose triphasic COC for 6 months, but the effects were not sufficient to alter glucose tolerance.[37]

In another large prospective observational cohort study of Latino women with prior GDM, Kjos et al found that COC use was not associated with risk of T2DM compared with women not using hormonal contraception during 7 years of follow-up.[38] To further our understanding of the effects of COCs in women with a history of GDM, more long-term studies are needed of COC use, preferably in ethnically diverse populations with detailed information on baseline metabolic risk factors and outcomes, and with attention to the specific types of OC and the androgenicity of the progestin component.

In general, evidence from existing studies of COCs in healthy populations, women with diabetes, and women with a history of GDM suggest that the use of low-dose COCs can be prescribed to women with prior GDM. However, formulations with the lowest dose ethinyl estradiol and the lowest dose and least androgenic progestin should be prescribed. If women have coexisting hypertension or other CVD risk factors than consideration should be given to nonestrogen containing methods. More information is needed to clarify whether certain types of COC are actually beneficial and others detrimental in terms of carbohydrate metabolism; this could have clinical implications for recommendations as to what types of COC to prescribe, especially for high risk women such as women with diabetes or a history of GDM. More studies are needed with large enough numbers to compare different types of COC and to examine whether the effects vary among obese vs. normal weight women.

21.9 Progestin-Only Oral Contraceptives

POCs are commonly used by women who are breastfeeding and women with contraindications to taking synthetic estrogens. POCs have no effects on maternal coagulation factors or blood pressure and do not affect milk supply in lactating women. However, POCs are more likely to cause break through bleeding which, in turn, could affect their acceptability and lead to poor compliance and hence higher pregnancy rates. POC efficacy has been estimated to be between 1.4 and 4.3 pregnancies per 100 woman-years of use.[39]

In a landmark study, Kjos et al examined a large cohort of 904 postpartum women with a recent history of GDM and found a threefold increased risk of developing type 2 diabetes among lactating women who were using POCs (0.35 mg of norethindrone) compared with low-dose COC and nonhormonal methods.[38] The magnitude of this risk increased with duration of uninterrupted use and was highest among women who used POCs for more than 8 months. Only breastfeeding women were prescribed POCs and therefore the question of whether non-breastfeeding women with prior GDM also have any increased risk with POC use could not be examined. The authors concluded that the observed adverse effects of unopposed progestins, may have been due to the combination of the hormonal effects of lactation, whereby endogenous estrogen is suppressed and combined with the underlying insulin resistance and a β-cell dysfunction in women with GDM.[38] There is currently no data available to determine whether POCs have similar adverse effects in nonlactating women. These findings have yet to be confirmed in other populations or ethnic groups or to see if these associations vary by obesity status in women with a history of GDM. Therefore, POCs may be a good contraceptive option for women with contraindications to COCs, such as women with hypertension, but more information is needed to confirm their safety in lactating women with a history of GDM.

21.10 Long-Acting Progestin Only Methods

Long-acting progestin contraceptive methods can be administered intramuscularly or subcutaneously. The subcutaneous levonorgestrel implant, Norplant, is no longer marketed in the US and will not be discussed. Little information is available on Implanon, an etonogestrel implant, although this implant contains much lower doses of progestin, suggesting it should have minimal effects on glucose metabolism and data from two small observational studies, one in diabetic women[40] and one in healthy women,[41] found it did not have meaningful effects on carbohydrate metabolism. DMPA is administered intramuscularly. It delivers a plasma concentration of 1 ng/mL medroxyprogesterone and its effects last 3 months.[42] DMPA is highly effective (≤0.3% pregnancies with typical use in the first year.[43] Similar to POCs, DMPA has no effects on maternal coagulation or blood pressure. However, a review of the effects of injectable or implantable POCs on insulin-glucose metabolism found 7 out of 8 studies with data from an oral glucose tolerance test found an approximately doubling of insulin at 2- or 3-h postchallenge test[6]; the effects on fasting, half-hour, or 1-h postchallenge insulin levels were less consistent. DPMA use has also been associated with increases in mean weight,[44, 45] which appears to be due to changes in adipose mass rather than fluid or lean tissue.[46]

The studies examining the effects of DMPA in populations at high risk for T2DM suggest that it may substantially increase the risk of progression to T2DM. In a case–control study of 284 women with diabetes and 570 controls conducted among a high-risk

Navajo population, Kim found that T2DM was 3.6 times more common in women who used DMPA compared with women who used COCs. Kim also found a dose–response association with longer duration of use, women who used DMPA for 1 year or more had an almost eightfold increased risk of diabetes compared with combination OC-users.[47] In an observational cohort study Xiang and colleagues[48] examined DMPA use compared with use of COCs on the risk of T2DM among Latino women with a history of GDM. After adjusting for covariates and weight gain during follow-up there was no increased risk of T2DM among DMPA users. However, in stratified analyses, use of DMPA among women with high baseline triglycerides or during breastfeeding did increase the risk of diabetes. Xiang and colleagues[49] also found that 1–2 years of treatment with DMPA was associated with greater weight gain compared with nonhormonal or COC users, but there were no significant differences in changes in lipids among the groups and women taking COCs experienced greater increases in systolic blood pressure. In general, data suggests that DMPA may cause adverse metabolic effects, which may be particularly concerning in women at high risk of T2DM or while breastfeeding. Therefore, it would not be recommended as a first-line choice for most women with a history of GDM. However, since DMPA has the advantage of requiring very little active involvement from the patient and since an additional pregnancy in women with prior GDM is associated with a threefold increased risk of developing T2DM,[5] it may be an option for patients who have a hard time with the compliance required to take daily medication and who do not desire an additional pregnancy. However, these women should be clinically monitored for adverse metabolic changes.

21.11 Intrauterine Devices

IUDs are a very effective form of reversible contraception. The two forms of IUDs currently used in the U.S. are predominantly copper (TCu380A) or levonorgestrel-releasing. The levonorgestrel-releasing IUD and to a slightly lesser extent the TCu380A IUD are extremely effective, with a cumulative pregnancy rate at 5 years of <0.5% for the levonorgestrel-releasing IUD and between 0.3 and 0.6% for the TCu380A IUD.[50] The currently available IUDs may be an ideal form of contraceptive for women with a history of GDM, because they do not appear to have substantial metabolic effects, especially the nonhormonal copper IUD. According to medical guidelines of the World Health Organization, the copper IUD is advised for women with diabetes mellitus with or without comorbidity.[51] However, side effects of copper IUDs including bleeding and pain cause removal of the device within the first year in up to 15% of users.[52] Therefore, the levonorgestrel IUD may be preferred in some women with a history of GDM as it has a low frequency of bleeding disturbances.

There have been no studies of IUD use in women with a history of GDM. A randomized trial of women with type 1 diabetes comparing levonorgestrel-releasing IUD to a copper T 380A IUD with respect to effects on glucose metabolism after 12 months of use found the levonorgestrel-releasing IUD had no effects on fasting glucose, glycosylated hemoglobin, or daily insulin doses.[53] One study[54] of levonorgestrel IUD use among 48 perimenopausal women suffering from menorrhagia found mean fasting plasma glucose levels increased, whereas mean diastolic blood pressure decreased after 12 months of use, however, this study was not a randomized trial and not a representative sample. In general, data to date suggest that both levonorgestrel and copper IUDs can be used in women with a history of GDM, however more studies on the effects of IUD use in women with a history of GDM are needed.

21.12 Contraceptive Vaginal Ring

The contraceptive vaginal ring is a flexible ring composed of ethinyl vinyl acetate and releases 15 μg of ethniyl estradiol and 120 μg of the third-generation progestin, etonogestrel, per day.[55] The delivery system had the advantage of avoiding first-pass metabolism through the liver and a once a month insertion. NuvaRing is the only vaginal ring available in the US and it is highly efficacious with an efficacy of 99.1%.[55] While there is limited information on the metabolic effects of the vaginal ring, the one small study to date found that the NuvaRing had less impact on carbohydrate metabolism and greater reduction in free androgen levels than a low dose COC pill.[56]

21.13 Surgical Sterilization

Operative sterilization is a nonreversible form of contraceptive that is an excellent choice for women with a history of GDM who have decided they do not want to have any more children. This option should be offered to parous women and can be performed during delivery among women who are undergoing cesarean section. Vasectomy is also a nonreversible form of contraceptive that can be performed with comparatively less morbidity and lower cost than either bilateral tubal ligation or microinsert coil insertion (Essure), both of which require a hysteroscopic or laparoscopic procedure.

21.14 Obesity and Contraception Use

Obesity is the strongest modifiable risk factor for GDM identified to date. Unfortunately, most of the studies to date on the metabolic effects of hormonal contraceptives were unable to examine whether the effects varied by obesity. Recent studies suggest that increased weight and body mass index (BMI) may affect steroid hormonal metabolism or sequestration in fat and can alter hormonal contraceptive effectiveness.[57, 58] A study of health plan enrolees who became pregnant while using hormonal contraceptives found that among consistent users (women who missed no pills in the reference month), the risk of pregnancy was more than doubled in women with a BMI greater than 27.3. More information is needed to clarify whether the metabolic effects of hormonal contraceptives vary by obesity status and to further clarify how obesity affects contraceptive efficacy in order to determine if overweight women need additional contraceptive methods.

21.15 Conclusions

Effective contraception with minimal metabolic side effects is essential for women both before and after a pregnancy complicated by GDM. Table 21.1 summarizes the recommendations in this chapter. In general, women with prior GDM have many contraception options and the benefits of most forms of contraception seem to outweigh the risks of an unwanted pregnancy. Existing evidence suggests progestin-only methods during lactation should be used with caution. Women with prior GDM should be given contraceptive options that meet their lifestyle and does not further increase their risk of developing diabetes. More rigorous studies examining the metabolic effects of the various hormonal contraceptive methods currently available could help clarify if some forms are actually beneficial and other detrimental to glucose metabolism.

Table 21.1 Summary of the types of contraception and the current recommendations based on their effects on glucose metabolism

Type of contraception	Recommendation
Combination OCPs	Safe; little known regarding fourth generation
Progestin-only OCPs	May increase glucose intolerance, particularly during breastfeeding
Depo-Provera (depot medroxyprogesterone acetate [DMPA])	May increase glucose intolerance, particularly during breastfeeding
Etonogestrel implants	Limited data, but appear to be safe
NuvaRing	Safe
IUDs(levonorgestrel, copper)	Safe
Condoms/diaphragm	Safe, although efficacy rates not as high as other methods
Lactation amenorrhea method	Safe temporary method while exclusively breastfeeding, but must be used accurately and it is recommended to use barrier method in addition for added efficacy

References

1. Ferrara A. Increasing prevalence of gestational diabetes mellitus: a public health perspective. *Diabetes Care*. 2007;30(suppl 2):S141-S146.
2. Kim C, Newton KM, Knopp RH. Gestational diabetes and the incidence of type 2 diabetes: a systematic review. *Diabetes Care*. 2002;25:1862-1868.
3. Ferrara A, Peng T, Kim C. Trends in postpartum diabetes screening and subsequent diabetes and impaired fasting glucose among women with histories of gestational diabetes mellitus. A report from the Translating Research Into Action for Diabetes (TRIAD) Study. *Diabetes Care*. 2009;32:269-274.
4. Wolff S, Legarth J, Vangsgaard K, Toubro S, Astrup A. A randomized trial of the effects of dietary counseling on gestational weight gain and glucose metabolism in obese pregnant women. *Int J Obes (Lond)*. 2008;32:495-501.
5. Peters RK, Kjos SL, Xiang A, Buchanan TA. Long-term diabetogenic effect of single pregnancy in women with previous gestational diabetes mellitus [see comments]. *Lancet*. 1996;347:227-230.
6. Kahn HS, Curtis KM, Marchbanks PA. Effects of injectable or implantable progestin-only contraceptives on insulin-glucose metabolism and diabetes risk. *Diabetes Care*. 2003;26:216-225.
7. Kay CR. Progestogens and arterial disease–evidence from the Royal College of General Practitioners' study. *Am J Obstet Gynecol*. 1982;142:762-765.
8. Darney PD. The androgenicity of progestins. *Am J Med*. 1995;98:104S-110S.
9. Boden G. Fuel metabolism in pregnancy and in gestational diabetes mellitus. *Obstet Gynecol Clin North Am*. 1996;23:1-10.
10. Hedderson MM, Ferrara A, Williams MA, Holt VL, Weiss NS. Androgenicity of progestins in hormonal contraceptives and the risk of gestational diabetes mellitus. *Diabetes Care*. 2007;30:1062-1068.
11. Kennedy KI, Rivera R, McNeilly AS. Consensus statement on the use of breastfeeding as a family planning method. *Contraception*. 1989;39:477-496.
12. Labbok MH, Hight-Laukaran V, Peterson AE, Fletcher V, von Hertzen H, Van Look PF. Multicenter study of the Lactational Amenorrhea Method (LAM): I. Efficacy, duration, and implications for clinical application. *Contraception*. 1997;55:327-336.
13. Kennedy KI, Visness CM. Contraceptive efficacy of lactational amenorrhoea. *Lancet*. 1992;339:227-230.
14. Trussel J, Warner DL, Hatcher R. Condom performance during vaginal intercourse: comparison of Trojan-Enz and Tactylon condoms. *Contraception*. 1992;45:11-19.
15. Petitti DB. Clinical practice. Combination estrogen-progestin oral contraceptives. *N Engl J Med*. 2003;349:1443-1450.
16. Spellacy WN, Buhi WC, Birk SA. The effect of estrogens on carbohydrate metabolism: glucose, insulin, and growth hormone studies on one hundred and seventy-one women ingesting Premarin, mestranol, and ethinyl estradiol for six months. *Am J Obstet Gynecol*. 1972;114:378-392.
17. Petersen KR. Pharmacodynamic effects of oral contraceptive steroids on biochemical markers for arterial thrombosis. Studies in non-diabetic women and in women with insulin-dependent diabetes mellitus. *Dan Med Bull*. 2002;49:43-60.
18. Damm P, Mathiesen ER, Petersen KR, Kjos S. Contraception after gestational diabetes. *Diabetes Care*. 2007;30(suppl 2):S236-S241.
19. Sitruk-Ware R. Pharmacology of different progestogens: the special case of drospirenone. *Climacteric*. 2005;8(suppl 3):4-12.
20. Godsland IF, Crook D, Simpson R, et al. The effects of different formulations of oral contraceptive agents on lipid and carbohydrate metabolism. *N Engl J Med*. 1990;323:1375-1381.

21. Godsland IF, Walton C, Felton C, Proudler A, Patel A, Wynn V. Insulin resistance, secretion, and metabolism in users of oral contraceptives. *J Clin Endocrinol Metab*. 1992;74:64-70.
22. Perlman JA, Russell-Briefel R, Ezzati T, Lieberknecht G. Oral glucose tolerance and the potency of contraceptive progestins. *J Chronic Dis*. 1985;38:857-864.
23. Wynn V, Godsland I. Effects of oral contraceptives on carbohydrate metabolism. *J Reprod Med*. 1986;31:892-897.
24. Kalkhoff RK. Relative sensitivity of postpartum gestational diabetic women to oral contraceptive agents and other metabolic stress. *Diabetes Care*. 1980;3:421-424.
25. Straznicky NE, Barrington VE, Branley P, Louis WJ. A study of the interactive effects of oral contraceptive use and dietary fat intake on blood pressure, cardiovascular reactivity and glucose tolerance in normotensive women. *J Hypertens*. 1998;16:357-368.
26. Lopez LM, Grimes DA, Schulz KF. Steroidal contraceptives: effect on carbohydrate metabolism in women without diabetes mellitus. *Cochrane Database Syst Rev*. 2007;(4):CD006133.
27. Gaspard U, Scheen A, Endrikat J, et al. A randomized study over 13 cycles to assess the influence of oral contraceptives containing ethinylestradiol combined with drospirenone or desogestrel on carbohydrate metabolism. *Contraception*. 2003;67:423-429.
28. Gaspard U, Endrikat J, Desager JP, Buicu C, Gerlinger C, Heithecker R. A randomized study on the influence of oral contraceptives containing ethinylestradiol combined with drospirenone or desogestrel on lipid and lipoprotein metabolism over a period of 13 cycles. *Contraception*. 2004;69:271-278.
29. Bullock LP, Bardin CW. Androgenic, synandrogenic, and antiandrogenic actions of progestins. *Ann N Y Acad Sci*. 1977;286:321-330.
30. Rimm EB, Manson JE, Stampfer MJ, et al. Oral contraceptive use and the risk of type 2 (non-insulin-dependent) diabetes mellitus in a large prospective study of women. *Diabetologia*. 1992;35:967-972.
31. Chasan-Taber L, Willett WC, Stampfer MJ, et al. A prospective study of oral contraceptives and NIDDM among U.S. women. *Diabetes Care*. 1997;20:330-335.
32. Morin-Papunen L, Martikainen H, McCarthy MI, et al. Comparison of metabolic and inflammatory outcomes in women who used oral contraceptives and the levonorgestrel-releasing intrauterine device in a general population. *Am J Obstet Gynecol*. 2008;199:529.
33. Petersen KR, Skouby SO, Sidelmann J, Molsted-Pedersen L, Jespersen J. Effects of contraceptive steroids on cardiovascular risk factors in women with insulin-dependent diabetes mellitus. *Am J Obstet Gynecol*. 1994;171:400-405.
34. Skouby SO, Molsted-Pedersen L, Kuhl C, Bennet P. Oral contraceptives in diabetic women: metabolic effects of four compounds with different estrogen/progestogen profiles. *Fertil Steril*. 1986;46:858-864.
35. Kjos SL, Shoupe D, Douyan S, et al. Effect of low-dose oral contraceptives on carbohydrate and lipid metabolism in women with recent gestational diabetes: results of a controlled, randomized, prospective study. *Am J Obstet Gynecol*. 1990;163:1822-1827.
36. Skouby SO, Kuhl C, Molsted-Pedersen L, Petersen K, Christensen MS. Triphasic oral contraception: metabolic effects in normal women and those with previous gestational diabetes. *Am J Obstet Gynecol*. 1985;153:495-500.
37. Skouby SO, Andersen O, Saurbrey N, Kuhl C. Oral contraception and insulin sensitivity: in vivo assessment in normal women and women with previous gestational diabetes. *J Clin Endocrinol Metab*. 1987;64:519-523.
38. Kjos SL, Peters RK, Xiang A, Thomas D, Schaefer U, Buchanan TA. Contraception and the risk of type 2 diabetes mellitus in Latina women with prior gestational diabetes mellitus. *JAMA*. 1998;280:533-538.
39. Chi I. The safety and efficacy issues of progestin-only oral contraceptives–an epidemiologic perspective. *Contraception*. 1993;47:1-21.

40. Vicente L, Mendonca D, Dingle M, Duarte R, Boavida JM. Etonogestrel implant in women with diabetes mellitus. *Eur J Contracept Reprod Health Care*. 2008;13:387-395.
41. Inal MM, Yildirim Y, Ertopcu K, Avci ME, Ozelmas I, Tinar S. Effect of the subdermal contraceptive etonogestrel implant (Implanon) on biochemical and hormonal parameters (three years follow-up). *Eur J Contracept Reprod Health Care*. 2008;13:238-242.
42. Kaunitz AM. Injectable depot medroxyprogesterone acetate contraception: an update for U.S. clinicians. *Int J Fertil Womens Med*. 1998;43:73-83.
43. Hatcher R, Trussell J, Stewart F, Nelson A. Contraceptive technology; New York: *Ardent Media Inc*. 1998.
44. Espey E, Steinhart J, Ogburn T, Qualls C. Depo-provera associated with weight gain in Navajo women. *Contraception*. 2000;62:55-58.
45. Risser WL, Gefter LR, Barratt MS, Risser JM. Weight change in adolescents who used hormonal contraception. *J Adolesc Health*. 1999;24:433-436.
46. Amatayakul K, Sivasomboon B, Thanangkul O. A study of the mechanism of weight gain in medroxyprogesterone acetate users. *Contraception*. 1980;22:605-622.
47. Kim C, Seidel KW, Begier EA, Kwok YS. Diabetes and depot medroxyprogesterone contraception in Navajo women. *Arch Intern Med*. 2001;161:1766-1771.
48. Xiang AH, Kawakubo M, Kjos SL, Buchanan TA. Long-acting injectable progestin contraception and risk of type 2 diabetes in Latino women with prior gestational diabetes mellitus. *Diabetes Care*. 2006;29:613-617.
49. Xiang AH, Kawakubo M, Buchanan TA, Kjos SL. A longitudinal study of lipids and blood pressure in relation to method of contraception in Latino women with prior gestational diabetes mellitus. *Diabetes Care*. 2007;30:1952-1958.
50. Thonneau PF, Almont T. Contraceptive efficacy of intrauterine devices. *Am J Obstet Gynecol*. 2008;198:248-253.
51. WHO 2004 Reproductive Health and Research. World Health Organization. *Medical eligibility criteria for contraceptive use*. Geneva; Switzerland: World Health Organization; 2004.
52. Trieman K, Liskin L, Kols A, Rinehart W. IUDs-an update. Populations Reports, Series B, No.6 Baltimore, Johns Hopkins School of Public Health, Population Information Program, December 1995.
53. Rogovskaya S, Rivera R, Grimes DA, et al. Effect of a levonorgestrel intrauterine system on women with type 1 diabetes: a randomized trial. *Obstet Gynecol*. 2005;105:811-815.
54. Kayikcioglu F, Gunes M, Ozdegirmenci O, Haberal A. Effects of levonorgestrel-releasing intrauterine system on glucose and lipid metabolism: a 1-year follow-up study. *Contraception*. 2006;73:528-531.
55. Madden T, Blumenthal P. Contraceptive vaginal ring. *Clin Obstet Gynecol*. 2007;50: 878-885.
56. Elkind-Hirsch KE, Darensbourg C, Ogden B, Ogden LF, Hindelang P. Contraceptive vaginal ring use for women has less adverse metabolic effects than an oral contraceptive. *Contraception*. 2007;76:348-356.
57. Holt VL, Scholes D, Wicklund KG, Cushing-Haugen KL, Daling JR. Body mass index, weight, and oral contraceptive failure risk. *Obstet Gynecol*. 2005;105:46-52.
58. Holt VL, Cushing-Haugen KL, Daling JR. Body weight and risk of oral contraceptive failure. *Obstet Gynecol*. 2002;99:820-827.

Lactation and Diabetes Among Women with a History of GDM Pregnancy

22

Erica P. Gunderson

22.1 Introduction

Lactation has been associated with more favorable cardiometabolic risk factor profiles during the postpartum period among women in general, and those with a history of gestational diabetes mellitus (GDM) during pregnancy.[1,2] Among women in general, evidence suggests that extended lactation may protect against future development of type 2 diabetes[3] and the onset of the metabolic syndrome in midlife.[4,5] However, among women with a history of GDM, evidence is based on two studies which have yielded inconsistent results. Studies examining increasing months of lactation have reported a null association with incident type 2 diabetes[3], and a 44 to 86% lower incidence of the metabolic syndrome.[6]

Evidence is also equivocal that breastfeeding influences the long-term health of the offspring of mothers with GDM during pregnancy. Breastfeeding has been associated with beneficial, adverse, or no effects on development of overweight and type 2 diabetes for the offspring of women with diabetes during pregnancy.[7] Early infant feeding practices and postnatal influences may be particularly important for offspring of mothers with GDM, because they are more likely to become overweight, and to develop impaired glucose tolerance, the metabolic syndrome, and type 2 diabetes later in life.[8–13]

In this chapter, we critically examine the available data that lactation influences the development of cardiometabolic risk factors, the metabolic syndrome, and type 2 diabetes among women in general and those with a history of GDM. In addition, we examine the evidence that breastfeeding may affect development of overweight and diabetes among the offspring of mothers with a history of GDM pregnancy. Finally, we provide recommendations for future research.

E.P. Gunderson, PhD
Division of Research, Epidemiology and Prevention Section,
Kaiser Permanente Northern California, Oakland, CA, USA
e-mail: epg@dor.kaiser.org

C. Kim and A. Ferrara (eds.), *Gestational Diabetes During and After Pregnancy*,
DOI: 10.1007/978-1-84882-120-0_22,

22.2 Lactation and Women's Health

22.2.1 Effects of Lactation on Cardiometabolic Risk Factors and Long-term Disease Risk

Lactation has favorable effects on cardiometabolic risk profiles during the postpartum period among women with and without a history of GDM. The maternal risk factors that may be influenced by lactation include plasma lipid, insulin and glucose profiles, body fat distribution and postpartum weight loss. Although the effects of lactation on cardiometabolic risk factors may persist postweaning, one study[6] provides direct biochemical evidence that these favorable changes in postpartum risk factor profiles persist years later to lower risk of incident disease in women later in life.

22.2.2 Studies of Risk Factors Among Women in General

Lower blood glucose and insulin concentrations, along with higher rates of glucose production and lipolysis, have been observed among lactating women compared with nonlactating women.[14] Moreover, plasma total cholesterol and triglyceride levels declined more rapidly from delivery to 3–5 months postpartum in lactating women,[15,16] and their lipid profiles were more favorable (i.e., lower plasma low-density lipoprotein cholesterol or LDL-C, triglycerides and higher high-density lipoprotein cholesterol or HDL-C) by 6 months postpartum.[17,18] However, these studies did not control for differences in preconception lipid profiles and obesity, postpartum weight loss, or lifestyle behaviors. Recently, in 67 Brazilian women given oral glucose tolerance tests at 12–18 months postpartum, increasing duration of lactation was inversely associated with the area under the insulin curve independent of body adiposity.[19] These data suggest that lactation may be an important factor in reversal of gestational hyperlipidemia and have lasting favorable effects on women's health. However, these studies do not provide evidence for lasting effects because they did not examine postweaning levels.

Gunderson et al[2] examined changes in cardiometabolic risk factors from preconception to an average of 13 months postweaning (range of 2–24 months) among women who gave birth during a 3-year interval. Postweaning levels of HDL-C were 6 mg/dL higher among women who lactated for 3 months or longer vs. less than 3 months ($p<0.01$), and parous women who did not lactate had a 2.6 uU higher fasting insulin postpartum ($p=0.06$) given similar preconception levels and weight gain.[2] These lasting effects on plasma HDL-C levels associated with lactation (i.e., postweaning) are important because low plasma HCL-C is a strong predictor of type 2 diabetes in women.

Obesity and weight gain contribute to development of type 2 diabetes. Yet, evidence is equivocal about whether lactation promotes greater loss in fat mass.[20] One study of body composition found a 2 kg greater loss in total body fat mass for lactating vs. nonlactating women that did not reach statistical significance.[21] Studies that measured body weight changes from before or during early pregnancy (not self-reported) consistently reported that lactating vs. nonlactating women had lower postpartum weight retention, greater weight loss, and more rapid return to pregravid weight within 6–12 months.[22–25] These studies carefully assessed lactation and demonstrate that both intensity and duration of lactation are important determinants of postpartum weight loss. Longer duration of lactation has also been associated with lower maternal weight gain 10–15 years later.[26,27]

22.2.3 Lactation and Future Diabetes Risk Among Women in General

To our knowledge, only two studies have examined lactation duration and future risk of diabetes among women in general. The Nurses' Health Study II (NHS II) found that lactation for 4–6 months and up to 2 years was associated with a 25–40% lower incidence of self-reported DM among women aged 24–43 yrs at baseline who reported a birth within the past 15 years of follow-up.[3] The association was independent of current BMI and other risk factors, and risk reductions were stronger with exclusive lactation.[3] In the Shanghai Women's Health Study, Villegas et al. found that lactation for 4 years or longer reported when women were aged 40–70 was associated with a 10–12% lower incidence of DM that varied by years since last birth and number of children.[28] However, plasma glucose levels were not measured before, during, and/or after pregnancy in either study of the long-term effects of lactation on development of diabetes in mid and late life.

22.2.4 Lactating versus Non-Lactating Women with a Recent GDM Pregnancy

Lactation also favorably affects maternal glucose tolerance and lipid profiles after GDM pregnancy. Fourteen lactating compared with 12 nonlactating women with previous GDM had higher insulin sensitivity, glucose effectiveness and first phase insulin response to glucose (AIRg) assessed by Bergman's Minimal Model, but statistical significance was not reached.[29] However, the disposition index (insulin sensitivity multiplied by AIRg) was 2.5 times higher (129.9 ± 26.0 vs. $53.4 \pm 18.0 \times 10^{(-4)}$ min$^{(-1)}$; $p < 0.05$) in lactating vs. nonlactating women matched for age, weight, postpartum weight loss, and exercise habits.[29] These data suggest that women who lactated after GDM pregnancy had improved insulin sensitivity and β-cell function.

A series of cross-sectional and follow-up studies (Table 22.1) of Latinas with history of GDM provide evidence that lactation influences glucose metabolism.[1,30–32] For example, lactating women had better glucose tolerance at 4–12 weeks postpartum; a lower total area under the glucose tolerance curve (AUC) (17.0 ± 4.2 vs. 17.9 ± 5.0 g/min/dL), and lower fasting serum glucose (93 ± 13 vs. 98 ± 17 mg/dL) and 2-h OGTT glucose levels (124 ± 41 vs. 134 ± 49 mg/dL) after controlling for BMI, maternal age and insulin use during pregnancy.[1] The prevalence of type 2 diabetes was lower for lactating (4.2%) vs. nonlactating

Table 22.1 Association of lactation status or lactation duration with Risk of Type 2 Diabetes Mellitus (DM) or the Metabolic Syndrome among Women with a history of GDM

Reference	Study design, years	*n*, GDM pregnancy	Study population	Lactation measure	Type 2 DM definition	Time since delivery	Type 2 DM outcome	Conclusion
Kjos et al[1]	Cross-sectional 1990–1991	809	Latinas attending family planning clinic	Yes/no at 4–16 weeks postpartum	2-h 75-g OGTT	4–16 weeks	Prevalence: 9.4% in nonlactating 4.2% in lactating	Lower prevalence of diabetes $p=0.01$ in lactating
Kjos et al[30]	Retrospective analysis 1987–1994	671	Latinas in central Los Angeles	Yes/no at 4–16 weeks postpartum	2-h 75-g OGTT	Variable follow-up, Within 7.5 years	Incidence rate: 1.1 cases/1,000 person-years (95%CI: 0.9–1.9)	No association of lactation with DM in bivariate analyses
Buchanan et al[31]	Cross-sectional 1993–1995	122 normal fasting glucose, diet-control	Latinas in central Los Angeles	Yes/no at 1–6 months	75-g OGTT and FSIGTs	1–6 months	Overall prevalence 10%	DM less likely to be lactating than non-DM (42% vs. 71%) $p=0.03$
Buchanan et al[32]	Longitudinal 1993–1997	91	Latinas in central Los Angeles	Yes/no at 11–26 months postpartum	75-g OGTT and FSIGTs	15-month interval, 11–26 months	Overall cumulative incidence 15%	No differences in lactation prevalence for DM vs. normal (25% vs. 15.4%) $p=0.41$
Stuebe et al[3]	Retrospective cohort 1989–2003	Not reported age 24–43 years in 1989	The Nurses' Health Study cohort	Total lifetime months of lactation for pregnancies	Self-report	Variable, up to 14 years	Incidence rate: 6.24 cases per 1000 person-years	No significant association
Gunderson[6]	Prospective Cohort 1985-2006	84, Aged 18–30 in 1985	CARDIA, Multi-center 50% White 50% Black	Total months of lactation, all pregnancies	Fasting and 75-g OGTT and other measures*	Average 8 years	Metabolic Syndrome Incidence rate*: 22.1 per 1,000 person-years	44% to 86% lower incidence; $p=0.03$ >1 to >9 months versus 0–1 month

DM diabetes mellitus; *GDM* gestational diabetes mellitus, *The Metabolic Syndrome instead of Type 2 DM

(9.4%) women with recent GDM.[1] Buchanan et al examined 122 Latinas with normal fasting glucose and no insulin use during GDM pregnancy and found that those diagnosed with diabetes within 6 months postpartum were less likely to be currently lactating (42%) than those with normal glucose tolerance (71%); $p=0.03$.[31] These data suggest that lactation may have favorable effects on glucose tolerance during the postpartum period.

22.2.5 Lactation and Future Diabetes Risk Among Women with a History of GDM

Less evidence is available to determine whether lactation has lasting effects on glucose metabolism to prevent development of type 2 diabetes in women with a history of GDM. Studies that examined lactation and incidence of diabetes among women with a history of GDM are shown in (Table 22.1). However, several studies assessed lactating versus non-lactating women at the early postpartum glucose tolerance test (i.e., 1–4 months postpartum) rather than lactation duration. Specifically, among Latinas in central Los Angeles, lactation at 4–16 weeks postpartum was not associated with development of type 2 diabetes within 7.5 years after delivery.[30] For 91 Latinas, lactation status (yes/no) at testing did not differ by type 2 diabetes diagnosis at 11–26 months after GDM pregnancy.[32] Only two studies have assessed lactation duration and disease incidence years later specifically among women with a history of GDM. A retrospective analysis of women with a history of GDM in the NHS cohort found no association between lifetime lactation or other lifestyle behaviors (i.e., diet, exercise habits) and incidence of type 2 diabetes several years after delivery.[3] However, limitations of these studies included retrospective analysis, limited assessment of lactation, nonuniversal postpartum screening for diabetes, no plasma glucose measurements before, during, or after pregnancy, self-report of subsequent type 2 diabetes, and no data on lifestyle behaviors. In the NHS cohort, diabetes screening was not conducted prospectively after delivery and diabetes status was ascertained by self-report. The Coronary Artery Risk Development in Young Adults (CARDIA) study,[6] measured cardiometabolic risk factors prospectively, both before and after pregnancies during 20 years of follow-up, and assessed lactation duration in relation to incidence of the metabolic syndrome among women with and without a history of GDM. In 702 nulliparas who went on to give birth during follow-up, increasing months of lactation was associated with lower incidence of the metabolic syndrome; 44 to 86% lower among women with a history of GDM and 39 to 56% lower among women with no history of GDM several years post-weaning. These findings suggest that lactation may have persistent favorable effects on women's cardiometabolic health, and effects may be stronger among women with a history of GDM.[6]

22.2.6 Lactogenesis and History of GDM

Effects of GDM pregnancy on lactogenesis have rarely been studied. One small clinical study of women with recent GDM reported no marked delays in lactogenesis based on similar concentration of lactose in the colostrum at 40–50 h postpartum for GDM women compared with control women.[33] However, GDM women had more difficulty expressing colostrum from their breasts during the first 2 days of lactation.[33] Moreover, maternal obesity may delay the onset of lactogenesis[34,35] due to lower physiological levels of prolactin in response to suckling.[34] Delayed milk production has been associated with lower rates of breastfeeding and shorter duration among obese women.[35] Furthermore, medical management of newborns that involves provision of supplemental milk feedings (i.e., neonatal hypoglycemia) may also interfere with maternal milk production.

Preliminary evidence suggests that lactation may confer long-term protection against development of type 2 diabetes later in life, among women in general. The evidence for an association between lactation and lower risk of cardiometabolic disease in women with a history of GDM is inconclusive given that prospective, population-based studies have not been conducted. Future studies should employ standardized screening methods for diabetes diagnosis at regular intervals, assess both lactation duration and exclusivity, and control for potential confounders including gestational glucose tolerance, maternal lifestyle and sociodemographics.

22.3 Breastfeeding and Health of the Offspring

22.3.1 General Population and Development of Overweight

In developed countries, evidence supports a robust protective association between breastfeeding and becoming overweight during childhood and adolescence, even after accounting for maternal obesity and family lifestyle behaviors.[36,37] In 2007, consensus expert panels concluded that breastfeeding reduces the risk of overweight by 22–24% in children and adolescents,[38,39] with attenuation after adjustment for parental anthropometry, socioeconomic status, and birth weight.[39] The consistency of these associations from infancy to adulthood, suggests that breastfeeding may have lasting protective effects independent of dietary intake and physical activity later in life.[37] Because studies have been conducted primarily in European and Caucasian populations, whether breastfeeding protects against overweight in childhood and adolescence among minority groups is unclear. A caveat arises from the observational data that breastfeeding may be a marker for more healthful behaviors in families rather than by exerting a true biological effect.

Nonetheless, biologic mechanisms may explain breastfeeding's protection against future overweight. Breast milk's unique biochemical constituents and nutrient composition may favorably affect infant growth and regulate energy balance. For example, relative to formula feeds, breast milk contains lower protein levels. Higher protein levels in early life have been linked to higher BMI later in life in some,[40,41] but not all studies.[42] Higher insulin levels have also been reported in formula fed compared with breastfed babies.[43] Behavioral aspects may also contribute the favorable effects of breastfeeding on optimal growth and development of energy balance.

22.3.2 Offspring of Mothers with Diabetes During Pregnancy: Development of Overweight

Evidence is equivocal that breastfeeding affects the future health of offspring whose mothers who had diabetes during pregnancy.[44] Of four studies (Table 22.2), the risk of childhood or adolescent overweight was higher,[45, 46] not different,[47] and lower[48] for breastfeeding vs. not breastfeeding among offspring whose mothers had diabetes (either GDM or pregestational diabetes) during pregnancy. One nonrandomized, longitudinal study compared early intake of breast milk from diabetic mothers (83 type 1 diabetes, 29 GDM) with banked donor breast milk during the first week of life[45] and during the second to fourth weeks of life, controlling for the first week.[46] Highest vs. lowest breast milk intake from diabetic mothers during the first week of life was associated with a twofold higher (OR=1.91; 95%CI:1.10–3.30) risk of overweight at age 2, defined as relative body weight above 110%. The association was strengthened (OR=2.59; 95%CI:1.32–5.04) after adjusting for age, sex, type of maternal diabetes, and maternal BMI.[45] The prevalence of impaired glucose tolerance was lower among 2-year-olds who were fed highest vs. lowest amounts of banked donor breast milk in the first week of life (OR=0.19; 95%CI:0.05–0.70).[45] In the same cohort, breast milk intake during the second to fourth weeks of life (OR=1.61; 95%CI:0.76–3.42) and duration of breastfeeding were not associated with risk of overweight or with impaired glucose tolerance at age 2 adjusted for early neonatal breast milk intake and other covariates.[46] However, study subjects were not randomized to donor-banked breast milk, which may have introduced selection bias and residual confounding. Further, the first study did not report the total volume of diabetic breast milk in the first week of life, and neither study assessed the severity of maternal gestational and postpartum hyperglycemia.[45]

Other studies found that breastfeeding protected against overweight during childhood and adolescence in the offspring of mothers with GDM. The NHS of Offspring examined youth aged 9–14 years whose mothers had diabetes during pregnancy (417 GDM, 56 pregestational diabetes) and found a lower, but nonsignificant association for ever vs. never breastfed with risk of overweight (OR=0.62; 95%CI:0.24–1.60).[47] Among German mothers with GDM and their offspring (*n*=324, aged 2–8 years), exclusive breastfeeding for 3 months or longer was associated with a lower risk of overweight (0.55; 95%CI:0.33–0.91), but only among offspring of obese mothers.[48]

These conflicting findings may be related to the differences in the age that overweight was ascertained for subjects (i.e., early ages of 2–3 years are much less predictive of overweight status than at older ages). Another limitation is that most studies involved heterogeneous samples where offspring of mothers with pregestational diabetes during pregnancy were included along with offspring of mothers with GDM. Further, none of the studies controlled for the intrauterine metabolism (i.e., degree of maternal glycemic control) or postnatal environment.

22.3.3 Offspring of Women with Diabetes during Pregnancy: Development of Type 2 Diabetes

Breastfeeding may be associated with a lower prevalence of type 2 diabetes in adulthood and lower incidence of type 2 diabetes in childhood (Table 22.3) among offspring whose mothers had diabetes during pregnancy. The studies included indigenous North American

Table 22.2 Association of breastfeeding with risk of overweight among offspring of mothers with diabetes during pregnancy

Author (reference)	Study design	*n*, mothers type of DM during pregnancy	Study population	Breastfeeding measure	Obesity definition	Offspring age range	OR 95% CI	Covariates adjusted
Mayer-Davis et al[47]	Retrospective cohort, 1996	GDM 417 PG 56 (self-report)	Nurses' Health Study, GUTS	Exclusive breastfeeding vs. exclusive formula	BMI ≥25 kg/m² (self-reported weight and height)	9–14 years in 1996	0.62 (0.24–1.60)	Age, sex, race, Tanner stage, maternal BMI, smoking, income, birth order, diet, physical activity, gestational age
Schaefer-Graf et al[48]	Prospective cohort, 1995–2000	GDM 324	Berlin, Germany	Retrospective duration >3 months vs. ≤3 months	BMI ≥90th percentile in cohort	2–8 years (mean 5.4 years)	0.55 (0.33–0.91)	Parental obesity, birth weight percentile
Rodekamp et al[46]	Lontitudinal 1980–1989	T1DM 83 GDM 26	Berlin, Germany	2nd–4th week of life, highest tertile of donor-banked breast milk	RW >110%	2 years	1.61 (0.76–3.42)	Diabetic breast milk volume 1–7 day life and other covariates from Plagemann et al[30]
Plagemann et al[45]	Longitudinal 1980–1989	T1DM 83 GDM 26	Berlin, Germany	1–7 days of life, highest tertile of donor-banked breast milk	RW >110%	2 years	2.59 (1.32–5.04)	Birth weight, gestational age, sex, maternal BMI, type of maternal diabetes

DM diabetes mellitus; *RW* relative weight; *T1DM* type 1 diabetes mellitus; *GDM* gestational diabetes mellitus; *BMI* body mass index; *PG* pregestational diabetes

Table 22.3 Association of breastfeeding with risk of type 2 diabetes or impaired glucose tolerance among offspring of mothers with diabetes during pregnancy (mixed GDM and pregestational diabetes)

Reference	Study design	*n*, Mother's type of DM during pregnancy	Study population	Breastfeeding measure	T2DM outcome definition	Offspring age range	OR (95%CI) or percent with DM	Covariates adjusted
Mayer-Davis et al[52]	Case–control	Any DM: Cases 16 Controls 8	SEARCH Diabetes in youth	Ever vs. Never BF	Provider diagnosed, T2DM 80 Control 167	10–21 years	0.43 (0.19–0.99)	Sex, age, race, family history DM, maternal attributes, child BMI z-score
Young et al[51]	Case–control 2000–2001	T1DM 14 GDM 22 None 102	Native Canadian, Manitoba	Duration >12 months vs. none	T2DM 46 Control 92 Diagnosis <18 years, FPG ≥126 mg/dl	<18 years	0.24 (0.13–0.99)	Age, sex-matched type of maternal diabetes
Pettit et al[50]	Longitudinal 1978	75-g OGTT during pregnancy GDM 21 None 551	Pima Indians	Exclusive BF for ≥2 months vs. none	75-g OGTT WHO criteria Child every 2 years since age 5 years	10–39 years	30.1 vs. 43.5%	None
Pettit et al[49]	Longitudinal 1978	Not measured during pregnancy $n=720$	Pima Indians	Exclusive BF for >2 months vs. none	75-g OGTT WHO criteria, Prevalent T2DM	10–39 years	0.41 (0.18–0.93)	Age, sex, birth year, parental diabetes, relative weight, birth weight
Plagemann et al[45]	Longitudinal nonrandomized 1980–1989	T1DM 83 GDM 29	Berlin, Germany	1st–7th days of life donor-banked breast milk vs. diabetic breast milk	IGT based on 2-h OGTT 1.75-g glucose/kg body weight	2 years	0.19 (0.05–0.70)	Birth weight, sex, age, gestational age, relative birth weight, maternal BMI, type of maternal DM
Rodekamp et al[46]	Longitudinal nonrandomized 1980–1989	T1DM 83 GDM 29	Berlin, Germany	2nd–4th week of life donor-banked breast milk	IGT based on 2-h OGTT 1.75-g glucose/kg body weight	2 years	0.66 (0.22–2.02)	Volume of diabetic breast milk in first week of life and others

OGTT oral glucose tolerance test; *IGT* impaired glucose tolerance; *BF* breastfed; *T1DM* type 1 diabetes mellitus; *T2DM* type 2 diabetes mellitus; *GDM* gestational diabetes mellitus populations with high prevalence of type 2 diabetes and a multiethnic US population. In Pima Indians, exclusive breastfeeding compared with exclusive bottle-feeding was associated with a lower prevalence of type 2 diabetes (OR = 0.41; 95%CI:0.18–0.93) among offspring 10–39 years of age adjusted for age, sex, parental diabetes, and birth weight,[49] but the study did not examine maternal diabetes during pregnancy. A subsequent analysis of Pima Indians found that exclusive breastfeeding (>2 months) vs. nonbreastfeeding was associated with a lower prevalence of type 2 diabetes (OR = 0.56; 95%CI:0.41–0.76) in 551 offspring of mothers without diabetes during pregnancy.[50] But no association was found for 21 offspring of Pima mothers with diabetes during pregnancy; prevalence of type 2 diabetes was 30.1% for exclusively breastfed and 43.5% for not breastfed adjusted for age, sex, birth weight, birth date, and the presence of DM in either parent.[50]

Case–control studies have consistently reported that breastfeeding is associated with lower rates of offspring diabetes. A case–control study of 46 Native Canadian children diagnosed with diabetes before age 18 years and 92 age- and sex-matched controls found a lower OR of type 2 diabetes among offspring who were breastfed 12 months or more vs. none (OR = 0.24;95% CI:0.13–0.84) adjusted for type of maternal diabetes during pregnancy (type 1 diabetes, GDM, or none).[51] A case–control study of African American, Hispanic, and non-Hispanic white youth with type 2 diabetes (n = 80) and 167 controls aged 10–21 years, SEARCH for Diabetes in Youth, found a protective association between breastfeeding duration and incidence of type 2 diabetes (OR = 0.43; 95%CI:0.19–0.99) adjusted for 12 covariates.[52]

Composition of the breast milk of diabetic mothers may vary based on glucose control. For example, higher and more variable glucose levels in breast milk have been found for moderately controlled diabetic women vs. nondiabetic women.[53] Based on these limited data, evidence is insufficient to determine whether breastfeeding prevents type 2 diabetes in the offspring of women with GDM, or whether breast milk from diabetic mothers has beneficial or detrimental effects on the growth and health of their infants.[44]

22.4 Conclusions

Lactation is a modifiable health behavior with the potential to beneficially affect the long-term health of women and their offspring. Whether lactation confers the same benefits to women with a history of GDM and their children has yet to be determined conclusively. The American Academy of Pediatrics recommends that all infants should be exclusively breastfed through 6 months of age and that breastfeeding should continue until the infant is 1 year of age.[54] Although 80% of US women initiate lactation, 45% report "any" breastfeeding at 6 months and less than 20% report "exclusively" breastfeeding their infants at 6 months. Thus, increasing lactation rates among women may have positive effects on both infant and maternal health in the general population.

Clinical and epidemiologic evidence support the hypothesis that lactation has lasting effects on maternal glucose tolerance for the general population. In the NHS, women who lactated for 4–6 months and up to 2 years experienced a 25–40% lower incidence of self-reported type 2 diabetes, and exclusive lactation was associated with a 35–40% lower risk. In the NHS retrospective analysis, similar associations were not found among women with GDM. In CARDIA, longer duration of lactation was associated with a 2- to 7-fold lower incidence of the metabolic syndrome within 8 years after delivery among both women with a history of GDM, and among women without at history of GDM. Lactation has favorable effects on maternal glucose tolerance during the postpartum period after GDM pregnancy, but evidence is insufficient to conclude that these effects endure post-weaning, or that lactation influences development of type 2 diabetes in women years later.

An abundance of evidence from developed countries supports a robust association between breastfeeding and lower risk of becoming overweight during childhood and adolescence, even after accounting for maternal obesity and family lifestyle behaviors. However, evidence is inconclusive that breastfeeding confers the same protection against obesity for offspring of women with a history of GDM as is reported in the general population. Since 1986, the American Diabetes Association has recommended that women with GDM be encouraged to breastfeed.[55,56] The Fourth International Workshop-Conference on Gestational Diabetes Mellitus recommended that women with previous GDM breastfeed, although it was acknowledged that data to demonstrate efficacy were lacking.[57] In 2007, the Fifth International Workshop-Conference made the same recommendation and stated the need for research on breastfeeding's effects on health of GDM offspring.[58] Identification of modifiable risk factors in early life that prevent childhood obesity is important among GDM offspring because they are more likely to become overweight, and develop impaired glucose tolerance, the metabolic syndrome, and type 2 diabetes.[8–13]

Prospective studies of women with a history of GDM and their offspring are needed to gather evidence related to breastfeeding and infant growth, as well as development of diabetes, controlling for parental attributes, intrauterine metabolic milieu, maternal postpartum glucose tolerance, and postnatal behavioral traits. Further research is needed to determine whether favorable effects of lactation persist years after delivery to influence development of type 2 diabetes in women. Specifically, biochemical measurements from before to after pregnancy may provide important clues to mechanisms related to lactation's influence on type 2 diabetes in women beyond the childbearing years. Breastfeeding is a modifiable health behavior that may play an important role in future disease risk for women with a history of GDM and their offspring.

Acknowledgments Supported by Career Development Award, Grant number K01 DK059944 from the National Institute of Diabetes, Digestive and Kidney Diseases, R01 HD050625 from the National Institute of Child Health and Human Development, and a Clinical Research Award from the American Diabetes Association.

References

1. Kjos SL, Henry O, Lee RM, Buchanan TA, Mishell DR Jr. The effect of lactation on glucose and lipid metabolism in women with recent gestational diabetes. *Obstet Gynecol.* 1993;82:451-455.
2. Gunderson EP, Lewis CE, Wei GS, Whitmer RA, Quesenberry CP, Sidney S. Lactation and changes in maternal metabolic risk factors. *Obstet Gynecol.* 2007;109:729-738.

3. Stuebe AM, Rich-Edwards JW, Willett WC, Manson JE, Michels KB. Duration of lactation and incidence of type 2 diabetes. *JAMA*. 2005;294:2601-2610.
4. Cohen A, Pieper CF, Brown AJ, Bastian LA. Number of children and risk of metabolic syndrome in women. *J Womens Health (Larchmt)*. 2006;15:763-773.
5. Ram KT, Bobby P, Hailpern SM, et al. Duration of lactation is associated with lower prevalence of the metabolic syndrome in midlife – SWAN, the study of women's health across the nation. *Am J Obstet Gynecol*. 2008;198:266-268.
6. Gunderson EP, Jacobs DR, Jr., Chiang V, et al. Duration of lactation and incidence of the metabolic syndrome in women of reproductive age according to gestational diabetes mellitus status: a 20-Year prospective study in CARDIA (Coronary Artery Risk Development in Young Adults). *Diabetes*. 2010;59:495-504.
7. Gunderson EP. Breast-feeding and diabetes: long-term impact on mothers and their infants. *Curr Diab Rep*. 2008;8:279-286.
8. Dabelea D, Pettitt DJ. Intrauterine diabetic environment confers risks for type 2 diabetes mellitus and obesity in the offspring, in addition to genetic susceptibility. *J Pediatr Endocrinol Metab*. 2001;14:1085-1091.
9. Franks PW, Looker HC, Kobes S, et al. Gestational glucose tolerance and risk of type 2 diabetes in young Pima Indian offspring. *Diabetes*. 2006;55:460-465.
10. Petitt DJ, Bennett PH, Knowler WC, Baird HR, Aleck KA. Gestational diabetes mellitus and impaired glucose tolerance during pregnancy. Long-term effects on obesity and glucose tolerance in the offspring. *Diabetes*. 1985;34(suppl 2):119-122.
11. Silverman BL, Rizzo T, Green OC, et al. Long-term prospective evaluation of offspring of diabetic mothers. *Diabetes*. 1991;40(suppl 2):121-125.
12. Gillman MW, Rifas-Shiman S, Berkey CS, Field AE, Colditz GA. Maternal gestational diabetes, birth weight, and adolescent obesity. *Pediatrics*. 2003;111:e221-e226.
13. Silverman BL, Rizzo TA, Cho NH, Metzger BE. Long-term effects of the intrauterine environment. The Northwestern University Diabetes in Pregnancy Center. *Diabetes Care*. 1998;21(suppl 2):B142-B149.
14. Tigas S, Sunehag A, Haymond MW. Metabolic adaptation to feeding and fasting during lactation in humans. *J Clin Endocrinol Metab*. 2002;87:302-307.
15. Qureshi IA, Xi XR, Limbu YR, Bin HY, Chen MI. Hyperlipidaemia during normal pregnancy, parturition and lactation. *Ann Acad Med Singapore*. 1999;28:217-221.
16. Darmady JM, Postle AD. Lipid metabolism in pregnancy. *Br J Obstet Gynaecol*. 1982;89: 211-215.
17. Kallio MJ, Siimes MA, Perheentupa J, Salmenpera L, Miettinen TA. Serum cholesterol and lipoprotein concentrations in mothers during and after prolonged exclusive lactation. *Metabolism*. 1992;41:1327-1330.
18. Butte NF, Hopkinson JM, Mehta N, Moon JK, Smith EO. Adjustments in energy expenditure and substrate utilization during late pregnancy and lactation. *Am J Clin Nutr*. 1999;69:299-307.
19. Diniz JM, Da Costa TH. Independent of body adiposity, breast-feeding has a protective effect on glucose metabolism in young adult women. *Br J Nutr*. 2004;92:905-912.
20. Gunderson EP, Abrams B. Epidemiology of gestational weight gain and body weight changes after pregnancy. *Epidemiol Rev*. 1999;21:261-275.
21. Butte NF, Hopkinson JM. Body composition changes during lactation are highly variable among women. *J Nutr*. 1998;128:381S-385S.
22. Olson CM, Strawderman MS, Hinton PS, Pearson TA. Gestational weight gain and postpartum behaviors associated with weight change from early pregnancy to 1 y postpartum. *Int J Obes Relat Metab Disord*. 2003;27:117-127.
23. Dewey KG, Heinig MJ, Nommsen LA. Maternal weight-loss patterns during prolonged lactation. *Am J Clin Nutr*. 1993;58:162-166.
24. Janney CA, Zhang D, Sowers M. Lactation and weight retention. *Am J Clin Nutr*. 1997; 66:1116-1124.

25. Ohlin A, Rossner S. Maternal body weight development after pregnancy. *Int J Obes*. 1990; 14:159-173.
26. Rooney BL, Schauberger CW. Excess pregnancy weight gain and long-term obesity: one decade later. *Obstet Gynecol*. 2002;100:245-252.
27. Linne Y, Dye L, Barkeling B, Rossner S. Weight development over time in parous women – the SPAWN study – 15 years follow-up. *Int J Obes Relat Metab Disord*. 2003;27:1516-1522.
28. Villegas R, Gao YT, Yang G, et al. Duration of breast-feeding and the incidence of type 2 diabetes mellitus in the Shanghai Women's Health Study. *Diabetologia*. 2008;51:258-266.
29. McManus RM, Cunningham I, Watson A, Harker L, Finegood DT. Beta-cell function and visceral fat in lactating women with a history of gestational diabetes. *Metabolism*. 2001;50: 715-719.
30. Kjos SL, Peters RK, Xiang A, Henry OA, Montoro M, Buchanan TA. Predicting future diabetes in Latino women with gestational diabetes. Utility of early postpartum glucose tolerance testing. *Diabetes*. 1995;44:586-591.
31. Buchanan TA, Xiang A, Kjos SL, et al. Gestational diabetes: antepartum characteristics that predict postpartum glucose intolerance and type 2 diabetes in Latino women. *Diabetes*. 1998;47:1302-1310.
32. Buchanan TA, Xiang AH, Kjos SL, Trigo E, Lee WP, Peters RK. Antepartum predictors of the development of type 2 diabetes in Latino women 11-26 months after pregnancies complicated by gestational diabetes. *Diabetes*. 1999;48:2430-2436.
33. Hartmann P, Cregan M. Lactogenesis and the effects of insulin-dependent diabetes mellitus and prematurity. *J Nutr*. 2001;131:3016S-3020S.
34. Rasmussen KM, Kjolhede CL. Prepregnant overweight and obesity diminish the prolactin response to suckling in the first week postpartum. *Pediatrics*. 2004;113:e465-e471.
35. Donath SM, Amir LH. Does maternal obesity adversely affect breastfeeding initiation and duration? *Breastfeed Rev*. 2000;8:29-33.
36. Arenz S, Ruckerl R, Koletzko B, von Kries R. Breast-feeding and childhood obesity – a systematic review. *Int J Obes Relat Metab Disord*. 2004;28:1247-1256.
37. Owen CG, Martin RM, Whincup PH, Smith GD, Cook DG. Effect of infant feeding on the risk of obesity across the life course: a quantitative review of published evidence. *Pediatrics*. 2005;115:1367-1377.
38. Agency for Healthcare Research and Quality. *Breastfeeding and Maternal and Infant Health Outcomes in Developed Countries*, Structured Abstract. AHRC Publication No. 07-E007; 2007 (GENERIC).
39. Ebbeling CB, Pearson MN, Sorensen G, et al. Conceptualization and development of a theory-based healthful eating and physical activity intervention for postpartum women who are low income. *Health Promot Pract*. 2007;8:50-59.
40. Rolland-Cachera MF, Deheeger M, Akrout M, Bellisle F. Influence of macronutrients on adiposity development: a follow up study of nutrition and growth from 10 months to 8 years of age. *Int J Obes Relat Metab Disord*. 1995;19:573-578.
41. Koletzko B, Broekaert I, Demmelmair H, et al. Protein intake in the first year of life: a risk factor for later obesity? The E.U. childhood obesity project. *Adv Exp Med Biol*. 2005;569:69-79.
42. Dorosty AR, Emmett PM, Cowin S, Reilly JJ. Factors associated with early adiposity rebound. ALSPAC Study Team. *Pediatrics*. 2000;105:1115-1118.
43. Lucas A, Boyes S, Bloom SR, Aynsley-Green A. Metabolic and endocrine responses to a milk feed in six-day-old term infants: differences between breast and cow's milk formula feeding. *Acta Paediatr Scand*. 1981;70:195-200.
44. Gunderson EP. Breastfeeding after gestational diabetes pregnancy: subsequent obesity and type 2 diabetes in women and their offspring. *Diabetes Care*. 2007;30(suppl 2):S161-S168.
45. Plagemann A, Harder T, Franke K, Kohlhoff R. Long-term impact of neonatal breast-feeding on body weight and glucose tolerance in children of diabetic mothers. *Diabetes Care*. 2002; 25:16-22.

46. Rodekamp E, Harder T, Kohlhoff R, Franke K, Dudenhausen JW, Plagemann A. Long-Term Impact of Breast-Feeding on Body Weight and Glucose Tolerance in Children of Diabetic Mothers: Role of the late neonatal period and early infancy. *Diabetes Care*. 2005;28:1457-1462.
47. Mayer-Davis EJ, Rifas-Shiman SL, Zhou L, Hu FB, Colditz GA, Gillman MW. Breast-feeding and risk for childhood obesity: does maternal diabetes or obesity status matter? *Diabetes Care*. 2006;29:2231-2237.
48. Schaefer-Graf UM, Hartmann R, Pawliczak J, et al. Association of breast-feeding and early childhood overweight in children from mothers with gestational diabetes mellitus. *Diabetes Care*. 2006;29:1105-1107.
49. Pettitt DJ, Forman MR, Hanson RL, Knowler WC, Bennett PH. Breastfeeding and incidence of non-insulin-dependent diabetes mellitus in Pima Indians. *Lancet*. 1997;350:166-168.
50. Pettitt DJ, Knowler WC. Long-term effects of the intrauterine environment, birth weight, and breast-feeding in Pima Indians. *Diabetes Care*. 1998;21(suppl 2):B138-B141.
51. Young TK, Martens PJ, Taback SP, et al. Type 2 diabetes mellitus in children: prenatal and early infancy risk factors among native Canadians. *Arch Pediatr Adolesc Med*. 2002;156:651-655.
52. Mayer-Davis EJ, Dabelea D, Lamichhane AP, et al. Breast-feeding and type 2 diabetes in the youth of three ethnic groups: the SEARCh for diabetes in youth case-control study. *Diabetes Care*. 2008;31:470-475.
53. Butte NF, Garza C, Burr R, Goldman AS, Kennedy K, Kitzmiller JL. Milk composition of insulin-dependent diabetic women. *J Pediatr Gastroenterol Nutr*. 1987;6:936-941.
54. Anonymous(1997) Breastfeeding and the use of human milk. American Academy of Pediatrics. Work Group on Breastfeeding. Pediatrics 100:1035–1039.
55. American Diabetes Association. Position statement on gestational diabetes mellitus. *Diabetes Care*. 1986;9:430-431.
56. American Diabetes Association. Gestational diabetes mellitus. *Diabetes Care*. 2004;27(suppl 1): S88-S90.
57. Metzger BE, Coustan DR. Summary and recommendations of the fourth international workshop-conference on gestational diabetes mellitus. The organizing committee. *Diabetes Care*. 1998;21(suppl 2):B161-B167.
58. Metzger BE, Buchanan TA, Coustan DR, et al. Summary and Recommendations of the Fifth International Workshop-conference on Gestational Diabetes Mellitus. *Diabetes Care*. 2007; 30:S251-S260.

Section VIII

GDM Interventions

Emerging Science: Interventions in Women at Risk of GDM During Pregnancy

23

Lisa Chasan-Taber

23.1 Introduction

As the prevalence of diabetes continues to rise worldwide,[1] it is increasingly important to identify high risk populations and to implement strategies to delay or prevent diabetes onset.[2,3] Women diagnosed with gestational diabetes mellitus (GDM) are at substantially increased risk of developing type 2 diabetes and obesity, both currently epidemic in the United States. Furthermore, there is evidence that the incidence of GDM and of postpartum type 2 diabetes following a diagnosis of GDM may both be increasing.[4–6] It has been estimated that, in some populations, women with a history of GDM may account for up to one-third of diabetes cases among parous women.[7] They are also more likely to display features of the insulin resistance syndrome which are linked to cardiovascular disease.[8] In the long term, their children are at increased risk of obesity and glucose intolerance.[9–11] GDM, therefore, identifies a population of women at high risk of developing type 2 diabetes and thus provides an excellent opportunity to intervene years before the development of this disorder.

The rapidly changing context of pregnancy brings opportunities for women to adopt and maintain healthy new behaviors which may be incorporated as lifestyle habits in the postpartum period. This chapter will summarize interventions which rely on lifestyle modifications to prevent GDM or mitigate the effects of GDM during pregnancy. Such modifications include changes in diet as well as physical activity, already established factors in the prevention and treatment of type 2 diabetes. The chapter concludes with recommendations for future intervention studies.

L. Chasan-Taber
Department of Public Health, University of Massachusetts, Amherst,
405 Arnold House, 715 North Pleasant Street, Amherst, MA 01003, USA
e-mail: LCT@schoolph.umass.edu

C. Kim and A. Ferrara (eds.), *Gestational Diabetes During and After Pregnancy*,
DOI: 10.1007/978-1-84882-120-0_23, © Springer-Verlag London Limited 2010

23.2 Interventions to Prevent GDM

Established GDM risk factors include race/ethnicity, elevated body mass index (BMI), history of GDM in a past pregnancy, >25 years of age, family history of diabetes mellitus, history of abnormal glucose metabolism, and history of poor obstetric outcome.[12] Maternal weight gain and diet are also likely to be important factors.[12] However, recognized risk factors for GDM are absent in up to half of affected women.[13] In addition, many of these factors, such as age and family history, are nonmodifiable. In the light of these facts, as well as the increasing prevalence of GDM, the need to assess strategies to prevent its onset is critical.

23.2.1 Exercise Interventions Designed to Prevent GDM

The hormonal changes of pregnancy reduce insulin sensitivity and glucose tolerance, which can result in the clinical presentation of GDM.[14] By increasing insulin sensitivity and improving glucose tolerance via several mechanisms, physical activity has a beneficial effect on many aspects of insulin resistance syndromes.[15–17] During physical activity, glucose uptake and utilization by working muscle are increased in direct proportion to the intensity of the exercise.[16] After physical activity, glucose tolerance is improved for 48–72 h by increasing cellular sensitivity to circulating insulin.[18, 19] Although the exact mechanism is still contentious, prior physical activity clearly upregulates the translocation of insulin-sensitive glucose transporters to the cell surface, facilitating glucose uptake from the blood.[20] Longer-term, even relatively modest increases in habitual physical activity induce adaptations that can have profound effects on glucose tolerance[18] and potentially reduce the risk for GDM.

Prior epidemiologic studies have suggested that prepregnancy physical activity may have a protective role in the development of GDM.[21–27] Studies examining activity during pregnancy have been less consistent with one case–control study[21] and one small cohort study[28] observing a significant protective effect and others supporting this trend, but not significantly so.[22, 23, 26, 27]

Engaging in 30 min of moderate intensity physical activity (e.g., brisk walking) during most days of the week has been adopted by the American College of Obstetricians and Gynecologists as a recommendation for pregnant women without medical or obstetrical complications.[29] This approach, which emphasizes the accumulation of physical activity (e.g., through 10-min sessions) may be more acceptable to pregnant women than traditional exercise recommendations. Individually-tailored, motivationally-matched exercise interventions have been found to be an effective, low-cost approach for enhancing physical activity participation among nonpregnant women in the community but have not been adequately evaluated among pregnant women.[30–32] Furthermore, the majority of pregnant women in the United States are inactive,[33] with minority women reporting lower levels of recreational physical activity during pregnancy as compared with nonminority women.[34]

To date, few primary prevention studies have intervened to test whether making a change in physical activity reduces risk of developing GDM among women at risk of this disorder. In one of the first studies, Dyck et al. examined the feasibility of early pregnancy exercise (<21 weeks gestation) in Aboriginal women in Saskatchewan with a prior history of GDM.[35] Participants were asked to exercise for 45 min, 3 times per week, at 70% of age predicted maximum. Failure to achieve targeted recruitment goals ($n = 10$) was attributed to lack of community-based participatory research techniques.

Mottola et al. conducted a pilot study, the Nutrition and Exercise Lifestyle Intervention Program (NELIP), among 23 overweight women (prepregnancy BMI ≥ 25 kg/m^2) at 16–20 weeks gestation. The intervention consisted of a mild walking program (30% of peak VO_2, 3–4 times/week) combined with nutritional control (8,350 kJ/day; 200 g carbohydrate/day).[36] None of the participants developed GDM, and oral glucose tolerance (OGTT) values at 34–36 weeks gestation were significantly lower than reference values for women diagnosed with GDM ($p < 0.05$). HbA_{1c} values and insulin areas under the curve remained within the normal range at 34–36 weeks. While provocative, this study was limited by lack of a control group.

The Behaviors Affecting Baby and You (BABY) Study is an ongoing intervention study in Western Massachusetts designed to investigate the effects of a motivationally-targeted, individually tailored physical activity intervention on risk of GDM among women at high risk of the disorder.[37] The B.A.B.Y. study was initiated in 2007 and plans to recruit a total of 364 women (49% will be from minority groups). Primary outcomes include GDM, serum biomarkers associated with insulin resistance (i.e., glucose, insulin, leptin, tumor necrosis factor alpha, resistin, C-reactive protein, and adiponectin), and the adoption and maintenance of exercise during pregnancy. Secondary goals are to investigate the impact of the intervention on gestational weight gain and selected birth outcomes (i.e., accelerated fetal growth, Apgar score).

Women are recruited in early pregnancy and randomized to either an exercise intervention or a comparison health and wellness intervention. Both interventions consist of 12-week programs ending at routine GDM screen (24–28 weeks gestation) with approximately 14 weeks of follow-up (ending at birth). The overall goal of the exercise intervention is to encourage pregnant women to achieve American College of Obstetricians and Gynecologists (ACOG) guidelines for physical activity during pregnancy (30 min or more of moderate-intensity activity on most days of the week) through increased walking and developing a more active lifestyle in one daily session or accumulated through 10-min sessions.[29] The health and wellness group receives high-quality, low-cost, self-help general health and wellness during pregnancy material, which is currently available to the public.

For both intervention groups, a baseline face-to-face session with individualized counseling is followed by weekly and biweekly mailed, print-based materials as well as telephone booster calls to provide motivationally-based individualized feedback. The face-to-face session takes place at the hospital or at the participant's home, according to the participant's preference. Physical activity is assessed via three 24-h recalls, 7-days of accelerometer monitoring, and the Pregnancy Physical Activity Questionnaire (PPAQ).[38] Dietary recalls are conducted in mid pregnancy and serum biomarkers are collected at baseline and at 24–28 weeks gestation. The intervention protocol can readily be translated into clinical practice in underserved and minority populations.

In summary, intervention studies utilizing exercise to prevent GDM are sparse and largely reflect pilot studies or recently initiated trials. Consistent with this finding, evidence-based physical activity prevention programs for GDM with guidelines for frequency, intensity, duration, and type of activity remain to be established.[39] Ongoing and future well-controlled intervention studies in this area will inform programs designed to prevent the incidence of GDM in women at risk of this disorder.

23.2.2 Dietary Interventions Designed to Prevent GDM

Dietary factors such as fat, fiber, and glycemic load (GL) have been associated with fasting insulin levels and obesity in adults[40] and a small number of prior studies suggest that they may also be related to GDM. In epidemiologic studies, GL prior to pregnancy was associated with the development of GDM in a large prospective cohort study of 21,765 nurses.[24] In contrast, GL during early pregnancy was not associated with risk of GDM in a cohort of 1,733 women enrolled in Project Viva.[41] High fat diets have been associated with the recurrence of GDM in future pregnancies[42] and the development of glucose abnormalities during pregnancy in some studies[43] but not in others.[41] The findings for fiber have also been inconsistent with some studies supporting a protective effect[42, 44] while others have not.[41,45,46]

The Cochrane Review recently reviewed randomized and quasi-randomized controlled trials including dietary strategies designed to prevent GDM in pregnant women.[47] One study assessed the effect of a high fiber diet[48] and two studies compared the impact of high and low glycemic index (GI) diets.[49, 50] In the first, Fraser et al. randomized 23 nonobese women at 27 weeks gestation to a high fiber diet group or a control group. The high fiber group received advice from a dietician to reduce intake of sucrose and white flour and to make as many high fiber substitutions as possible. The control group was given standard dietary advice. There was no significant difference in mean OGTT results at 35 weeks between the groups (mean difference −0.36, 95% CI −0.90–0.18). However, there was a significant attenuation of postprandial insulin secretion in the high fiber group.

The two studies which evaluated GI randomly assigned a small number of women (ranging from $n=20$ to $n=62$) to either a low GI or high GI diet in early pregnancy.[49,50] In terms of maternal outcomes, the one study that assessed GDM observed only one case in the high GI group and none in the low GI group.[50] This study also found an RR of 0.09 for large-for-gestational age (LGA) infants among women in the low GI diet as compared to women on the high GI diet (95% CI 0.01–0.69). For both studies, maternal fasting blood glucose was lower on the low GI diet (weighted mean difference −0.28 mmol/L, 95% CI −0.54 to −0.02) and infants born to women on the low GI diet had better outcomes with respect to birth weight and ponderal index. However, while a low GI diet was beneficial for these selected maternal and child outcomes, results from the review were inconclusive. Neither study reported on other prespecified neonatal outcomes including macrosomia, perinatal mortality, shoulder dystocia, neonatal hypoglycemia, or maternal outcomes such as preeclampsia.

In summary, exercise and diet are promising approaches in the prevention of GDM but intervention studies are sparse. The three studies meeting the Cochrane review criteria included a limited number of outcome variables and included small numbers of participants. Further trials with larger sample sizes and longer follow-up are required to reach more definitive conclusions and to inform clinical practice.

23.3 Interventions to Treat GDM Among Women Diagnosed with GDM

There is controversy regarding the management of GDM and impaired glucose tolerance (IGT) in pregnancy. The majority of women diagnosed with GDM undergo intensive treatment regimens with the goal of preventing pregnancy complications, the most common of which is macrosomia.[51] However, other factors such as maternal weight and ethnicity may be more important predictors of birth weight than GDM. Further complicating treatment decisions are recent findings suggesting that there may be a continuum of risk with respect to glucose levels and birth weight.[52] In spite of these factors, lifestyle modifications, including physical activity and diet in response to the GDM diagnosis, have potential long-term implications for maternal and fetal health. In addition, such behavioral changes made during pregnancy may also be sustained after pregnancy, thus independently reducing risk of type 2 diabetes.

23.3.1 Dietary-Based Treatment Interventions After Diagnosis of GDM

Dietary advice has long been part of a standard regimen of GDM treatment. In 2003, the Cochrane review evaluated randomized controlled trials of alternative management strategies, including diet, for women with GDM and IGT in pregnancy.[51] Inclusion criteria were strict and many studies were excluded due to the variation in diagnostic criteria or because they contained an additional screening step that selected from within the population of women with GDM. Trials with GDM as an outcome did not meet the criteria, and only one dietary intervention study with IGT as the primary outcome was included.[53] In this study, Langer et al. randomized 126 women with IGT to a treated and untreated group. All participants monitored capillary blood glucose 7 times/day. In addition, the treated group was managed according to a protocol which included dietary advice determined by prepregnancy BMI and insulin treatment. The untreated group continued normal eating patterns. There was no difference in the percentage of cesarean sections, NICU admissions, or the gestational age at delivery between the treated and untreated groups. However, the authors observed a lower incidence of neonatal hypoglycemia (RR=0.13, 95% CI 0.02–0.97) as well as a significant reduction in macrosomia (RR=0.27, 95% CI 0.09–0.76) in the treated group as compared with the untreated group.

While this review failed to show any benefit from dietary intervention in women with GDM, a review of observational and clinical studies conducted from 1995 to 2001 determined that although a number of the studies were of poor quality, findings in general supported the effectiveness of dietary advice as a means of improving maternal hyperglycemia and reducing the risk of accelerated fetal growth.[54] However, the evidence supporting energy restriction, as well as the optimal balance of dietary carbohydrate and fat intake remain controversial.

Since the publication of these reviews, the Australian Carbohydrate Intolerance Study in Pregnancy (ACHOIS) completed a multicenter, blinded, randomized controlled trial to determine whether treatment of mild GDM, including a dietary strategy, would reduce perinatal complications and improve maternal outcomes, mood, and quality of life ref 72. A total of 1,000 women were enrolled at 14 sites in Australia and four sites in the United Kingdom. Between 24 and 34 weeks gestation, women were randomly assigned to receive individualized dietary advice, blood glucose monitoring, and insulin therapy as required for glycemic control ($n=490$); or to routine care ($n=510$).

The authors found that the rate of serious perinatal complications was significantly lower among the infants in the intervention group (1% vs. 4%, RR=0.33; 95% C.I. 0.14–0.75). There were no differences in the rate of cesarean section between groups, however infants of women in the intervention group had higher neonatal intensive care unit admissions and labor induction rates as compared with women in the routine care group. This difference may have been due to physician awareness and response to GDM diagnosis.[55] Infants born to mothers in the intervention group were less likely to be LGA as compared with the routine care group. This is important, as infants who are LGA are prone to impaired glucose tolerance or diabetes later in life and have an increased risk of GDM.[56, 57] This study, therefore, provides critical evidence that GDM treatment, including dietary advice, can reduce the risk of adverse perinatal outcomes.

In summary, while recommendations for GDM management have long included nutritional counseling, areas of continued controversy include defining the appropriate glucose levels to initiate such therapy. Further intervention studies are required to assess the impact of dietary management on pregnancy outcomes in women with GDM, as well as the impact on long-term maternal and fetal outcomes.

23.3.2 Exercise-Based Treatment Interventions After Diagnosis of GDM

Although dietary strategies have been the mainstay of therapy for women with GDM, many of these women will experience fasting and/or postprandial hyperglycemia despite dietary interventions. Insulin is typically prescribed for these patients.[58] However, insulin corrects the hyperglycemia without affecting the peripheral insulin resistance.[58] Thus, physical activity, which affects insulin resistance, may be the preferable intervention in the absence of either medical or obstetric complications. Indeed, exercise has long been accepted as an adjunctive intervention in the management of diabetes in nonpregnant subjects.[39]

In 1985, Artal et al conducted the first pilot study on the efficacy and safety of an exercise program in 13 insulin-requiring pregnant women with GDM and 42 control women.[59] The authors did not observe significant changes in plasma glucose, epinephrine, glucagon, or free-fatty-acid levels with low-level exercise, however plasma norepinephrine significantly increased with exercise. These findings were reflected in the Second International Workshop-Conference on GDM, which recommended that women with an active lifestyle continue a program of moderate exercise under medical supervision during pregnancy.[60]

In 2006, the Cochrane Review reviewed randomized controlled trials comparing any exercise program to no specific exercise program among pregnant women with GDM.[61] A total of four trials met the eligibility criteria.[62-65] In these studies, women were recruited during the third trimester and the exercise intervention was performed for approximately 6 weeks. Programs consisted of exercising 3–4 times weekly on a cycle ergometer at 70% VO_2 max for 30 min,[64] cycling for 45 min 3 times weekly at 50% VO_2 max,[63] 20 min training on an arm ergometer 3 times/week,[62] and 30 min circuit type resistance training 3 times/week.[65] The review found no significant differences between the exercise and control groups for all the outcomes evaluated and concluded that there is insufficient evidence to recommend, or advise against, enrolling diabetic pregnant women in exercise programs. However, in combination with other small treatment studies which did not qualify for the review, findings suggest that women receiving an exercise intervention had greater glycemic control, lower fasting and postprandial glucose concentrations, and improved cardiorespiratory fitness as compared with those receiving a standard dietary intervention.[66]

In one of the most well known randomized trials, Jovanovic-Peterson et al. randomized 19 women to an arm ergometry exercise program in combination with a dietary intervention, or to a standard diet for 6 weeks.[62] The exercise program consisted of 20 min of arm ergometry 3 times per week at 50% of VO_2 max. The intervention group had greater glycemic control, lower fasting and postprandial glucose concentrations, and improved cardiorespiratory fitness as compared with the control group. However, glycemic levels did not diverge between the groups until week 4 of the intervention.

More recently, Artal et al. conducted an intervention study to assess whether a weight gain restriction regimen with or without exercise would impact glycemic control, pregnancy outcome, and total pregnancy weight gain among obese subjects with GDM.[67] A total of 39 subjects were self enrolled in the exercise and diet group and 57 subjects self enrolled in a diet only group according to contraindications or lack of personal preference for exercise. Exercise subjects were prescribed an exercise routine equivalent to 60% of VO_2 max. Although glucose control was not reported, weight gain per week was significantly lower in the exercise group (0.1 ± 0.4 kg vs. 0.3 ± 0.4 kg, $p < 0.05$) as compared to the diet only group; pregnancy and fetal outcomes were similar in both groups. Findings suggest that a diet plus exercise intervention is successful at limiting excessive weight gain in women with GDM as compared to diet alone. However the lack of randomization precludes attributing results to the exercise intervention alone; the two groups may have differed on factors also related to weight change.

Most recently, Davenport et al. conducted a pilot project to determine the effectiveness of a structured low intensity walking protocol on capillary glucose control in women with GDM.[68] Women were randomized to conventional management of diet and insulin therapy plus a low intensity walking program ($n = 10$) or to conventional management alone ($n = 20$). The walking program consisted of 3–4 exercise sessions per week at 30% of heart rate reserve, increasing gradually from 25 min of walking to 40 min of walking from the time of GDM diagnosis to delivery. The groups were matched on BMI, age, and insulin usage. In the week prior to delivery, the intervention group had significantly lower mean glucose concentrations in the fasted state, and 1-h after meals, achieved with fewer units of insulin per day than the comparison group. Findings suggest an effective role for a practical, structured walking program for women with GDM.

In summary, exercise intervention studies suggest that moderate exercise may be effective in lowering maternal glucose concentrations in women with GDM but are limited by small sample size, lack of well controlled or reported exercise intensity, and differences in the type, intensity, and duration of the training programs.[39, 69] Despite endorsements by professional organizations,[29, 70, 71] exercise for patients with GDM has not been widely prescribed or practiced and exercise remains an adjunctive therapy.[39] Additional controlled clinical trials are necessary to determine the effectiveness of structured exercise programs as well as to identify the appropriate type, duration, and intensity of such exercise.[39]

23.4 Conclusion

Physical inactivity and poor diet are important risk factors for obesity and type 2 diabetes, currently at epidemic rates in the United States. There is substantial evidence that targeting at-risk groups for type 2 diabetes prevention is effective, if lifestyle changes are made. For example, the Diabetes Prevention Program found that intensive lifestyle modification over 4 years with diet and exercise reduced the incidence of type 2 diabetes by more than 50%.[19] In light of these observations, the potential for lifestyle interventions integrating appropriate diet and physical activity to reduce such GDM risk factors as overweight, obesity, and excessive maternal weight gain is high. In addition to being a tool for GDM prevention, the bulk of evidence from observational and clinical studies supports a protective role for diet and physical activity in the treatment of GDM. However, to date, randomized controlled clinical trials have been insufficient to conclusively demonstrate that treatment of women with GDM or IGT with diet, physical activity, and/or insulin improves maternal (e.g., preeclampsia) or fetal outcomes (e.g., birthweight, perinatal morbidity, and mortality).

Evidence-based exercise intervention studies should be designed to evaluate the frequency, intensity, duration, and type of physical activity necessary to optimize maternal and fetal outcomes among women with GDM or at risk for GDM. For example, such programs should evaluate the effect of exercise programs of differing intensities as well as active living activities such as walking, gardening, and household activities.[39] Further dietary intervention studies are critical to assess the effects of a low GI diet on both GDM prevention as well as GDM treatment. The effectiveness of dietary interventions for overweight or obese women should also be assessed.[47] Finally, given that each subsequent pregnancy is associated with greater postpartum weight retention, coupled with the increasing incidence of maternal obesity and GDM, a greater focus should be placed on evaluating the impact of diet and exercise interventions on excessive maternal weight gain.[67]

To date, randomized trials have not evaluated whether treatment with dietary strategies and/or exercise reduce the long-term risks associated with GDM including obesity and type 2 diabetes in the offspring.[55] Such trials would add weight to the ACHOIS findings which supported the use of treatment, including a dietary strategy, in a population similar to the US in terms of ethnicity and obesity.[72] The success of these future intervention studies relies, in part, on the achievement of consensus regarding the threshold for diagnosis and treatment of carbohydrate intolerance during pregnancy.

With this purpose in mind, the hyperglycemia and adverse pregnancy outcome (HAPO) study was designed to identify the diagnostic threshold between maternal hyperglycemia and adverse perinatal outcomes (i.e., cesarean section rates, fetal size, neonatal hypoglycemia, and fetal hyperinsulinemia).[73] This 7-year prospective observational study enrolled 25,505 nondiabetic pregnant women in nine countries. However, no specific threshold was identified as findings suggested a consistent, continuous increase in risk of adverse pregnancy outcomes over the range of maternal blood glucose levels.

The ongoing Maternal Fetal Medicine Unit (MFMU) trial may also inform the threshold for diagnosis and treatment of carbohydrate intolerance during pregnancy.[74,75] This multicenter randomized controlled trial randomizes women in the United States with mild GDM (fasting glucose <95 mg/dL) to formal nutritional counseling and dietary therapy along with insulin as required or to no specific treatment.[74,75] Perinatal outcomes will be compared between the two groups.

In conclusion, dietary advice and physical activity reinforcement should continue beyond pregnancy. Women should be informed of their risks and empowered to make lifestyle changes. As long-term follow-up studies reveal that a significant proportion of women with GDM go on to develop diabetes outside of pregnancy, especially during the first decade after the index pregnancy, GDM offers an important opportunity for the development, testing, and implementation of clinical strategies for diabetes prevention.[76] Pregnant women more readily seek medical care and are highly motivated to make healthy lifestyle changes, making pregnancy a critical opportunity for both short- and long-term behavior modification.

References

1. King H, Aubert RE, Herman WH. Global burden of diabetes, 1995-2025: prevalence, numerical estimates, and projections. *Diabetes Care*. 1998;21(9):1414-1431.
2. Reichard P, Nilsson BY, Rosenqvist U. The effect of long-term intensified insulin treatment on the development of microvascular complications of diabetes mellitus. *N Engl J Med*. 1993;329(5):304-309.
3. Anonymous. Intensive blood-glucose control with sulphonylureas or insulin compared with conventional treatment and risk of complications in patients with type 2 diabetes (UKPDS 33). UK Prospective Diabetes Study (UKPDS) Group. *Lancet*. 1998;352(9131):837-853.
4. Cheung NW, Byth K. Population health significance of gestational diabetes. *Diabetes Care*. 2003;26(7):2005-2009.
5. Dabelea D, Snell-Bergeon JK, Hartsfield CL, Bischoff KJ, Hamman RF, McDuffie RS. Increasing prevalence of gestational diabetes mellitus (GDM) over time and by birth cohort: Kaiser Permanente of Colorado GDM Screening Program. *Diabetes Care*. 2005;28(3):579-584.
6. Ferrara A, Kahn HS, Quesenberry CP, Riley C, Hedderson MM. An increase in the incidence of gestational diabetes mellitus: Northern California, 1991-2000. *Obstet Gynecol*. 2004;103(3): 526-533.
7. Kim C, Newton KM, Knopp RH. Gestational diabetes and the incidence of type 2 diabetes: a systematic review. *Diabetes Care*. 2002;25(10):1862-1868.
8. Buchanan TA, Xiang AH. Gestational diabetes mellitus. *J Clin Invest*. 2005;115(3):485-491.
9. Pettitt DJ, Knowler WC. Long-term effects of the intrauterine environment, birth weight, and breast-feeding in Pima Indians. *Diabetes Care*. 1998;21(suppl 2):B138-B141.

10. Silverman BL, Rizzo TA, Cho NH, Metzger BE. Long-term effects of the intrauterine environment. The Northwestern University Diabetes in Pregnancy Center. *Diabetes Care.* 1998;21(suppl 2):B142-B149.
11. Vohr BR, McGarvey ST, Tucker R. Effects of maternal gestational diabetes on offspring adiposity at 4-7 years of age. *Diabetes Care.* 1999;22(8):1284-1291.
12. Berkowitz GS, Lapinski RH, Wein R, Lee D. Race/ethnicity and other risk factors for gestational diabetes. *Am J Epidemiol.* 1992;135(9):965-973.
13. Coustan DR, Nelson C, Carpenter MW, Carr SR, Rotondo L, Widness JA. Maternal age and screening for gestational diabetes: a population-based study. *Obstet Gynecol.* 1989;73(4):557-561.
14. Sepe SJ, Connell FA, Geiss LS, Teutsch SM. Gestational diabetes. Incidence, maternal characteristics, and perinatal outcome. *Diabetes.* 1985;34(suppl 2):13-16.
15. Sato Y, Iguchi A, Sakamoto N. Biochemical determination of training effects using insulin clamp technique. *Horm Metab Res.* 1984;16(9):483-486.
16. Regensteiner JG, Shetterly SM, Mayer EJ, et al. Relationship between habitual physical activity and insulin area among individuals with impaired glucose tolerance. The San Luis Valley Diabetes Study. *Diabetes Care.* 1995;18(4):490-497.
17. Helmrich SP, Ragland DR, Leung RW, Paffenbarger RS Jr. Physical activity and reduced occurrence of non-insulin-dependent diabetes mellitus. *N Engl J Med.* 1991;325(3):147-152.
18. Kelley DE, Goodpaster BH. Effects of physical activity on insulin action and glucose tolerance in obesity. *Med Sci Sports Exerc.* 1999;31(11 Suppl):S619-S623.
19. Knowler WC, Barrett-Connor E, Fowler SE, et al. Reduction in the incidence of type 2 diabetes with lifestyle intervention or metformin. *N Engl J Med.* 2002;346(6):393-403.
20. Ivy JL, Zderic TW, Fogt DL. Prevention and treatment of non-insulin-dependent diabetes mellitus. *Exerc Sport Sci Rev.* 1999;27:1-35.
21. Dempsey JC, Butler CL, Sorensen TK, et al. A case-control study of maternal recreational physical activity and risk of gestational diabetes mellitus. *Diabetes Res Clin Pract.* 2004; 66(2):203-215.
22. Dempsey JC, Sorensen TK, Williams MA, et al. Prospective study of gestational diabetes mellitus risk in relation to maternal recreational physical activity before and during pregnancy. *Am J Epidemiol.* 2004;159(7):663-670.
23. Oken E, Ning Y, Rifas-Shiman SL, Radesky JS, Rich-Edwards JW, Gillman MW. Associations of physical activity and inactivity before and during pregnancy with glucose tolerance. *Obstet Gynecol.* 2006;108(5):1200-1207.
24. Zhang C, Solomon CG, Manson JE, Hu FB. A prospective study of pregravid physical activity and sedentary behaviors in relation to the risk for gestational diabetes mellitus. *Arch Intern Med.* 2006;166(5):543-548.
25. Iqbal R, Rafique G, Badruddin S, Qureshi R, Cue R, Gray-Donald K. Increased body fat percentage and physical inactivity are independent predictors of gestational diabetes mellitus in South Asian women. *Eur J Clin Nutr.* 2006;61(6):736-742.
26. Dyck R, Klomp H, Tan LK, Turnell RW, Boctor MA. A comparison of rates, risk factors, and outcomes of gestational diabetes between aboriginal and non-aboriginal women in the Saskatoon health district. *Diabetes Care.* 2002;25(3):487-493.
27. Dye TD, Knox KL, Artal R, Aubry RH, Wojtowycz MA. Physical activity, obesity, and diabetes in pregnancy. *Am J Epidemiol.* 1997;146(11):961-965.
28. Chasan-Taber L. Physical activity and gestational diabetes mellitus among Hispanic Women. *J Women's Health.* 2008;17(6):999-1008.
29. ACOG Committee Obstetric Practice. ACOG Committee opinion. Number 267, January 2002: Exercise during pregnancy and the postpartum period. *Obstet Gynecol.* 2002;99(1):171-173.
30. Marcus BH, Bock BC, Pinto BM, Forsyth LH, Roberts MB, Traficante RM. Efficacy of an individualized, motivationally-tailored physical activity intervention. *Ann Behav Med.* 1998;20(3):174-180.

31. Marcus BH, Emmons KM, Simkin-Silverman LR, et al. Evaluation of motivationally tailored vs. standard self-help physical activity interventions at the workplace. *Am J Health Promot.* 1998;12(4):246-253.
32. Marcus BH, Banspach SW, Lefebvre RC, Rossi JS, Carleton RA, Abrams DB. Using the stages of change model to increase the adoption of physical activity among community participants. *Am J Health Promot.* 1992;6(6):424-429.
33. Zhang J, Savitz DA. Exercise during pregnancy among US women. *Ann Epidemiol.* 1996; 6(1):53-59.
34. Evenson KR, Savitz DA, Huston SL. Leisure-time physical activity among pregnant women in the US. *Paediatr Perinat Epidemiol.* 2004;18(6):400-407.
35. Dyck RF. Preventing NIDDM among aboriginal people: is exercise the answer? Description of a pilot project using exercise to prevent gestational diabetes. *Int J Circumpolar Health.* 1998;57(suppl 1):375.
36. Mottola MF, Lander S, Giroux I, Hammond J, Lebrun C. Glucose and insulin responses in women at risk for GDM before and after a nutrition, exercise & lifestyle intervention program (NELIP). *Med Sci Sports Exerc.* 2005;37(5 suppl):S309-S310.
37. Chasan-Taber L, Marcus BH, Stanek E, et al. A randomized controlled trial of prenatal physical activity to prevent gestational diabetes: design and methods. *J Women's Health.* 2009; 18:851-859.
38. Chasan-Taber L, Schmidt MD, Roberts DE, Hosmer D, Markenson G, Freedson PS. Development and validation of a Pregnancy Physical Activity Questionnaire. *Med Sci Sports Exerc.* 2004;36(10):1750-1760.
39. Mottola MF. The role of exercise in the prevention and treatment of gestational diabetes mellitus. *Current sports medicine reports.* 2007;6(6):381-386.
40. Marshall JA. High saturated fat and low starch and fibre are associated with hyperinsulinaemia in a non-diabetic population: the San Luis Valley Diabetes Study. *Diabetologia.* 1997; 40(4):430.
41. Radesky JS, Oken E, Rifas-Shiman SL, Kleinman KP, Rich-Edwards JW, Gillman MW. Diet during early pregnancy and development of gestational diabetes. *Paediatr Perinat Epidemiol.* 2008;22(1):47-59.
42. Moses RG, Shand JL, Tapsell LC. The recurrence of gestational diabetes: could dietary differences in fat intake be an explanation? *Diabetes Care.* 1997;20(11):1647-1650.
43. Saldana TM, Siega-Riz AM, Adair LS. Effect of macronutrient intake on the development of glucose intolerance during pregnancy. *Am J Clin Nutr.* 2004;79(3):479-486.
44. Zhang C. Dietary fiber intake, dietary glycemic load, and the risk for gestational diabetes mellitus. *Diabetes Care.* 2006;29(10):2223.
45. Bo S, Menato G, Lezo A, et al. Dietary fat and gestational hyperglycaemia. *Diabetologia.* 2001;44(8):972-978.
46. Wang Y, Storlien LH, Jenkins AB, et al. Dietary variables and glucose tolerance in pregnancy. *Diabetes Care.* 2000;23(4):460-464.
47. Tieu J. Dietary advice in pregnancy for preventing gestational diabetes mellitus. *Cochrane Database Syst Rev.* 2008;2:CD006674.
48. Fraser RB. A controlled trial of a high dietary fibre intake in pregnancy–effects on plasma glucose and insulin levels. *Diabetologia.* 1983;25(3):238.
49. Clapp JF. Maternal carbohydrate intake and pregnancy outcome. *Proc Nutr Soc.* 2002;61(1):45.
50. Moses RG. Effect of a low-glycemic-index diet during pregnancy on obstetric outcomes. *Am J Clin Nutr.* 2006;84(4):807.
51. Tuffnell DJ, West J, Walkinshaw SA. Treatments for gestational diabetes and impaired glucose tolerance in pregnancy. *Cochrane Database Syst Rev.* 2003;(3):CD003395.
52. Metzger BE. Hyperglycemia and adverse pregnancy outcomes. *New Engl J Med.* 2008; 358(19):1991.

53. Langer O. Management of women with one abnormal oral glucose tolerance test value reduces adverse outcome in pregnancy. *Am J Obstetr Gynecol.* 1989;161(3):593.
54. Dornhorst A. The principles of dietary management of gestational diabetes: reflection on current evidence. *J Hum Nutr Diet.* 2002;15(2):145.
55. Greene MF, Solomon CG. Gestational diabetes mellitus – time to treat. *N Engl J Med.* 2005;352(24):2544-2546.
56. Innes KE, Byers TE, Marshall JA, Baron A, Orleans M, Hamman RF. Association of a woman's own birth weight with subsequent risk for gestational diabetes. *JAMA.* 2002;287(19):2534-2541.
57. Silverman BL, Metzger BE, Cho NH, Loeb CA. Impaired glucose tolerance in adolescent offspring of diabetic mothers. Relationship to fetal hyperinsulinism. *Diabetes Care.* 1995; 18(5):611-617.
58. Artal R. Exercise: the alternative therapeutic intervention for gestational diabetes. *Clin Obstet Gynecol.* 2003;46(2):479-487.
59. Artal R, Wiswell R, Romem Y. Hormonal responses to exercise in diabetic and nondiabetic pregnant patients. *Diabetes.* 1985;34(suppl 2):78-80.
60. Artal R, Bellman O, Dekest T, et al. Summary and recommendations of the second international workshop-conference on gestational diabetes mellitus: therapeutic strategies. *Diabetes.* 1985;34:125.
61. Ceysens G, Rouiller D, Boulvain M. Exercise for diabetic pregnant women. *Cochrane Database Syst Rev.* 2006;3:CD004225.
62. Jovanovic-Peterson L, Durak EP, Peterson CM. Randomized trial of diet versus diet plus cardiovascular conditioning on glucose levels in gestational diabetes. *Am J Obstet Gynecol.* 1989;161(2):415-419.
63. Bung P, Artal R, Khodiguian N, Kjos S. Exercise in gestational diabetes. An optional therapeutic approach? *Diabetes.* 1991;40(suppl 2):182-185.
64. Avery MD, Leon AS, Kopher RA. Effects of a partially home-based exercise program for women with gestational diabetes. *Obstet Gynecol.* 1997;89(1):10-15.
65. Brankston GN. Resistance exercise decreases the need for insulin in overweight women with gestational diabetes mellitus. *Am J Obstetr Gynecol.* 2004;190(1):188.
66. Dempsey JC, Butler CL, Williams MA. No need for a pregnant pause: physical activity may reduce the occurrence of gestational diabetes mellitus and preeclampsia. *Exerc Sport Sci Rev.* 2005;33(3):141-149.
67. Artal R, Catanzaro RB, Gavard JA, Mostello DJ, Friganza JC. A lifestyle intervention of weight-gain restriction: diet and exercise in obese women with gestational diabetes mellitus. *Appl Physiol Nutr Metab.* 2007;32(3):596-601.
68. Davenport MH, Mottola MF, McManus R, Gratton R. A walking intervention improves capillary glucose control in women with gestational diabetes mellitus: a pilot study. *Appl Physiol Nutr Metab.* 2008;33(3):511-517.
69. Anonymous. Impact of physical activity during pregnancy and postpartum on chronic disease risk. *Med Sci Sports Exer.* 2006;38(5):989.
70. American Diabetes Association AD. Gestational diabetes mellitus. *Diabetes Care.* 2004; 27(suppl 1):S88-S90.
71. Metzger BE. Summary and recommendations of the Fifth International Workshop-Conference on Gestational Diabetes Mellitus. *Diabetes Care.* 2007;30(suppl 2):S251.
72. Crowther CA, Hiller JE, Moss JR, et al. Effect of treatment of gestational diabetes mellitus on pregnancy outcomes. *N Engl J Med.* 2005;352(24):2477-2486.
73. HAPO Study Cooperative Research Group, Metzger BE, Lowe LP, Dyer AR, Trimble ER, Chaovarindr U, et al. Hyperglycemia and adverse pregnancy outcomes. *N Engl J Med.* 2008;358(19):1991-2002.
74. Landon MB. A planned randomized clinical trial of treatment for mild gestational diabetes mellitus. *J Maternal-Fetal Neonatal Med.* 2002;11(4):226.

75. Landon MB, Thom E, Spong CY, et al. The National Institute of Child Health and Human Development Maternal-Fetal Medicine Unit Network randomized clinical trial in progress: standard therapy versus no therapy for mild gestational diabetes. *Diabetes Care*. 2007;30 (suppl 2):S194-S199.
76. Buchanan TA. What is gestational diabetes? *Diabetes Care*. 2007;30(suppl 2):S105.

Diabetes Prevention Interventions for Women with a History of GDM

24

Assiamira Ferrara and Samantha F. Ehrlich

24.1 Women with a History of GDM: Interventions to Prevent Type 2 Diabetes

24.1.1 Introduction

Women with a history of gestational diabetes (GDM) are at increased risk of later developing type 2 diabetes. Lifestyle modification interventions promoting weight loss and pharmacotherapy interventions to improve insulin sensitivity have been shown to be effective in preventing or delaying the onset of type 2 diabetes in older women with impaired glucose tolerance and/or a previous pregnancy complicated by GDM.

This chapter reviews interventions aimed at reducing the incidence of type 2 diabetes in women with a history of GDM. The chapter also presents the few available, small-scale lifestyle interventions for weight management during pregnancy and/or during the early postpartum period; these potential interventions could be applied to women soon after a diagnosis of GDM in order to reduce their lifetime risk of developing type 2 diabetes.

We present evidence supporting a lifestyle modification intervention that would begin during pregnancy and continue through the postpartum period, as pharmacotherapy interventions may not be appropriate for pregnant women or women of reproductive age who may intend to become pregnant. However, young women with GDM may not be aware of their diabetes risk and may perceive difficulty in changing lifestyle behaviors. Thus, novel approaches are necessary to translate lifestyle modifications previously proven effective in older women with impaired glucose tolerance to younger women with a recent history of GDM, particularly those with normal glucose tolerance postpartum. Directions for future research include randomized clinical trials assessing the effectiveness of lifestyle modification interventions targeting women with current GDM or a recent pregnancy complicated by GDM. Understanding the barriers to increasing physical activity and adopting a healthy

A. Ferrara (✉)
Division of Research, Kaiser Permanente Northern California, Oakland, CA, USA
e-mail: Assiamira.Ferrara@nsmtp.kp.org

C. Kim and A. Ferrara (eds.), *Gestational Diabetes During and After Pregnancy*,
DOI: 10.1007/978-1-84882-120-0_24,

diet, and learning how preventative lifestyle modifications may best be integrated into the busy schedules of young women caring for young children, are crucial.

24.2 The Risk of Type 2 Diabetes in Women with a History of Gestational Diabetes: Why, When, and for Whom Should we Intervene?

Screening for GDM may identify up to 31% of parous women who will develop type 2 diabetes at some point in their lifetime[1] and has the added advantage of identifying a vast majority of these women prior to the development of abnormal glycemia in a nonpregnant state. Thus, women with a history of GDM are excellent candidates for interventions that aim to prevent the development of type 2 diabetes.[2,3] Estimates of the relative risk for developing type 2 diabetes among women with a history of GDM range from 3 to 20, which are comparable in magnitude to the risks observed among individuals with impaired glucose tolerance, impaired fasting glucose, or both (3.5–8.6, 5.1–9.9 and 5.5–20.1, respectively).[4] A recent meta-analysis reports that women with GDM have 7.4 times the risk of developing type 2 diabetes relative to women with normoglycemic pregnancies.[2] In the Diabetes Prevention Program, the estimated cumulative incidence of diabetes was 38.4% for women with a history of GDM and 25.7% for parous women without a history of GDM.[5] Thus, despite both groups having similar levels of impaired glucose tolerance at study entry, and women with a history of GDM being younger, women with a history of GDM had a 71% increased incidence rate compared with women without such a history.[5] These data suggest that a pregnancy complicated by GDM adds additional risk.

Studies conducted among a broad distribution of ethnicities and geographical locations have all reported an increased risk for post-delivery development of diabetes among women with a history of GDM.[6] Women with GDM have reduced insulin secretion during pregnancy[7] and the postpartum risk of type 2 diabetes has been shown to increase with decreasing insulin secretion in response to an oral glucose tolerance test in the pregnant state.[8,9] This reduction in insulin secretion is likely to contribute to the later development of type 2 diabetes, particularly among women with behavioral factors that further decrease insulin sensitivity, such as excessive gestational weight gain, pregnancy weight retention, physical inactivity and increased caloric intake.

A systematic review[6] of studies investigating the incidence of postpartum type 2 diabetes in women with a history of GDM reported that 5–10% of women with a history of GDM develop type 2 diabetes during the first year postpartum, while 50% develop type 2 diabetes in the 5 years following delivery.[6] After controlling for variable testing rates and lengths of follow up between and within studies, progression to type 2 diabetes increased steeply in the first 5 years postpartum and then appeared to plateau.[6] These data suggest that women with GDM would benefit most from intervention strategies to prevent or delay the onset of type 2 diabetes that are initiated soon after a diagnosis of GDM rather than years later. Early intervention also makes sense physiologically. In women with a history of GDM, the development of type 2 diabetes is correlated with progressive pancreatic β-cell failure to compensate for ongoing insulin resistance.[5] Thus, for optimal success, interventions aimed at preventing or delaying the development of type 2 diabetes should be initiated as early as possible to avoid prolonged exposure to insulin resistance and the resulting β-cell deterioration.

Although the carbohydrate intolerance brought on by pregnancy usually resolves after delivery,[10, 11] approximately one third of women diagnosed with GDM will be diagnosed with impaired fasting glucose or impaired glucose tolerance at postpartum screening.[12, 13] Women with a history of GDM with normal postpartum screening results (i.e., those not diagnosed with impaired glucose tolerance or impaired fasting glucose in the postpartum) may be at lower risk for developing type 2 diabetes in the short term, but remain at increased risk for developing type 2 diabetes in the long term when compared with women without a history of GDM.[2,4] In fact, although 64.1% of women with GDM have normal postpartum screening and 21.8% have either impaired fasting glucose or impaired glucose tolerance,[12,13] up to 50% will develop type 2 diabetes in the 5 years after delivery.[6] Therefore, all women with a history of GDM should be targeted for prevention strategies aimed at reducing the risk of developing type 2 diabetes later in life.

24.3 Women with a History of Gestational Diabetes: How Should we Intervene?

This section focuses on evidence supporting early initiation of prevention efforts, evidence from clinical trials investigating the effectiveness of prevention strategies, and offers suggestions for future directions of research.

Several observational studies provide evidence supporting a lifestyle intervention that starts soon after the diagnosis of GDM, and continues into the postpartum period. In women with GDM, antepartum predictive factors for future type 2 diabetes are elevated glucose levels, reduced insulin secretion, and obesity.[9, 14–20] The combination of prepregnancy obesity and reduced insulin secretion during pregnancy is associated with an eightfold increased risk of developing type 2 diabetes in the 5 years following a pregnancy complicated by GDM.[8] Postpartum predictors of type 2 diabetes include elevated postpartum glucose levels that are below the diagnostic threshold for type 2 diabetes,[15] obesity, and postpartum weight gain.[21,22] O'Sullivan[21] found that after 23 years of follow-up on women with a history of GDM, type 2 diabetes was present in 61% of the women who were obese prior to pregnancy, in 42% of the women who had gained weight since pregnancy, and in only 28% of the women who were not obese or had lost weight since pregnancy. Peters[22] also found that, among 666 Latino women with a recent history of GDM, postpartum weight gain of 4.5 kg was independently associated with a twofold increase in the risk of developing type 2 diabetes. Therefore, preventing weight gain and helping overweight/obese women with GDM to lose weight in the postpartum period might decrease their risk of developing type 2 diabetes.

Most women, including those with GDM, retain some of the weight they gained during pregnancy in the postpartum period. The 1988 National Maternal and Infant Health Survey[23] demonstrates that pregnancy weight retention at 10–18 months postpartum is common, even among women who were not overweight prior to pregnancy.

Among normal weight women (prepregnancy BMI 19.8–26.0) whose pregnancy weight gain met the Institute of Medicine's (IOM) 1990 guidelines, only 28.9% returned to below their prepregnancy weight, while 51% retained between 0 and 3.63 kg, and 20.1% retained 4.08 kg or more of the weight they had gained during pregnancy. The same data[23] show greater pregnancy weight retention among women who were overweight prior to pregnancy (prepregnancy BMI 26.1–29.0) and who had also gained within the IOM 1990 guidelines[24]: 31.6% returned to below their prepregnancy weight and 32% retained between 0 and 3.63 kg, but 36.3% retained 4.08 kg or more. The authors also reported that pregnancy weight retention was higher (median value 2.6 kg) among women with gestational gains above the IOM recommendations.[24]

A study[25] conducted among women with a history of GDM suggests that pregnancy weight retention is also of concern in this population. Among women with a history of GDM who had a prepregnancy BMI greater than 25.0, only 18% lost weight (≥5 kg) while 33% gained weight (≥5 kg) within the median observation time of 24 months post delivery.

Excessive weight gain during pregnancy (beyond the IOM guidelines) is a major risk factor for pregnancy weight retention in the postpartum period. In fact, the best predictor of pregnancy weight retention is excessive weight gain during pregnancy.[26] In addition, pregnancy weight retention is associated with a woman being overweight in the long term[27,28] and overweight is a well established risk factor for developing type 2 diabetes. Preventing excessive gestational weight gain is also beneficial to women with GDM in terms of pregnancy outcomes.[29,30] Therefore, an intervention for women with GDM that aims to avoid excessive gestational weight gain and help women to return to their prepregnancy weight in the postpartum period, or lose additional weight if overweight prior to pregnancy, has the potential to prevent type 2 diabetes in both the short and long term. Given the pregnant and early postpartum state, behavioral interventions are preferred to pharmacological interventions, since the latter has the potential to harm developing fetuses or breastfeeding infants.

However, no lifestyle intervention trials among women with GDM that start during pregnancy or the early postpartum have been conducted and only a few small trials have focused on weight management, diet, or physical activity during pregnancy and/or early postpartum; only one of these focused on women with GDM.

24.4 Pregnancy Lifestyle Interventions

In a trial by Polley et al,[31] 120 normal weight and overweight women were randomized to either a behavioral intervention or usual care by 20 weeks gestation. The intervention women received education on pregnancy weight gain, healthy eating, and exercise and individual graphs of their weight gain progress. If they nevertheless exceeded their weight goals (i.e., gained more than the IOM recommendation for a given gestational week[24]), the intervention women received additional individualized nutrition and behavioral counseling. The intervention significantly decreased the percentage of normal weight women who exceeded the Institute of Medicine's recommendations for total pregnancy weight gain.

However, there was a nonsignificant effect in the opposite direction among overweight women, suggesting the need for additional support to promote appropriate pregnancy weight gain in that population.

On the other hand, in a randomized clinical trial conducted among obese women without GDM ($n=73$), Wolff et al[32] found that an intervention delivered through ten counseling sessions with a dietician with restriction of total energy intake was effective in reducing gestational weight gain (6.6 kg in women in the intervention group vs. 13.3 kg in the control group, $p=0.002$).

A small non randomized study conducted among obese women with GDM compared a weight gain restriction program with and without supplemental physical activity and found that weight gain per week was significantly lower in the exercise group as compared with the diet-only group.[33] However, women ($n=96$) in this study selected their group assignments,[33] so the observed difference in gestational weight gain could be attributed to factors other than physical activity. Although larger randomized clinical trials among women with GDM are needed, the results of these studies suggest that a pregnancy intervention combining diet and physical activity might be successful in limiting gestational weight gain in this population.

24.5 Early Postpartum: Lifestyle Interventions

Returning to prepregnancy weight soon after delivery, or below, if the woman was obese or overweight prior to pregnancy, might lower a woman's risk for type 2 diabetes by reducing her risk of being overweight. Unfortunately, there are only a few, small randomized studies[34–37] examining behavioral interventions for weight loss in the early postpartum period, and none are specific to women with a history of GDM.

Lovelady et al[37] randomized 33 previously sedentary women who were 6–8 weeks postpartum and exclusively breastfeeding to a 12-week exercise program or to a control group. The exercise program consisted of 45 min a day of aerobic exercise, performed 5 days a week. The authors found a significant decline in weight and percent body fat for the entire study population, but no significant differences between the exercise and the control groups. Although women in the exercise group had higher energy expenditure, they compensated with higher energy intake. The results of this study suggest that aerobic exercise alone, without diet modification, is insufficient to promote postpartum weight loss. Lovelady et al[36] conducted another trial in which 40 overweight, exclusively breastfeeding postpartum women were randomized at 4 weeks postpartum to either a diet and exercise intervention group or a control group. The diet and exercise program lasted for 10 weeks, during which time the women were instructed to reduce their energy intake by 500 kcal/day and to exercise for 45 min a day, 4 days a week. Women in the intervention group lost significantly more weight and fat mass than control women; 48% of the women in the diet and exercise group were within 1 kg of their prepregnancy weight by the end of the study period, compared with 21% of the women in the control group. Although women in the diet and exercise group decreased their energy intake more than women in the control group, the difference was not statistically significant, which could be due to the small sample size. Taken together, the results of the two Lovelady studies[36,37] suggest that an intervention which combines diet and physical activity may be the best strategy for achieving postpartum weight loss.

O'Toole et al[34] conducted a randomized trial that investigated a diet and physical activity intervention for weight loss in the first year postpartum among overweight women. The 13 women in the intervention group experienced significant weight loss (7.3 kg on average) by 1 year postpartum, while the 10 women in the control group had only a small, nonsignificant reduction in weight (1.3 kg on average). Leermakers et al[35] randomized 90 women who had given birth in the previous 3–12 months to either a no-treatment control group or a behavioral weight loss intervention that focused on a low-fat/low-calorie diet and increasing physical activity. Women in the behavioral intervention group lost significantly more weight than controls (7.8 kg vs. 4.9 kg). The amount of weight retained at baseline emerged as the single strongest predictor of how close a woman came to reaching her prepregnancy weight. These results provide additional support for initiating lifestyle modification interventions early in the postpartum period, in order to maximize success.

Behavioral interventions targeting postpartum women, including those with a history of GDM, are particularly challenging to implement due to the considerable life changes that occur in the postpartum period. Previous trials[34,35] evaluating behavioral interventions for postpartum women, which incorporated education, goal setting, counseling, and follow-up via telephone or mailings, obtained only modest success in helping women reach their weight and physical activity goals. A number also saw high attrition rates: 42[34] and 31%.[35] Compliance with behavioral interventions, which typically include multiple counseling sessions and extended periods of follow-up, may be inherently difficult for women with infants or young children.

Albright et al[38] conducted a small observational study among postpartum women to compare pre-intervention to post-intervention minutes of moderate and vigorous leisure-time physical activity. The 2-month intervention relied primarily on email and weekly telephone counseling contacts to promote physical activity; all participants also received a pedometer to provide them with an objective measure of the number of steps they accumulated each day. At baseline, participants reported a mean of 3 ± 13.4 min/week of moderate and vigorous leisure-time physical activity. Minutes per week were significantly higher post-intervention: 85.5 ± 76.4 min/week ($p < 0.001$), leading the authors to conclude that a telephone/email intervention tailored to the needs of postpartum women effectively increased levels of physical activity. Project Viva,[39] which explored longitudinal changes in physical activity from prepregnancy to the postpartum period, reported that women decreased their moderate and vigorous physical activity but maintained levels of walking. A small study assessing the exercise beliefs of women with GDM found that the most common barrier to exercise in the postpartum period was a lack of time.[40] A diet and physical activity intervention, administered through telephone and email contacts that emphasizes walking or other forms of physical activity that can be done with an infant, may be more effective in this population.

24.6 Late Postpartum: Lifestyle and Pharmacotherapy Interventions

The Diabetes Prevention Program (DPP)[41] was a randomized, controlled clinical trial conducted among men and women with impaired glucose tolerance, elevated fasting blood glucose levels, and a BMI >24 (or >22 among Asians), including women with a history of GDM. The DPP[41] investigated the efficacy of metformin therapy and an intensive lifestyle intervention versus placebo in delaying or preventing the development of diabetes. The intensive lifestyle intervention aimed to achieve and maintain: (1) weight reduction of at least 7% of initial body weight through healthy eating and physical activity, and (2) at least 150 min/week of moderate intensity physical activity, such as walking or bicycling.[41] The intensive lifestyle intervention included training on diet, exercise, and behavior modification skills and was delivered through a structured protocol that included strategies for individually tailoring the intervention, in an attempt to maximize participant success. In analyses conducted among the entire DPP study population, the intensive lifestyle intervention significantly reduced the incidence of diabetes by 58% relative to the placebo control group, while metformin plus the standard lifestyle intervention reduced the incidence by 31%.[41]

The Diabetes Prevention Program Research Group also conducted subgroup analyses comparing parous women enrolled in the DPP with a history of GDM to parous women enrolled in the DPP without a history of GDM.[5] The two groups of women were comparable with respect to parity, BMI, fasting glucose, 2-h post-load glucose, glycosylated hemoglobin, insulin sensitivity, and insulin secretion at randomization, but differed in age: women with a history of GDM were significantly younger than parous women without a history of GDM (43 vs. 51 years, on average).

The results of this study also suggest that, among women with history of GDM, intensive lifestyle intervention and metformin are equally effective in decreasing the risk of developing type 2 diabetes.[5] In women with a history of GDM, the intensive lifestyle intervention resulted in a significant 53% reduction in risk when compared with placebo, whereas metformin resulted in a statistically significant 50% reduction in risk. Among women without a history of GDM, those in the intensive lifestyle intervention experienced a statistically significant 49% reduction in risk when compared with the placebo group; those taking metformin had a statistically significant 14% reduction in risk. Thus, the reduction in risk afforded by metformin was modified by history of GDM (50% in women with a history of GDM vs. 14% in those without, interaction $p=0.06$). The greater effectiveness of metformin in women with history of GDM might be related to their younger age, since the analyses that included all DPP participants also suggested that metformin was more effective in younger men and women.[41]

However, women with a history of GDM were less successful in adhering to the intensive lifestyle intervention in the long-term than were women without a GDM history. Although women both with and without a history of GDM who were randomized to the intensive lifestyle intervention increased their physical activity by approximately 1.5 h/week in the first year, this increase was not sustained among women with a history of GDM, who fell to less than 30 min of increased physical activity per week by year 3 of the study. There were also differences in weight loss by history of GDM. Women with a history of GDM lost weight in the first 6 months of the intervention (maximum achieved weight loss: 5.13±0.43 kg, mean ± SD), after which they began to steadily gain weight. Women without a history of GDM achieved most of their weight loss by 6 months but continued to lose weight at a lower rate through 1 year, after which they too, began to steadily gain weight (maximum achieved weight loss: 6.40±0.20 kg). Thus, women with a history of GDM had a mean weight loss of only 1.60 kg (SD 0.80 kg) by year 3 of the study while those without a history of GDM had a mean weight loss of 4.03 kg (SD 0.40 kg) in the same interval ($p=0.021$ for differences in weight at year 3). The intensive lifestyle intervention may have been more effective in preventing or delaying the development of type 2 diabetes among women with a history of GDM if they had been more able to adhere to the prescribed physical activity and weight loss. Again, it is possible that the lower level of adherence to physical activity and weight loss observed among women with a history of GDM was due to their younger age and presumably, busier postpartum lives.

It should be noted that an average of 12 years elapsed between the participants' first GDM pregnancies and enrollment in the DPP. Since participation in the DPP also required impaired glucose tolerance with elevated fasting glucose, women with GDM who developed diabetes in the first few years following delivery were ineligible. The results of these subgroup analyses may only apply to a select group of women with a history of GDM: those who remained free of diabetes for 12 years, on average, following a pregnancy complicated by GDM.

The Troglitazone in Prevention of Diabetes (TRIPOD)[42] was the first randomized control trial to examine the effectiveness of a pharmacotherapy intervention in delaying or preventing the development of diabetes among women with a history of GDM. Women were eligible for the trial if they had had a pregnancy complicated by GDM in the prior 4 years and if they were at high risk for developing type 2 diabetes in the subsequent 5 years, based on the results of a 75-g oral glucose tolerance test performed postpartum.[15] A total of 266 high risk Hispanic women were randomized to receive either placebo or 400 mg/day of troglitazone, a thiazolidinedione. Thiazolidinediones improve insulin sensitivity and short-term treatment with troglitazone had been previously shown to reduce the secretory demands that insulin resistance places on pancreatic β-cells.[43] The TRIPOD study[42] aimed to test whether chronic treatment of insulin resistance with troglitazone could preserve β-cell function and delay or prevent type 2 diabetes.

After 28–30 months of follow up, the authors found a significantly lower cumulative incidence of diabetes among women receiving troglitazone as compared with women who received placebo (5.4 vs. 12.1%).[42] Among the 236 women who returned for at least one follow up visit, troglitazone had reduced the incidence of diabetes by over 50%. However, protection required an initial increase in whole body insulin sensitivity; troglitazone therapy was most effective among women who responded to that increase with a large reduction in insulin output. One-third of the women in the troglitazone group failed to demonstrate initial increases in whole body insulin sensitivity, and relative to the placebo group, these women were not protected from diabetes. These non-responders were similar to women who did demonstrate initial increases in whole body insulin sensitivity in terms of baseline characteristics and compliance with troglitazone therapy. Thus, the authors were unable to identify any clinical or metabolic characteristics that could distinguish those who would be protected by troglitazone therapy from those who would not.

The TRIPOD trial[42] was discontinued in March of 2000 when troglitazone was withdrawn from the market due to reports of hepatotoxicity. Eighty-four of the 102 women who reached the end the trial without developing diabetes returned for post-trial testing (40 in the placebo group and 44 in the troglitazone group). Returnees in the troglitazone group had an average annual incidence rate of diabetes of 3.1% in the post-trial period, while returnees from the placebo group had a significantly higher average annual incidence rate of 21.2%. Thus, the drug's protective effect persisted for approximately 8 months after discontinuation of therapy. These findings led the authors to suggest that troglitazone had fundamentally transformed the underlying metabolic changes leading to the development of diabetes. They proposed that troglitazone therapy provided indirect protection that was mediated through improved whole body insulin sensitivity and resulted in β-cell rest.

24.7 Directions for Future Research

Lifestyle modification interventions that begin shortly after a diagnosis of GDM and continue into the postpartum period have the greatest potential for success in reducing the incidence of type 2 diabetes among all women with GDM. However, young women with a recent history of GDM may not appreciate their future risk of type 2 diabetes[44] and may perceive difficulty in starting to exercise. Thus, unique approaches will be required to translate the prevention strategies shown to be effective among older patients with impaired glucose tolerance[45] to younger women with a history of GDM. Interventions targeting this group must take into consideration the demands of being a new parent and the physical activity barriers specific to postpartum women, particularly the perceived lack of time to exercise[40] and a lack of childcare.[39] Interventions that utilize the telephone, text messaging, a MP3 player, email, or an interactive Web site may be more effective for achieving lifestyle change in young women with a recent history of GDM due to the unique barriers faced by postpartum women. Qualitative studies in the target population would help identify the preferred modalities of intervention delivery. Future interventions for weight management in women with a recent history of GDM should also provide a theoretical basis attempting to explain the mechanism by which the intervention is designed to work.[46] Attention to the cultural, social, and contextual factors established in descriptive research would also improve intervention design and implementation.[46]

Lifestyle modification interventions for women with a recent history of GDM may be preferred to pharmacotherapy interventions for several reasons. As both intervention strategies are intended for women of reproductive age, the use of daily pharmacotherapy agents may be recommended only for women who will not become pregnant. Lifestyle modification interventions also have the potential to positively impact the children and families of women who participate: counseling women to increase their physical activity and make healthy dietary changes may potentially impact the health behaviors of the entire family. Research investigating the secondary, family-level effects of lifestyle modification interventions targeting postpartum women has yet to be conducted.

References

1. Cheung NW, Byth K. Population health significance of gestational diabetes. *Diab Care.* 2003;26:2005-2009.
2. Bellamy L, Casas JP, Hingorani AD, Williams D. Type 2 diabetes mellitus after gestational diabetes: a systematic review and meta-analysis. *Lancet.* 2009;373:1773-1779.
3. Bentley-Lewis R. Gestational diabetes mellitus: an opportunity of a lifetime. *Lancet.* 2009; 373:1738-1740.
4. England LJ, Dietz PM, Njoroge T, et al. Preventing type 2 diabetes: public health implications for women with a history of gestational diabetes mellitus. *Am J Obstet Gynecol.* 2009;200:365-368.
5. Ratner RE, Christophi CA, Metzger BE, et al. Prevention of diabetes in women with a history of gestational diabetes: effects of metformin and lifestyle interventions. *J Clin Endocrinol Metab.* 2008;93:4774-4779.
6. Kim C, Newton KM, Knopp RH. Gestational diabetes and the incidence of type 2 diabetes: a systematic review. *Diab Care.* 2002;25:1862-1868.
7. Nicholls JS, Chan SP, Ali K, Beard RW, Dornhorst A. Insulin secretion and sensitivity in women fulfilling WHO criteria for gestational diabetes. *Diabet Med.* 1995;12:56-60.
8. Metzger BE, Cho NH, Roston SM, Radvany R. Prepregnancy weight and antepartum insulin secretion predict glucose tolerance five years after gestational diabetes mellitus. *Diab Care.* 1993;16:1598-1605.
9. Damm P, Kuhl C, Bertelsen A, Molsted-Pedersen L. Predictive factors for the development of diabetes in women with previous gestational diabetes mellitus. *Am J Obstet Gynecol.* 1992;167:607-616.
10. Kaaja RJ, Greer IA. Manifestations of chronic disease during pregnancy. *JAMA.* 2005;294: 2751-2757.
11. Buchanan TA, Xiang AH. Gestational diabetes mellitus. *J Clin Invest.* 2005;115:485-491.
12. Ferrara A, Peng T, Kim C. Trends in postpartum diabetes screening and subsequent diabetes and impaired fasting glucose among women with histories of gestational diabetes mellitus. A report from the Translating Research Into Action for Diabetes (TRIAD) Study. *Diab Care.* 2008;32(2):269-274.
13. Schaefer-Graf UM, Buchanan TA, Xiang AH, Peters RK, Kjos SL. Clinical predictors for a high risk for the development of diabetes mellitus in the early puerperium in women with recent gestational diabetes mellitus. *Am J Obstet Gynecol.* 2002;186:751-756.
14. Kjos SL, Buchanan TA, Greenspoon JS, Montoro M, Bernstein GS, Mestman JH. Gestational diabetes mellitus: the prevalence of glucose intolerance and diabetes mellitus in the first two months post partum. *Am J Obstet Gynecol.* 1990;163:93-98.
15. Kjos SL, Peters RK, Xiang A, Henry OA, Montoro M, Buchanan TA. Predicting future diabetes in Latino women with gestational diabetes. Utility of early postpartum glucose tolerance testing. *Diabetes.* 1995;44:586-591.
16. Lam KS, Li DF, Lauder IJ, Lee CP, Kung AW, Ma JT. Prediction of persistent carbohydrate intolerance in patients with gestational diabetes. *Diab Res Clin Pract.* 1991;12:181-186.
17. Catalano PM, Vargo KM, Bernstein IM, Amini SB. Incidence and risk factors associated with abnormal postpartum glucose tolerance in women with gestational diabetes. *Am J Obstet Gynecol.* 1991;165:914-919.

18. Coustan DR, Carpenter MW, O'Sullivan PS, Carr SR. Gestational diabetes: predictors of subsequent disordered glucose metabolism. *Am J Obstet Gynecol.* 1993;168:1139-1144.
19. Steinhart JR, Sugarman JR, Connell FA. Gestational diabetes is a herald of NIDDM in Navajo women. High rate of abnormal glucose tolerance after GDM. *Diab Care.* 1997;20:943-947.
20. Kaufmann RC, Schleyhahn FT, Huffman DG, Amankwah KS. Gestational diabetes diagnostic criteria: long-term maternal follow-up. *Am J Obstet Gynecol.* 1995;172:621-625.
21. O'Sullivan JB. Gestational diabetes: factors influencing the rates of subsequent diabetes. In: Sutherland HW, Stowers JM, eds. *Carbohydrate Metabolism During Pregnancy and the Newborn 1978.* Berlin, Germany: Springer; 1979:425-435.
22. Peters RK, Kjos SL, Xiang A, Buchanan TA. Long-term diabetogenic effect of single pregnancy in women with previous gestational diabetes mellitus [see comments]. *Lancet.* 1996; 347:227-230.
23. Keppel KG, Taffel SM. Pregnancy-related weight gain and retention: implications of the 1990 Institute of Medicine guidelines. *Am J Public Health.* 1993;83:1100-1103.
24. Institute of Medicine, National Academy of Sciences, Food and Nutrition Board. *Nutrition During Pregnancy. Part I Weight Gain.* Washington, DC: National Academy Press; 1990.
25. Stage E, Ronneby H, Damm P. Lifestyle change after gestational diabetes. *Diab Res Clin Pract.* 2004;63:67-72.
26. Greene GW, Smiciklas-Wright H, Scholl TO, Karp RJ. Postpartum weight change: how much of the weight gained in pregnancy will be lost after delivery? *Obstet Gynecol.* 1988;71:701-707.
27. Linne Y, Dye L, Barkeling B, Rossner S. Weight development over time in parous women–the SPAWN study–15 years follow-up. *Int J Obes Relat Metab Disord.* 2003;27:1516-1522.
28. Linne Y, Dye L, Barkeling B, Rossner S. Long-term weight development in women: a 15-year follow-up of the effects of pregnancy. *Obes Res.* 2004;12:1166-1178.
29. Hedderson MM, Weiss NS, Sacks DA, et al. Pregnancy weight gain and risk of neonatal complications: macrosomia, hypoglycemia, and hyperbilirubinemia. *Obstet Gynecol.* 2006;108: 1153-1161.
30. Cheng YW, Chung JH, Kurbisch-Block I, Inturrisi M, Shafer S, Caughey AB. Gestational weight gain and gestational diabetes mellitus: perinatal outcomes. *Obstet Gynecol.* 2008;112: 1015-1022.
31. Polley BA, Wing RR, Sims CJ. Randomized controlled trial to prevent excessive weight gain in pregnant women. *Int J Obes Relat Metab Disord.* 2002;26:1494-1502.
32. Wolff S, Legarth J, Vangsgaard K, Toubro S, Astrup A. A randomized trial of the effects of dietary counseling on gestational weight gain and glucose metabolism in obese pregnant women. *Int J Obes (Lond).* 2008;32:495-501.
33. Artal R, Catanzaro RB, Gavard JA, Mostello DJ, Friganza JC. A lifestyle intervention of weight-gain restriction: diet and exercise in obese women with gestational diabetes mellitus. *Appl Physiol Nutr Metab.* 2007;32:596-601.
34. O'Toole ML, Sawicki MA, Artal R. Structured diet and physical activity prevent postpartum weight retention. *J Womens Health (Larchmt).* 2003;12:991-998.
35. Leermakers EA, Anglin K, Wing RR. Reducing postpartum weight retention through a correspondence intervention. *Int J Obes Relat Metab Disord.* 1998;22:1103-1109.
36. Lovelady CA, Garner KE, Moreno KL, Williams JP. The effect of weight loss in overweight, lactating women on the growth of their infants. *N Engl J Med.* 2000;342:449-453.
37. Lovelady CA, Nommsen-Rivers LA, McCrory MA, Dewey KG. Effects of exercise on plasma lipids and metabolism of lactating women. *Med Sci Sports Exerc.* 1995;27:22-28.
38. Albright CL, Maddock JE, Nigg CR. Increasing physical activity in postpartum multiethnic women in Hawaii: results from a pilot study. *BMC Womens Health.* 2009;9:4.
39. Pereira MA, Rifas-Shiman SL, Kleinman KP, Rich-Edwards JW, Peterson KE, Gillman MW. Predictors of change in physical activity during and after pregnancy: Project Viva. *Am J Prev Med.* 2007;32:312-319.

40. Symons DD, Ulbrecht JS. Understanding exercise beliefs and behaviors in women with gestational diabetes mellitus. *Diab Care*. 2006;29:236-240.
41. Knowler WC, Barrett-Connor E, Fowler SE, et al. Reduction in the incidence of type 2 diabetes with lifestyle intervention or metformin. *N Engl J Med*. 2002;346:393-403.
42. Buchanan TA, Xiang AH, Peters RK, et al. Preservation of pancreatic beta-cell function and prevention of type 2 diabetes by pharmacological treatment of insulin resistance in high-risk hispanic women. *Diabetes*. 2002;51(9):2796-2803.
43. Buchanan TA, Xiang AH, Peters RK, et al. Response of pancreatic beta-cells to improved insulin sensitivity in women at high risk for type 2 diabetes. *Diabetes*. 2000;49:782-788.
44. Kieffer EC, Carman WJ, Gillespie BW, Nolan GH, Worley SE, Guzman JR. Obesity and gestational diabetes among African-American women and Latinas in Detroit: implications for disparities in women's health. *J Am Med Womens Assoc*. 2001;56:181-187,196.
45. Tuomilehto J, Lindstrom J, Eriksson JG, et al. Prevention of type 2 diabetes mellitus by changes in lifestyle among subjects with impaired glucose tolerance. *N Engl J Med*. 2001;344(18):1343-1350.
46. Keller C, Records K, Ainsworth B, Permana P, Coonrod DV. Interventions for weight management in postpartum women. *J Obstet Gynecol Neonatal Nurs*. 2008;37:71-79.

Section IX

Diabetes Control Programs and Policy

Diabetes Control Programs and Policy 25

Lois Jovanovic

25.1 Introduction

Gestational diabetes mellitus (GDM) is most accurately defined as "a transient abnormality of glucose tolerance during pregnancy."[1, 2] This definition does not include type 2 diabetes that is diagnosed during pregnancy.[2] In 1997 the American Diabetes Association (ADA) defined GDM as diabetes diagnosed during pregnancy.[3] This definition lead to a broad range of screening, diagnostic, treatment, and postpartum screening plans. Medical organizations have developed their own courses of action to deal with GDM. While the broad points of management are generally agreed upon, controversy does exist.

The ADA, The American College of Obstetricians and Gynecologists (ACOG), and the World Health Organization (WHO) are three of the primary medical organizations regarding GDM. In this chapter, we will focus on the overlap in these organizations' GDM guidelines.

The ADA is a nonprofit health organization that supports diabetes research, provides information, and engages in advocacy. The mission of the ADA is to prevent and cure diabetes and to improve the lives of all people affected by diabetes. To fulfill this mission, the ADA funds research, publishes scientific findings, and provides information and other services to individuals with diabetes, and to their families, health professionals, and the public.[4] ACOG supports measures to ensure healthy outcomes for mother and child. ACOG advocates a range of programs that support medical research and translates research into information that can be used to provide direct care for women. GDM is but one area of women's health that ACOG focuses upon.[5] WHO is the directing and coordinating authority for health within the United Nations system. It is responsible for providing leadership on global health matters, shaping the global health research agenda, setting norms and standards, articulating evidence-based policy options, providing technical support to countries, and monitoring and assessing health trends.[6] GDM is also but one of numerous medical conditions that WHO addresses.

L. Jovanovic
Department of Research, Sansum Diabetes Research Institute,
2219 Bath Street, Santa Barbara, CA 93105, USA
e-mail: ljovanovic@sansum.org

C. Kim and A. Ferrara (eds.), *Gestational Diabetes During and After Pregnancy*,
DOI: 10.1007/978-1-84882-120-0_25,

25.1.1 Screening and Diagnosis

Screening for GDM is a highly controversial topic. Differences between medical organizations are also discussed in the two other chapters on screening and the one chapter on prevalence of GDM. Broadly speaking, North America and Europe use two different methods for GDM screening.[7] A universal method for screening and diagnosis does not exist. Organizations such as the ADA and the WHO set their own clinical guidelines. Recent studies conducted by the United States Preventative Task Force (USPSTF) and the Canadian Task Force on Preventative Health Care both have agreed that there is insufficient evidence to recommend that all pregnant women undergo screening for GDM.[7,8] The purpose of the USPSTF review was to determine if the benefits of screening for GDM outweighed the harms. The review found that screening combined with treatment for hyperglycemia could reduce macrosomia in newborns, but the panel concluded that better scientific evidence was needed to determine if universal screening reduces adverse health outcomes for mothers and their infants.[7]

The ADA recommends that women who are at very high risk for GDM should be screened at the first prenatal visit.[9] Very high risk criteria are:

- Severe obesity
- Prior history of GDM or delivery of large-for-gestational-age (LGA) infant
- Presence of glycosuria
- Diagnosis of polycystic ovarian syndrome
- Strong family history of type 2 diabetes

All women at 24–28 weeks gestation, including those that were not found to have diabetes early in pregnancy, should be screened unless they are considered low risk. Women must have all of the following criteria to be considered low risk:

- Age less than 25 years
- Weight normal before pregnancy
- Member of an ethnic group with a low prevalence of diabetes i.e., non-Hispanic white women
- No known diabetes in first-degree relatives
- No history of abnormal glucose tolerance
- No history of poor obstetrical outcome

As recommended by the ADA, GDM screening at this stage is performed using a two-step approach. The first step is a 50-g glucose challenge test (GCT). Plasma glucose is measured 1-h after the 50-g glucose load is given. A value of 140 mg/dL (7.8 mmol/L) and above identifies approximately 80% of women with GDM, and a value of 130 mg/dL (7.2 mmol/dL) and above identifies approximately 90% of women with GDM.[9] If the threshold is exceeded, women are given a 100 or 75-g oral glucose tolerance test (OGTT) on a separate day. The threshold values recommended by the ADA for the 75 and 100-g OGTT at fasting, 1-h, and 2-h are exactly the same. The 25-g glucose difference between the 75- and 100-g glucose challenges is not addressed by the ADA. The OGTT is preformed in the morning following an 8-h overnight fast. Diagnosis of GDM requires at least two of the following plasma glucose levels:

100-g

Fasting: above 95 mg/dL (5.3 mmol/L)
1-h: above 180 mg/dL (10.0 mmol/L)
2-h: above 155 mg/dL (8.6 mmol/L)
3-h: above 140 mg/dL (7.8 mmol/L)

75-g

Fasting: above 95 mg/dL (5.3 mmol/L)
1-h: above 180 mg/dL (10.0 mmol/L)
2-h: above 155 mg/dL (8.6 mmol/L)

Studies have identified problems associated with the above guidelines. One study showed that only 20% of women who exceeded the threshold value on the GCT also exceeded the threshold value on the OGTT.[10] Therefore, the specificity of the text is extremely low. Another study tested the reliability of the GCT.[11] It showed that 30% of women with GDM had ambiguous GCT results on repetitive testing.

The National Diabetes Data Group (NDDG) and the Expert Committee on the Diagnosis and Classification of Diabetes Mellitus recommend OGTT cut-off values that are higher, and therefore less stringent, than those of the ADA.[12] They recommend the following cut-off values:

Fasting: glucose 105 mg/dL (5.8 mmol/L)
1-h: 190 mg/dL (10.6 mmol/L)
2-h: 165 mg/dL (9.2 mmol/L)
3-h: 145 mg/dL (8.1 mmol/L)[3]

Threshold OGTT values from the NDDG and the ADA are both considered acceptable by ACOG.[13] ACOG also states that women who are considered low risk by ADA guidelines need not undergo screening, however they do recognize that universal screening is the most sensitive and practical approach.[13]

WHO uses a different screening approach. Its approach, adopted in many countries outside of North America, uses identical diagnostic criteria for pregnant and nonpregnant women. WHO uses a 2-h 75-g OGTT. GDM is diagnosed if the fasting glucose is 126 mg/dL (7.0 mmol/L) and above, or if the 2-h glucose is 140 mg/dL (11.1 mmol/L) and above.[14]

The Hyperglycemia and Adverse Pregnancy Outcomes Study Cooperative Research Group (HAPO) conducted a prospective cohort study of 23,325 women.[15] Women and clinicians blinded to test results were tested at 24–32 weeks gestation for glucose tolerance using the 75-g OGTT. Four primary adverse pregnancy outcomes were examined: birth weight above the 90th percentile for gestational age, primary cesarean delivery, clinically diagnosed neonatal hypoglycemia, and cord-blood serum C-peptide level above the

90th percentile. Six secondary outcomes were examined: delivery before 37 weeks of gestation, shoulder dystocia or birth injury, need for intensive neonatal care, hyperbilirubinemia, and preeclampsia. Women were unblinded if their OGTT results were extremely elevated, so study results focus on women with relatively mild gestational hyperglycemia. Ten of 12 analyses of primary outcomes and 12 of 15 analyses of secondary outcomes showed significant positive correlation with increased plasma glucose levels. Analyses of the primary outcomes showed the strongest correlations between increasing maternal glucose levels at fasting, 1-h, and 2-h, and two primary adverse outcomes: birth weight above the 90th percentile and cord-blood serum C-peptide level above the 90th percentile.[15] Of note, Schrader and colleagues also showed significant correlation in women with a fasting plasma glucose above 90 mg/dL and increased delivery rates of macrosomic infants.[16]

Therefore, the investigators of both studies concluded that significant associations between adverse outcomes and higher levels of maternal glucose existed within what is currently considered a nondiabetic range, and lower gestational glycemic cut-offs needed to be defined.

The ADA did not address screening and diagnosis of GDM during the Fifth International Workshop-Conference on Gestational Diabetes but does plan on addressing the issue at the Sixth Workshop-Conference.[17] Until a gold standard diagnostic criterion is reached, controversy will continue to surround the issue of screening and diagnosis of GDM.

25.1.2 Monitoring, Management, Treatment, and Postpartum Screening

Organizations that have published guidelines on GDM also recommend different approaches to monitoring, management, treatment, and postpartum screening. As with diagnostic criteria for the identification of GDM, discrepancies exist between organizations regarding management guidelines. Many of these discrepancies stem from the lack of a consensus diagnostic criterion for GDM.

25.1.2.1 Monitoring

The ADA recommends a basic plan for monitoring GDM.[9] The plan includes maternal metabolic surveillance to determine if blood glucose levels are high enough to cause risks to the fetus. Metabolic surveillance consists of glucose self-monitoring by the gravida, with periodic checks by the health care provider. The ADA does not recommend a daily monitoring schedule but does acknowledge that postprandial measurements are more important than preprandial measurements. Maternal glucose levels should not be monitored from the urine. The ADA also advises closer maternal and fetal surveillance in pregnant women with a fasting glucose of 95 mg/dL (5.3 mmol/L) and above, or pregnancies that are post dates. This surveillance should consist of additional monitoring and possibly ultrasonography, to determine if asymmetric abnormal fetal growth is present, especially in the early third trimester.[9] Asymmetric abnormal fetal growth is defined as abdominal circumference greater than head circumference.[18]

25.1.2.2 Medical Nutritional Therapy

Medical nutritional therapy (MNT) should be given to all women with GDM. The ADA advises registered dietitians to deliver MNT, consistent with its guidelines.[9] Nonobese women with GDM should consume enough energy to allow for normal weight gain during pregnancy. The ADA recommends food choices be made to accomplish three main goals: appropriate weight gain, normoglycemia, and absence of urine ketones.[19] Women who are diagnosed with GDM should be placed on individualized diets that result in normal blood glucose levels. Quantity, type, and frequency of carbohydrate intake depends directly on individual responses of blood glucose levels. Glucose level consistency is very important because the fetus is constantly drawing blood from the mother. Women are encouraged to keep daily records of foods consumed and subsequent blood glucose levels. Change in carbohydrate intake and insulin dosage can be made based on these records. Obese women with a body mass index (BMI) over 30 kg/m^2 are encouraged to reduce caloric intake by 30%. This caloric reduction can improve blood glucose control and avoid ketonuria.[19] ACOG states that better evidence is needed to recommend for or against caloric restriction in obese women. If caloric restriction is used for obese women, ACOG recommends that it should not be restricted by more than 33%.[13]

In the Australian Carbohydrate Intolerance in Pregnancy (ACHOIS) trial, Crowther and colleagues examined whether treatment of GDM with dietary advice, blood glucose monitoring, and insulin therapy vs. routine care reduced the risk of perinatal complications.[20] Participants were randomly assigned to receive GDM treatment or routine care. Primary outcomes were infant death, shoulder dystocia, bone fracture, nerve palsy, admission to the neonatal nursery, jaundice requiring phototherapy, induction of labor, cesarean birth, and maternal anxiety, depression, and health status. Infants of the 490 women who received GDM treatment were found to have significantly lower perinatal complications than the 510 infants whose mothers received routine care. The relative risk was 1 vs. 4%, respectively, after adjustment for maternal age, race or ethnic group, and parity.[20]

Major and colleagues demonstrated the effect of carbohydrate restriction on perinatal outcomes in women with diet-controlled GDM.[21] Women were nonrandomly assigned to two groups: low dietary carbohydrate group vs. high dietary carbohydrate group. Women in the low carbohydrate group less frequently required the addition of insulin to control glucose, and also had fewer LGA infants and cesarean deliveries for cephalopelvic disproportion and macrosomia.[21] Jovanovic and colleagues examined women who were placed on insulin because they could not maintain fasting blood glucose values below 90 mg/dL and 1-h postprandial glucose levels below 120 mg/dL with diet modification alone. These women had significantly lower infant birth weights.[22]

ADA guidelines advise women with GDM to set the following glycemic thresholds:

Fasting whole blood glucose of 95 mg/dL (5.3 mmol/L) and below
1-h postprandial whole blood glucose of 140 mg/dL (7.8 mmol/L) and below
2-h postprandial whole blood glucose of 120 mg/dL (6.7 mmol/L) and below[9]

ACOG recommends similar glycemic goals, except for a slightly different postprandial threshold at 1-h of 130–140 mg/dL (7.2–7.8 mmol/L). Of note, these thresholds are higher than those found in HAPO and by Jovanovic and colleagues to be associated with fetal outcomes.[22]

25.1.2.3 Insulin Therapy

Insulin therapy is recommended by the ADA when MNT does not maintain threshold blood glucose levels.[9] Basal and prandial insulin injections provide the best results. Neutral Protamine Hagedorn insulin or NPH is recommended for basal insulin injections and should be injected 2–4 times daily. At the first prenatal visit or before pregnancy, women who are taking one daily dose of insulin should switch to multiple NPH injections daily. Another possible option for basal insulin is by continuous subcutaneous insulin infusion (CSII) of rapid-acting insulin. Prandial insulin amount should be determined by premeal blood glucose, anticipated activity, and carbohydrate intake. Lispro and aspart are the only two rapid-acting insulin analogs recommended for CSII and prandial insulin usage. Women using CSII need to know how to operate their insulin delivery devices and must frequently check blood glucose levels.[9]

Langer and colleagues examined whether insulin treatment significantly reduced adverse perinatal outcomes in women with GDM.[23] Key factors in LGA infants were found to be fasting plasma glucose and treatment modality. Four hundred and seventy-one women were randomized to either insulin treatment or dietary therapy only, to optimize glycemic control. In women with a fasting glucose <95 mg/dL (5.3 mmol/L), insulin treatment resulted in 3.5% LGA neonates vs. 5.3% LGA neonates in dietary therapy. In women with a fasting glucose of 95–105 mg/dL (5.3–5.8 mmol/L), insulin treatment resulted in 10.3% LGA neonates vs. 28.6% LGA neonates in dietary therapy. Obese women with a fasting glucose of 95–105 mg/dL (5.3–5.8 mmol/L) who received dietary therapy only had a fourfold increase in LGA neonates compared with the insulin treated group. The study concluded that women with a fasting glucose >95 mg/dL (5.3 mmol/L) should be given insulin treatment to optimize blood glucose levels.[23]

25.1.2.4 Physical Activity

Moderate physical exercise programs are encouraged by the ADA for women with GDM.[9] These programs have been shown to lower maternal blood glucose levels.[9] Exercise guidelines for women with GDM are based on three randomized studies. Bung and colleagues compared women with GDM in an exercise treatment group vs. an insulin treatment group. Both groups had similar prevalence of macrosomia and mean glucose values during pregnancy.[24] Another randomized study of women with GDM determined that diet combined with exercise vs. diet alone significantly reduced fasting plasma glucose and blood glucose levels 1-h after a 50-g GCT.[25] The third study did not find significant benefits in maternal blood glucose control but did find a significant benefit on cardiorespiratory fitness.[26] It also showed exercise programs are safe in women with GDM.[26] All three studies were limited by small patient populations.

ACOG recommends that women who are pregnant and do not have any contraindications exercise 30 min per day.[27] The exercise should be moderate-intensity aerobic physical activity. Blood glucose levels need to be monitored closely around times of exercise and women must be hydrated adequately for individual exercise programs. GDM patients who use insulin should adjust insulin requirements and carbohydrate intake according to blood glucose measurements with exercise. Supine position and activities in which loss of balance could cause fetal trauma are highly discouraged during exercise.[27] Women should stop exercising and seek medical attention when any of the following occur: vaginal bleeding, faintness, decreased fetal activity, or low back pain.[28]

25.1.2.5 Oral Hypoglycemic Agents

The use of oral glucose-lowering agents has not been approved by the United States Food and Drug Administration during pregnancy, and neither the ADA nor ACOG recommend the use of these agents for GDM.[9, 13] Clinical trials are needed to establish their safety. Glyburide is an oral glucose-lowering agent that one study found to be effective.[29] Langer and colleagues assigned 404 women with GDM into two groups: an insulin treatment group and a glyburide treatment group. The primary outcome was optimal glycemic control, with secondary outcomes including a wide range of maternal and neonatal complications. The study found that there were no significant differences in primary outcomes and only one secondary outcome that was significantly different. Additionally, glyburide was not found in the cord serum of any infant in the glyburide treatment group. Although this study did show promising data, the sample size of the clinical trial was not large enough to conclude that glyburide was safe and effective during pregnancy.[30] Trends toward poorer outcomes such as neonatal hypoglycemia, higher birth weights, macrosomia, lung complications, and hyperbilirubinemia were not significant in the trial, but might potentially be observed in larger trials.[30] At the time ACOG published its practice bulletin, this was the only randomized trial on glyburide and therefore the bulletin did not recommend it.[13] The ADA also did not recommend glyburide use at the Fifth International Workshop, awaiting further data of its efficacy.[17] A 2008 USPSTF review of three glyburide and insulin randomized trials and four observational studies also found insufficient evidence to support its use.[31] Many physicians ignore these organizations' recommendations and prescribe glyburide because it is much easier to use, as compared with insulin.[32] Metformin is currently not recommended by the ADA or ACOG until further clinical trials are conducted[13, 17]; the Metformin in Gestational Diabetes, or MiG trial, is discussed in further detail in the accompanying chapter on pharmacological management during a GDM pregnancy.

25.1.2.6 Antepartum Assessment and Delivery

ACOG recommends beginning antepartum fetal assessment at 32 weeks gestation for women who have poor glycemic control, require insulin therapy, or have other perinatal risk factors such as hypertension.[13] The type of antepartum test should be determined by local practice. ACOG states that evidence of antepartum testing regimens in women with controlled blood glucose levels, who do not use insulin, and who do not have any other perinatal risk factors, are insufficient.[13] The ACOG Practice Bulletin states that women who have good glycemic control and do not have any maternal or fetal complications should not have routine delivery before 40 weeks of gestation.[13] In their 2008 review, the USPSTF found insufficient evidence to recommend elective cesarean delivery or timing of induction.[31] One randomized study of insulin-requiring women compared induced labor at 38 weeks gestation to expectant management of delivery.[33] Significant differences in rates of shoulder dystocia and cesarean delivery were not found between the two groups. The study did find that there was an increase in the prevalence of LGA infants in the expectant delivery group. The rates were 23% for the expectant delivery group and 10% for the induced labor group. ACOG recommends discussion with the patient about possible cesarean delivery if the estimated fetal weight is ≥4,500 g. At 4,000–4,500 g other factors need to be considered in the mode of delivery. These factors include: patient's past delivery history, clinical pelvimetry, and progress during the pregnancy.[13] Amniocentesis is recommended if delivery is planned before 39 weeks gestation, in order to confirm pulmonary maturity.[13]

25.1.3 Postpartum Screening

A consensus on the follow-up test of choice and frequency does not exist for women with prior GDM. The ADA recommends screening women with GDM 6–12 weeks postpartum.[34] The diagnosis criterion that the ADA recommends for women with prior GDM is the same criteria used to diagnosis all adults with diabetes in a nonpregnant state.[12] These consist of a fasting glucose of 126 mg/dL (7.0 mmol/L), and if a 2-h OGTT is performed, a 2-h glucose of 200 mg/dL (11.1 mmol/L). However, ADA states that a fasting test is preferred, due to ease of administration and reduced cost. ACOG guidelines were revised in 2009 to approximate those of the ADA, although previous guidelines[13] stated little data existed that established the benefit of screening; this discrepancy is discussed further in the accompanying chapter on Postpartum Diabetes Risk.

Women with prior GDM should be educated as to their risk for developing diabetes and the best ways to prevent its onset.[9] Exercise and diet modifications to maintain normal body weight are highly encouraged for all women. These women should not use medications that increase insulin resistance.[9] Women who plan to have more children should be taught the importance of maintaining glycemic control both between and throughout pregnancies to avoid the adverse effects of hyperglycemia. The ADA recommends combination estrogen-progestogen pills as contraception if no contraindications exist.[9] The lowest dose of hormones should be used to achieve the desired effect.[17] When combined with breastfeeding, progestin-only pills have been shown to increase the risk of developing type 2 diabetes in women with prior GDM,[35] and therefore are not the agent of first choice in high-risk women. Intrauterine devices are also considered a safe and effective contraceptive method[36]; family planning methods are discussed further in the accompanying chapter on contraceptive options.

25.1.4 Recommendations

Our recommendations for women with GDM are the following:

- Universal screening at 24–28 weeks gestation for all women.
- Carbohydrate restricted diet.
- MNT and moderate exercise programs as the initial approach to treatment.
- Self blood glucose monitoring to evaluate effectiveness of treatment.
- Insulin therapy when MNT and moderate exercise cannot maintain glycemic control.
- No oral-hypoglycemic agents.
- Postpartum screening for all women with previous GDM.

Clearly, a single gold standard GDM diagnostic criterion needs to be agreed upon and implemented. We are optimistic that the dissemination of the HAPO results will lead to such a consensus. After the definition of GDM is established, assessment of postpartum risk can occur, and guidelines for postpartum screening can be formulated. In the meantime, further work on the safety of glyburide during pregnancy should be done to examine the effects of medication on neonatal outcomes, particularly anoxia and birth trauma. Ongoing studies of metformin should answer some of the questions regarding the use of metformin for GDM.

References

1. O'Sullivan J. Gestational diabetes and its significance. In: Camerini-Davalos R, Cole HS, eds. *Early Diabetes*. Academic Press: New York; 1970:339-344.
2. Omori Y, Jovanovic L. Proposal for the reconsideration of the definition of gestational diabetes. *Diabetes Care*. 2005;28:2592-2593.
3. The Expert Committee on the Diagnosis and Classification of Diabetes Mellitus. Report of the Expert Committee on the Diagnosis and Classification of Diabetes Mellitus. *Diabetes Care*. 1997;20:1183-1197.
4. American Diabetes Association. About Us. http://www.diabetes.org/aboutus.jsp?WTLPromo=HEADER_aboutus&vms=274312743154; 2008. Accessed 8.08.08.
5. *Proposed Legislative Priorities. 110th Congress – 2nd Session*. American College of Obstetricians and Gynecologists; 2008.
6. World Health Organization. About WHO. http://www.who.int/about/en; 2008. Accessed 8.08.08.
7. U.S. Preventive Services Task Force. Screening for Gestational Diabetes Mellitus: U.S. Preventive Services Task Force Recommendation Statement. *Ann Intern Med*. 2008;148:759-765.
8. Examination PH. Screening for gestational diabetes mellitus. Canadian Task Force on the Periodic Health Examination. *CMAJ*. 1992;147:435.
9. American Diabetes Association. Gestational diabetes mellitus (Position Statement). *Diabetes Care*. 2003;26(suppl 1):S103-S105.
10. Bartha J, Martinez-Del-Fresno P, Comino-Delgado R. Gestational diabetes mellitus diagnosed during early pregnancy. *Am J Obstet Gynecol*. 2000;182:346-350.
11. Harlass F, Brady K, Read J. Reproducibility of the oral glucose tolerance test in pregnancy. *Am J Obstet Gynecol*. 1991;164:564-568.

12. Anon. Report of the Expert Committee on the Diagnosis and Classification of Diabetes Mellitus. *Diabetes Care*. 2000;23(suppl 1):S4.
13. Practice Bulletin ACOG. Clinical management guidelines for obstetrician-gynecologists. Number 30 (replaces Technical Bulletin Number 200, December 1994). *Obstet Gynecol*. 2001;98:525-538.
14. World Health Organization. *Definition, diagnosis, and classification of diabetes mellitus and its complications: report of a WHO consultation. Part 1. Diagnosis and classification of diabetes mellitus*. Geneva, World Health Organization; 1999.
15. Metzger B, Lowe L, Dyer A, et al. Hyperglycemia and adverse pregnancy outcomes. *N Engl J Med*. 2008;358:1991-2002.
16. Schrader H, Jovanovic-Peterson L, Bevier W, et al. Fasting plasma glucose and glycosylated protein at 24 to 28 weeks of gestation predict macrosomia in the general obstetric population. *Am J Perinatol*. 1995;12:247-251.
17. Metzger B, Buchanan T, Coustan D, et al. Summary and recommendations of the Fifth International Workshop-Conference on Gestational Diabetes Mellitus. *Diabetes Care*. 2007;30(suppl 2): S251-S260.
18. Anon. Proceedings of the 4th International Workshop-Conference on Gestational Diabetes Mellitus Chicago, Illinois, USA. 14-16 March 1997. *Diabetes Care*. 1998;21(suppl 2):B1.
19. American Diabetes Association. Nutrition recommendations and interventions for diabetes (Position Statement). *Diabetes Care*. 2008;31(suppl 1):S61-S78.
20. Crowther C, Hiller J, Moss J, et al. Effect of treatment of gestational diabetes mellitus on pregnancy outcomes. *N Engl J Med*. 2005;352:2477-2486.
21. Major C, Henry M, DeVeciana M, et al. The effects of carbohydrate restriction in patients with diet-controlled gestational diabetes. *Obstet Gynecol*. 1998;91:600-604.
22. Jovanovic-Peterson L, Bevier W, Peterson C. The Santa Barbara County Health Care Services Program: birth weight change concomitant with screening for and treatment of glucose-intolerance of pregnancy: a potential cost-effective intervention? *Am J Perinat*. 1997;14: 221-227.
23. Langer O, Berkus M, Brustman L, et al. Rationale for insulin management in gestational diabetes mellitus. *Diabetes*. 1991;40(suppl 2):186-190.
24. Bung P, Artal R, Khodiguian N, et al. Exercise in gestational diabetes: an optional therapeutic approach? *Diabetes*. 1991;40:182-185.
25. Jovanovic-Peterson L, Durak E, Peterson C. Randomized trial of diet versus diet plus cardiovascular conditioning on glucose levels in gestational diabetes. *Am J Obstet Gynecol*. 1989;161: 415-419.
26. Avery M, Leon A, Kopher R. Effects of a partially home-based exercise program for women with gestational diabetes. *Obstet Gynecol*. 1997;89:10-15.
27. Committee ACOG. Opinion no. 267: exercise during pregnancy and the postpartum period. *Obstet Gynecol*. 2002;99:171-173.
28. Harris G. Exercise and the pregnant patient: a clinical overview. *Women Health Primary Care*. 2005;8:79-86.
29. Langer O, Conway D, Berkus, et al. A comparison of glyburide and insulin in women with gestational diabetes mellitus. *N Engl J Med*. 2000;343:1134-1138.
30. Jovanovic L. The use of oral agents during pregnancy to treat gestational diabetes. *Curr Diab Rep*. 2001;1:69-70.
31. Hillier T, Vesco K, Pedula K, et al. Screening for gestational diabetes mellitus: a systematic review for the U.S. Preventive Services Task Force. *Ann Intern Med*. 2008;148:766-775.
32. Turok D, Ratcliffe S, Baxley E. Management of gestational diabetes mellitus. *Am Fam Physician*. 2003;68:1767-1772.

33. Kjos S, Henry O, Montoro M, et al. Insulin-requiring diabetes in pregnancy: a randomized trial of active induction of labor and expectant management. *Am J Obstet Gynecol*. 1993;169:611-615.
34. American Diabetes Association. Standards of medical care in diabetes. *Diabetes Care*. 2008; 31(suppl 1):S12-S54.
35. Kjos S, Peters R, Xiang A, et al. Contraception and the risk of type 2 diabetes mellitus in Latina women with prior gestational diabetes mellitus. *JAMA*. 1998;280:533-538.
36. Molsted-Pedersen L, Skouby S, Damm P. Preconception counseling and contraception after gestational diabetes. *Diabetes*. 1991;40(suppl 2):147-150.

Index